EPIDEMIOLOGY – CURRENT PERSPECTIVES ON RESEARCH AND PRACTICE

Edited by **Nuno Lunet**

Epidemiology – Current Perspectives on Research and Practice
Edited by Nuno Lunet

Published by InTech

Janeza Trdine 9, 51000 Rijeka, Croatia

Publishing Process Manager Dragana Manestar

Technical Editor Teodora Smiljanic

Cover Designer InTech Design Team

Additional hard copies can be obtained from orders@intechopen.com

Epidemiology – Current Perspectives on Research and Practice, Edited by Nuno Lunet
p. cm.
ISBN 978-953-51-0382-0

For EU product safety concerns:
IN TECH d.o.o., Prolaz Marije Krucifikse Kozulić 3, 51000 Rijeka, Croatia,
info@intechopen.com or visit our website at intechopen.com.

Meet the editor

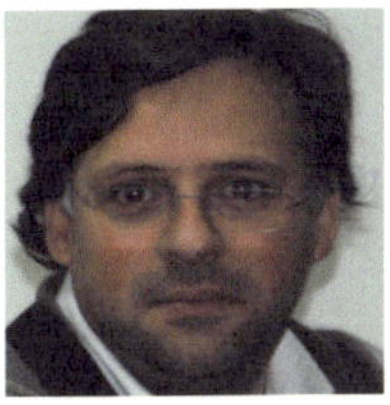

Nuno Lunet, PharmD, MPH, PhD, has been Assistant Professor of Epidemiology in the Department of Clinical Epidemiology, Predictive Medicine and Public Health of the University of Porto Medical School since 2006. He teaches and supervises students of several Master and PhD programs of the University of Porto. His main research interests are in public health and epidemiology, mainly descriptive and analytic cancer epidemiology, pharmacoepidemiology and systematic review and meta-analysis. He has authored/co-authored more than 100 articles in national and international journals with peer-review. He has been the director of the Master in Health Education of the University of Porto since 2009, a member of the Board of Directors of the Institute of Public Health, University of Porto since 2007, a member of the Editorial Board of the medical journal Arquivos de Medicina since 2003 and of the National Ethics Committee for Clinical Investigation since 2007.

Contents

Preface

The dictionary of epidemiology of the International Epidemiological Association defines epidemiology as "the study of the occurrence and distribution of health-related states or events in specified populations, including the study of the determinants influencing such states, and the application of this knowledge to control the health problems". This definition is currently well accepted and encompasses the activities that characterize epidemiology as an autonomous scientific discipline, as well as the use of epidemiological knowledge and tools to support the evidence based practice of public health and medicine.

The contribution of epidemiology to discoveries with a major impact on the health of the populations led to the recognition of its importance by the remaining scientific community and lay people, and to the anticipation for new discoveries. This poses stimulant intellectual challenges and research objectives that require the use of ever finer methodologies and longer times than the competing scientific disciplines and the public opinion may be willing to concede for their accomplishment. In parallel, the epidemiologists' tools and way of understanding health and disease are applied to resolve the everyday concerns of deciders in different health-related areas, and a sound and proficient use of the epidemiological methods is needed to meet their expectations.

This special issue resulted from the invitation made to selected authors to contribute with an overview of a specific subject of their choice, and is based on a collection of papers chosen to exemplify some of the interests, uses and views of the epidemiology across different areas of research and practice. Rather than the comprehensiveness and coherence of a conventional textbook, readers will find a set of independent chapters, each of them of a great interest in their own specialized areas within epidemiology. Taken together, they illustrate the contrast between the attempt to extend the limits of applicability of epidemiological research, and the "regular" scientific activity in this field or an applied epidemiology.

I believe that epidemiologists with different levels of expertise and interests will be able to find informative and inspiring readings among the chapters of this book.

Nuno Lunet
Department of Clinical Epidemiology, Predictive Medicine and Public Health,
University of Porto Medical School,
Institute of Public Health – University of Porto (ISPUP),
Portugal

1

Changing Contexts in Epidemiologic Research – Thoughts of Young Epidemiologists on Major Challenges for the Next Decades

Ana Azevedo[1], Leda Chatzi[2],
Tobias Pischon[3] and Lorenzo Richiardi[4]*
[1]University of Porto Medical School & Institute of Public Health of the University of Porto,
[2]Department of Social Medicine, Faculty of Medicine, University of Crete,
[3]Department of Epidemiology, German Institute of Human Nutrition Potsdam-Rehbruecke,
[4]Cancer Epidemiology Unit, CeRMS and CPO-Piemonte, University of Turin,
[1]Portugal
[2]Greece
[3]Germany
[4]Italy

1. Introduction

Since the second half of the last century, epidemiology has made key contributions to the identification of the causes of common chronic diseases, from cancers to cardiovascular and respiratory diseases, paving the way to effective prevention measures. In the process sophisticated epidemiologic methodologies have been developed for both observational and interventional studies in humans that have become the basis of "evidence-based" medicine and public health.

---

*On behalf of: Miia Artama[5], Ana Azevedo[1], Julia Bohlius[6], Marta Cabanas[7], Leda Chatzi[2], Anne-Sophie Evrard[8], Andrej Grjibovski[9], Emily Herrett[10], Raquel Lucas[1], Anouk Pijpe[11], Tobias Pischon[3], Lorenzo Richiardi[4], Gunnar Toft[12] and Piret Veerus[13]

[1]University of Porto Medical School & Institute of Public Health of the University of Porto, Portugal
[2]Department of Social Medicine, Faculty of Medicine, University of Crete, Greece,
[3]Department of Epidemiology, German Institute of Human Nutrition Potsdam-Rehbruecke, Germany
[4]Cancer Epidemiology Unit, CeRMS and CPO-Piemonte, University of Turin, Italy
[5]National Institute for Health and Welfare, Finland
[6]Institute of Social and Preventive Medicine, University of Bern, Switzerland
[7]IDIAP Jordi Gol, Spain
[8]Radiation Group, International Agency for Research on Cancer, Lyon, France
[9]Department of Infectious Diseases Epidemiology, Norwegian Institute of Public Health, Norway & International School of Public Health, Northern State Medical University, Russia
[10]Department of Epidemiology and Population Health, London School of Hygiene and Tropical Medicine, UK
[11]Department of Epidemiology, Netherlands Cancer Institute – Antoni van Leeuwenhoek Hospital, Netherlands
[12]Department of Occupational Medicine, Aarhus University Hospital, Denmark
[13]Department of Epidemiology and Biostatistics, National Institute for Health Development, Estonia

Two major developments have changed the scientific and societal contexts in which epidemiology operates: the extraordinary advances in molecular genetics, cell and developmental biology and a shift towards social philosophies in which individual values largely dominate over collective values. These developments affect on one side the aims, methods and contents of epidemiology as a research approach to health and disease and on the other side the public health perspective that confers a practical value to epidemiology.

Within this frame, a growing number of young epidemiologists, whose professional life will project over the next thirty or forty years, are involved in research, as indicated by the increasing number of epidemiology publications in the peer-reviewed literature. Less visible are, however, their activities concerning the medium and long term orientation and evolution of epidemiology, its role within public health and medicine and, ultimately, its ability to make a real difference to population health.

European Young Epidemiologists (EYE) is a network of young epidemiologists within the International Epidemiological Association - European Epidemiology Federation (IEA-EEF), founded in 2004, after the European Congress of Epidemiology. EYE aims to establish contact among young epidemiologists in Europe in order to facilitate future collaboration in scientific research, to engage in the development of epidemiological research methods, to foster the appropriate use of epidemiological research in the domains of public health and clinical medicine, and mainly to discuss and intervene in the future of epidemiologic research.

In 2011, a worldwide group of Early Career Researchers (ECR group) emerged within the International Epidemiological Association with representatives from all continents, and the chairman of EYE is the European representative at the worldwide group. This initiative reflects the felt need to network, promoting the discussion on what the future of epidemiology is and what it should be, by putting emerging epidemiologists' voices on the map about how to make health research work towards scientific and societal development, ultimately contributing to improve populations' health.

In this context, it seemed timely to us to share this chapter, which summarizes major topics that emerged from a 3-day workshop held in Turin, Italy, in 2008, to explore and debate the long term orientation and evolution of epidemiology. The workshop was organized by the European Educational Programme in Epidemiology in collaboration with the International Epidemiological Association and European Young Epidemiologists group and counted on the participation of 14 early career epidemiologists from different European countries and 7 experienced epidemiologists as discussants. This text does not intend to resuscitate a debate on the identity and role of epidemiology as a discipline, much less to offer a solution to these fundamental questions, but instead simply asks some questions about how epidemiology will respond to what we see as two major developments, as identified above - the inexorable rise of molecular biology and the shift from collectivist to individualist philosophy, which resonates with epidemiology's role as the basic science serving public health.

2. Development of epidemiology and its role in research

The importance of epidemiology as a scientific discipline has been steadily increasing over the past decades. In etiologic research this is partly driven by the intention to disentangle the independent effects of risk factors for the predominant chronic diseases in Western civilizations, including cardiovascular diseases and cancer. These complex diseases are caused by many different factors, including genetic and non-genetic (diet, lifestyle, occupation, environment), where each factor is usually related to only small changes in risk. Consequently, the identification of risk factors usually requires the study of large samples with sophisticated analytic techniques, making this the prototype of epidemiologic research.

Epidemiology has evolved into several different subdisciplines which are focused on specific areas of research, such as cardiovascular epidemiology, cancer epidemiology, genetic epidemiology, clinical epidemiology or nutritional epidemiology. What is noteworthy, though, is that the advancement of epidemiology often seems to be driven by developments in these other specific areas of research (and, equally important, by researchers in these other disciplines), rather than by epidemiology itself (or epidemiologists themselves). For example, the search for genetic variants that may be associated with increased health risk has led to the creation of large databases and to the conduct of genome wide association studies (GWAS). Partly because of the large number of variants examined, GWAS have a high risk of providing false-positive results. This has led to discussions and suggestions about how to conduct and interpret results of such studies in the fields of genetics and genetic epidemiology (Hattersley & McCarthy, 2005), although the question of how to appropriately deal with false-positive results is essentially a genuine general question in epidemiology. Another example comes from the field of clinical epidemiology, where a majority of pertinent studies are performed by clinicians, although the questions addressed in these studies are mostly those that traditionally fall in the field of epidemiology.

One concern that applies to epidemiology as well as to other areas of scientific research is that advancements may in some instances simply be driven by the pure availability of new technologies or by advances in existing technology rather than by research questions pertinent to the area of research. An example is the development of various "-omics" technologies, which provides promising tools to allow large-scale biomarker studies, including discovery-oriented as well as hypothesis-testing investigations (Vineis & Perera, 2007). However, there may also be an inherent risk, i.e. that the research agenda is dictated by the ability to have novel or advanced technologies instead of having sound scientific questions or hypotheses. Thus, epidemiology may be "vulnerable" to the focus on novel technologies by a tendency to "enrich" studies with these technologies in an attempt to obtain higher impact without critical reflections about their usefulness. Importantly, a fact that may be neglected is that the use of novel technologies is often vulnerable to similar shortcomings as are the more traditional approaches, and may even add complexity to the interpretation of results. For example, with regard to the use of biomarker technologies it was succinctly cautioned that "biochemical measures are almost always subject to the same problems of misclassification and bias [as answers provided by humans and their interviewers]" (Hunter, 1998). Also, it must be stressed that several of the major breakthroughs in epidemiology, including case-control and cohort studies that led to the discovery of the role of smoking as the major risk factor for lung cancer, serum cholesterol and smoking as risk factors for coronary heart disease and folate deficiency as a determinant of neural tube defects, in fact came from a rather "old-fashioned", black box approach (Susser & Susser, 1996). Although it may seem self-evident, it is important to reiterate that the research agenda in epidemiology should be driven by questions that primarily address topics that fall within the definition of epidemiology, rather than by technical details of related disciplines. Taking molecular epidemiology as an example, McMichael stated in an editorial more than 10 years ago, "…we do not need a new 'molecular' subdiscipline, with an inevitable inbuilt tendency to reductionism. Rather, we should critically incorporate the emerging array of molecular biologic measurements into mainstream epidemiologic research and thus broaden its scope. Good science will come from a synthesis that transcends disciplines and techniques" (McMichael, 1994). A successful example of the exploitation of genetic technology by epidemiologists to study exposures that are difficult to measure is Mendelian randomization, a method of direct value to understanding the environmental causes of common diseases using genetic variants as proxies (Davey Smith & Ebrahim, 2003).

As indicated further in the next paragraphs, the future will probably bring the need to create and analyze even larger databases, implementing new technologies, and unraveling the complex interplay between environmental and genetic factors in disease etiology. What role will epidemiologists play in such endeavors? What is the relationship of epidemiology to other disciplines (genetics, clinical medicine, etc.) in the context of the creation and analysis of such databases? Will epidemiology be a method and will epidemiologists be the database managers? Or will epidemiology be a field that takes a leading role in shaping the research agenda? These are important questions which epidemiologists have to face for the future.

By providing their specific expertise epidemiologists need to make sure that they form an essential part of that process. This means that they need to be integrated in all parts of research, including the formulation of hypotheses, development of study designs, establishment and conduction of studies, analysis and interpretation of data, and translation into public health settings. For this reason it is of course essential for epidemiologists to have detailed knowledge of their areas of interest. However, while the creation of subdisciplines is an enrichment of the field of epidemiology, it is important to keep in mind the global aim of epidemiology, that is, to study "the occurrence and distribution of health-related states or events in specified populations, including the study of the determinants influencing such states, and the application of this knowledge to control the health problems"(Porta, 2008); nothing more, nothing less.

3. The research agenda of an epidemiologist

The question that we would like to address here is: "What are the determinants of the choice of our area of research in epidemiology?"; in other words: "Based on which criteria do epidemiologists decide on which research to follow?". Even when a researcher has a complete independent status, the choice is the result of several forces and not restricted to the appreciation of which are the best scientific questions. In addition to scientific curiosity and public health relevance, many other factors have an implicit or explicit role.

Previous research experiences have great impact on our own research agenda. Changing one's own specific area of research can be challenging, not only because of the need of new skills and knowledge but also because of the lack of national and international recognition and networking in the new research area, with consequent difficulties in being involved in collaborative research and having access to funding. Thus a change in area of research cannot be achieved in short time, while it needs long-term programming and a supportive research environment and infrastructure.

The research environment, the interaction with colleagues and their expertises and the facilities available at the research institute are obvious strong determinants of the research agenda.

Facilities also include the availability of large databases, an issue that will be discussed in the next section. Here we emphasize that the availability of administrative large databases has increased dramatically the opportunities for epidemiological research. Sometimes, however, the availability of data may also shape the research questions. As opposed to already available databases, collection of new data can be specifically targeted at emerging research hypotheses, but it may be hampered by cost and organisational constraints. Often, we favour a research question that can be answered using already available data as opposed to a research question that needs time- and resource-intensive studies. This approach may allow the risk of testing hypotheses with lower *a priori* likelihood of providing a consistent answer that is reproduced in other studies, standing the test of time; these hypotheses would otherwise not be approached, at least not immediately, thus possibly creating opportunities for discovery (Vandenbroucke, 2008). It is difficult to know what combination of the two approaches, use of available data and new collections, maximizes the possibilities of progress in scientific knowledge.

Hot topics are more likely to be published in more important journals, which, in turn, enhance the opportunities to reach the scientific community as well as lay people through the media. More important journals have also higher impact factor, that, although being criticized (Hernán, 2008), is still affecting researchers' careers and access to funding. For their scientific and public health relevance as well for the reasons just described, hot topics are more likely to stimulate new research and to be considered as a research priority. This can translate in fast scientific progress and public health impact but, on the other hand, this process can divert resources and efforts from new developing fields.

A new field can emerge only if funding agencies are giving it adequate support. Indeed, funding agencies have a central role in shaping the research agenda, and, therefore, the transparency of their selection process is a fundamental issue. However, even a transparent selection that is strictly based on quality, public health implications and scientific relevance of the submitted projects does not limit the influence of the agencies. Often, funding agencies open specific calls for research aiming at *a priori* decided objectives. We feel that the extent of the role of public and private funding agencies in shaping research agenda should be measured and monitored over time, including an assessment of the process that leads to the definition of the specific calls and the actual societal impact of funded projects.

We started this section by considering an epidemiologist who has complete independence. The issue of independence has been studied and discussed in the epidemiological literature at length, mainly with reference to influences from the industry and, to a lesser extent, from governments (Pearce, 2008). Even assuming independence, however, we are aware of the fact that we all have *a priori* beliefs, we receive a salary from an institution or a funding agency, and we live in a community. It is widely accepted that epidemiologists should aim at giving priority to the research questions with the highest scientific interest and/or public health impact. This is however not a trivial task and we should recognise that the decision on what to study is affected by a large number of factors, many of which are not under our direct control.

4. Emerging opportunities and challenges in epidemiology: Large databases and use of secondary data

The twenty-first century undoubtedly provides new horizons regarding the availability and use of data sources. In the last decade a growing number of public databases for depositing data have emerged. Much of the impetus for this growing trend was given by the paradigm shift we witnessed in genetic research, which has moved from a candidate gene approach focused on few genes to GWAS, which require multifaceted linked databases of larger populations (Ioannidis et al., 2006; Kaiser, 2002; Wylie & Mineau, 2003). Although less common, similar trends in data storing and sharing occurred in other areas of epidemiology as well. One example is the Pharmacogenomics Knowledge of Base of PharmGKB (www.pharmgkb.org) that was established to store, manage and make available molecular data in addition to phenotype data obtained from pharmacogenetic studies. In the field of classical epidemiology, multi-centric collaborative studies and pooled analyses are becoming more and more common. Moreover, systematic reviews and meta-analyses try to integrate and synthesize existing research studies in an attempt to derive new information by quantitative statistical analysis. By examining the totality of data available about an issue, systematic review can identify inconsistencies in existing data and point to areas of research needed, reduce the potential for erroneous findings occurring by chance, and more accurately define the benefit and possible adverse effects of management strategies.

We feel that future epidemiological research will benefit greatly from the exchange of ideas between researchers and across disciplines/subdisciplines. This not only refers to concrete research results but also to approaches to the study of new areas. Existing studies could establish efficient routes of communication and co-ordination that allow a quick and detailed identification and promotion of common research areas. New studies could add protocols designed for specific purposes, preferably specialized rather than general, and study selected populations of special interest. A collaborative basis may in certain areas of research increase statistical power, ensure efficient design with large study populations, allow geographical comparisons and the replication of results, and give the possibility to study sub-groups or rare exposures (a crucial aspect of epidemiology) (Kogevinas et al., 2004).

Questions about ownership, custody and rights of access to data are major issues and determine restrictions to data sharing and collaborative research. These questions focus mainly on protection of privacy (the ability to control information about oneself) and confidentiality (the obligation of a second party to not reveal private information about an individual to a third party without the permission of the person concerned) (Willison, 1998). Confidentiality and privacy issues are emerging limiting factors (for both new data collection and use of available databases) that can have important effects on shaping research agenda and public health surveillance (Cuttini et al., 2009). At present, in many countries, legislations on confidentiality are defined with little consideration on their impact on medical and public health research, thus favouring personal privacy above societal benefits. The four principles of protection of a research participant are autonomy (self-determination), beneficence (maximal benefit), nonmalfeasance (minimal harm), and justice (distribution of benefits and harms across groups in society) (National Commission for Protection of Human Subjects of Biomedical and Behavioral Research, 1979). Although these principles focused on experimental studies in the past, it is essential that we follow established ethical guidelines also in observational studies that are perceived to have minimal harm. In the past, these issues have primarily been raised with regard to clinical trials where the intervention itself may do harm to the research subject. In observational studies, however, the concern about harm is not so much about the fact that the study procedures may do harm to the research subject (which is usually minimal because of the observational nature) but more about the fact that the results of that research may (indirectly) harm the participants or a group thereof. For example, results of a genetic study may reveal that individuals with a certain genetic variation may have a higher risk of disease. Should researchers report these results to their study subjects? If yes, then such reporting could harm the self-determination of these subjects because they may not have asked for that specific test. If not, then the researcher may withhold important information from that person. If results with potential clinical significance are delivered to individual participants, the communication should be made in close collaboration with clinicians who should be part of the research group from the beginning of the project. In addition, if researchers decide to disclose the results, participants should have the opportunity at the time of enrolment to give their consent to receive information about incidental findings or not, and should receive explanations on how incidental information will be handled. Often these two requirements are not met or are unfeasible in a specific research project. Partly based on these concerns, some countries already adopted new laws or regulations, such as the Genetic Information Nondiscrimination Act in the United States in the year 2008 (Hudson et al., 2008).

As large electronic databases have been developed, several management models have been designed [*e.g.*, the RGE (Resource for Genetic and Epidemiological Research) model, the Sweeney's model, the deCODE Genetics model and others] focusing on confidentiality versus research use, as well as public versus private access (Wylie & Mineau, 2003). Individual rights of subjects must be respected at all times, but should not be misused by data collecting institutions as an argument to restrict access of other researchers. A balance between individual rights to privacy and the societal benefit of research must be established (Bergmann et al., 2008).

Another important issue when examining large databases is the frequent lack of explicit reports on the methods followed for the collection of the data from different sources, the completeness of this information, and a discussion of limitations of the data source. This may also be driven by the strict space limits of most journals as investigators may have had appropriately described everything in the methods section but word count limitations led to the deletion of this information. There are examples of large collaborative studies where all the methods and quality have been specified and assured (Tunstall Pedoe, 2003). There is a crucial need for researchers and journal editors to become aware that guidelines have been developed on how to conduct and how to report results of epidemiologic studies (International Epidemiological Association, 2007; von Elm et al., 2007).

The next step will be to enhance the availability of methods for easily depositing data and to provide tools for ensuring the sustainability of the databases. Large databases may benefit from widely available electronic search tools listing available studies on a specific topic and they should encompass both published and deposited data. A research environment that promotes and rewards by publishing only results that reach statistical significance is likely to foster data dredging and will create a distorted literature with very low credibility

(Easterbrook et al., 1991; Ioannidis, 2005). The scientific community will also have to discuss issues of authorship, data property, and funding of secondary analyses.

The study of demographic, genetic, medical and environmental data from different populations may create an exciting and promising approach to identify the causes of common diseases and create effective preventive measures. "If you have large, accurate data sets on the health and death of human beings, what else do you need to improve the health of the public other than sound scientific method, cautious inference and a dialogue between science and policy?" (Coleman, 2007). Our knowledge of health and disease will certainly be greatly enhanced when the use of this immense amount of information is made available through the application of solid epidemiological principles. We are aware that there are problems to solve and agreements to reach within the field of large databases and use of secondary data. In addition, large databases and secondary analyses may not be useful to answer all new research questions, but they may be a (powerful) tool for epidemiological research.

5. Epidemiology and society: How each influences the other

Epidemiology tells us what we want to know about the human condition and, often, how it might be improved, in a way which no other science can offer (Coleman, 2007). This is a great challenge and a major reason why we find it so attractive and intellectually rewarding.

Throughout history, society has conditioned and channelled science. Societal reaction also influences the translation of epidemiology into public health. Many of the 20th century beliefs regarding the relation between epidemiology and society turned out to be only half-truths: 1) epidemiology would lead to prevention, 2) prevention was better than cure, 3) social justice would be achieved through prevention and 4) epidemiology would pervade clinical medicine and change its practice. We now recognize that success in epidemiology has not necessarily implied public health achievements (*e.g.* evidence on tobacco vs. economic interests) and health inequalities tend to increase instead of decrease.

The present loss of credibility before the society (and other fields of science) regarding risk factor epidemiology is partly a consequence of a reductionist view, i.e., a focus on associations between a single exposure and a single outcome, which frequently originates inconsistent messages (the same exposure may be publicized either as risk or protective factor on different adverse outcomes). Also, conflicting results regarding the same association might raise the question of how much evidence is needed to intervene or to advocate intervention (Taubes, 1995). Publication of small amounts of information without considering implications contributes to incomplete knowledge and in our view reflects some degree of irresponsibility. Publication drive may result in objective dishonesty that must be fought against. Introspection should be carried out before publication: are we honestly convinced by our findings?

Etiological epidemiology has mostly been looking at individual susceptibility and the distribution of disease in the population has been undervalued. The growing emphasis on genetic/molecular research contributes to direct epidemiology towards individual-based prevention as opposed to population level approaches. Concern with individual susceptibility has neglected the distribution of disease in the population, leading to the "type III error" - a good study to answer the wrong question. While an increased interplay between biotechnology, infrastructures and methods may be the future of epidemiologic research, translational research must be promoted, starting from the population and responding to its needs, with special attention being required towards understudied groups (*e.g.* migrants).

Political stability is an important basis for public health. Inequalities in health and research between countries, even within Europe, emphasize the need for a) one epidemiology for all societies in the 21st century, b) more quality research from less rich countries, c) stronger political will to translate evidence into action.

The reinforcement of epidemiologists' professional image with society in general is needed. The importance given to individual values such as the right to privacy has risen barriers to research that in our view do not benefit society as a whole while in fact the risk of disrespect for individual rights is smaller than its theoretical maximum. There is the need to distinguish between the risk to personal autonomy from the use of identifiable data without consent to select a given individual for prurient interest or unauthorized disclosure (moving from population data to the individual) and the far smaller risk posed by aggregating individual data for research in order to draw general conclusions about society (from individual data to the population) (Coleman, 2007). Striking the right balance between the confidentiality of identifiable health data and the need for medical research to improve public health is now an issue in many countries (Coleman et al., 2003). Though it is not necessarily straightforward where the line should be drawn, the societal pendulum needs to swing back towards the collective responsibility for medical research and public health surveillance. Current regulatory climate risks to refrain the scientific community from using available data to control health problems and improve population health.

We feel the need for a strengthening of the link between epidemiologic research and society, in order to translate findings into the effective improvement of population health. Part of this process should be the reinforcement of epidemiologists' professional image in the society in general to win its trust.

6. Conclusion

Research has been strongly influenced by a random and passive intersection between biotechnology, infrastructures and available methods. Young epidemiologists must reinforce their knowledge on the substantive issues they are researching and promote an active interaction between biology and society. Translational research is needed to use relevant laboratory research resources in population-based studies and to make the results of epidemiological studies useful to an individualized and predictive medical practice.

Professionals need to be prepared to collate data. Questions about ownership, custody and rights of access to data are major and determine restrictions to research. Individual rights of subjects must be respected at all times, but should not be misused by institutions that collected data as an argument to restrict access of other researchers. More than new information, we need to use the information we already have. A balance between individual rights to privacy and the societal benefit of research must be encountered.

In order to gain the possibility of playing a more active role in their research agenda, epidemiologists must improve their communication skills, both regarding risk communication to the population and scientific dialogue with other researchers and clinicians. Also, they need to conquer a position in funding agencies and as consultants for policy makers, and be available for these tasks over time.

The need to reinforce the professional image of epidemiologists could be met by as good a formal education as possible along with good epidemiologic practices. Epidemiological expertise will continue to be required for the attempt to set rational priorities for the control of disease and health promotion. This challenge is as breathtaking as we need to keep us on track to contribute to design the future of epidemiology.

7. Acknowledgment

This work was supported by Compagnia di S. Paolo, to whom the authors gratefully acknowledge all the material conditions for the workshop "Epidemiology in the new century: a perspective from the young european epidemiologists", held in Turin, Italy, in May 2008.

The liveliness of the discussions at the workshop and its output would not have been possible without the generous contribution of the senior epidemiologists who attended - Shah Ebrahim, Hans-Werner Hense, Franco Merletti, Jorn Olsen, Susanna Sans, Rodolfo Saracci, Paolo Vineis. The authors want to particularly thank Rodolfo Saracci for his intellectual input, as well as his initiative and enthusiasm in the organisation of this event, which were a *sine qua non* condition for the workshop and all the outputs thereafter.

8. References

Bergmann, M. M.,Gorman, U. & Mathers, J. C. (2008). Bioethical considerations for human nutrigenomics. *Annu Rev Nutr*, Vol.28, pp.447-467, 0199-9885 (Print).

Coleman, M. P. (2007). Commentary: Is epidemiology really dead, anyway?A look back at Kenneth Rothman's 'the rise and fall of epidemiology, 1950–2000 ad'. *Int J Epidemiol*, Vol.36, No.4, pp.719-723.

Coleman, M. P.,Evans, B. G. & Barrett, G. (2003). Confidentiality and the public interest in medical research--will we ever get it right? *Clin Med*, Vol.3, No.3, pp.219-228, 1470-2118.

Cuttini, M.,Marini, C.,Bruzzone, S.,Prati, S. & Saracci, R. (2009). Protection of health information in Italy: A step too far? *Int J Epidemiol*, Vol.38, No.6, pp.1739-1740.

Davey Smith, G. & Ebrahim, S. (2003). 'Mendelian randomization': Can genetic epidemiology contribute to understanding environmental determinants of disease? *Int J Epidemiol*, Vol.32, pp.1-22.

Easterbrook, P. J.,Berlin, J. A.,Gopalan, R. & Matthews, D. R. (1991). Publication bias in clinical research. *Lancet*, Vol.337, No.8746, pp.867-872, 0140-6736 (Print).

Hattersley, A. T. & McCarthy, M. I. (2005). What makes a good genetic association study? *Lancet*, Vol.366, No.9493, pp.1315-1323, 0140-6736.

Hernán, M. (2008). Epidemiologists (of all people) should question journal impact factors. *Epidemiology*, Vol.19, pp.366-368.

Hudson, K. L.,Holohan, M. K. & Collins, F. S. (2008). Keeping pace with the times -- the genetic information nondiscrimination act of 2008. *N Engl J Med*, Vol.358, No.25, pp.2661-2663.

Hunter, D. (1998). Biochemical indicators of dietary intake, In: *Nutritional epidemiology*. W. Willet. pp. 174-243, Oxford University Press, ISBN 978-0195122978, New York.

International Epidemiological Association. (2007). "Good epidemiological practice (GEP) IEA guidlines for proper conduct in epidemiologic research." 2009, from http://www.dundee.ac.uk/iea/GEP07.htm.

Ioannidis, J. P. (2005). Why most published research findings are false. *PLoS Med*, Vol.2, No.8, pp.e124, 1549-1676 (Electronic).

Ioannidis, J. P.,Gwinn, M.,Little, J.,Higgins, J. P.,Bernstein, J. L.,Boffetta, P.,Bondy, M.,Bray, M. S.,Brenchley, P. E.,Buffler, P. A.,Casas, J. P.,Chokkalingam, A.,Danesh, J.,Smith, G. D.,Dolan, S.,Duncan, R.,Gruis, N. A.,Hartge, P.,Hashibe, M.,Hunter, D. J.,Jarvelin, M. R.,Malmer, B.,Maraganore, D. M.,Newton-Bishop, J. A.,O'Brien, T. R.,Petersen, G.,Riboli, E.,Salanti, G.,Seminara, D.,Smeeth, L.,Taioli, E.,Timpson, N.,Uitterlinden, A. G.,Vineis, P.,Wareham, N.,Winn, D. M.,Zimmern, R. & Khoury, M. J. (2006). A road map for efficient and reliable human genome epidemiology. *Nat Genet*, Vol.38, No.1, pp.3-5, 1061-4036 (Print).

Kaiser, J. (2002). Biobanks: Population databases boom, from Iceland to the U.S. *Science*, Vol.298, No.5596, pp.1158-1161.

Kogevinas, M.,Andersen, A. & Olsen, J. (2004). Collaboration is needed to co-ordinate european birth cohort studies. *Int J Epidemiol*, Vol.33, pp.1172-1173.

McMichael, A. J. (1994). Invited commentary--"Molecular epidemiology": New pathway or new travelling companion? *Am J Epidemiol*, Vol.140, No.1, pp.1-11.

National Commission for Protection of Human Subjects of Biomedical and Behavioral Research. (1979). "The belmont report." from http://www.hhs.gov/ohrp/humansubjects/guidance/belmont.htm.

Pearce, N. (2008). Corporate influences on epidemiology. *Int J Epidemiol*, Vol.37, No.1, pp.46-53.

Porta, M. (2008). *A dictionary of epidemiology* (Fifth edition), Oxford University Press, ISBN 9780195314496, New York.

Susser, M. & Susser, E. (1996). Choosing a future for epidemiology: I. Eras and paradigms. *Am J Public Health*, Vol.86, pp.668-673.

Taubes, G. (1995). Epidemiology faces its limits. *Science*, Vol.269, No.5221, pp.164-169, 0036-8075.

Tunstall Pedoe, H. (2003). *Monica project. Monica monograph and multimedia sourcebook: World's largest study of heart disease, stroke, risk factors and population trends 1979-2002* World Health Organization, Geneva.

Vandenbroucke, J. P. (2008). Observational research, randomised trials, and two views of medical science. *PLoS Med*, Vol.5, No.3, pp.e67.

Vineis, P. & Perera, F. (2007). Molecular epidemiology and biomarkers in etiologic cancer research: The new in light of the old. *Cancer Epidemiol Biomarkers Prev*, Vol.16, No.10, pp.1954-1965.

von Elm, E.,Altman, D. G.,Egger, M.,Pocock, S. J.,Gotzsche, P. C. & Vandenbroucke, J. P. (2007). The strengthening the reporting of observational studies in epidemiology (strobe) statement: Guidelines for reporting observational studies. *Lancet*, Vol.370, No.9596, pp.1453-1457, 1474-547X (Electronic).

Willison, D. J. (1998). Health services research and personal health information: Privacy concerns, new legislation and beyond. *CMAJ*, Vol.159, No.11, pp.1378-1380, 0820-3946 (Print).

Wylie, J. E. & Mineau, G. P. (2003). Biomedical databases: Protecting privacy and promoting research. *Trends Biotechnol*, Vol.21, No.3, pp.113-116, 0167-7799.

2

Frameworks for Causal Inference in Epidemiology

Raquel Lucas
Department of Clinical Epidemiology, Predictive Medicine and Public Health, University of Porto Medical School and Institute of Public Heath of the University of Porto, Portugal

1. Introduction

In 1884, Robert Luedeking, Professor at the St. Louis Medical College and member of the St. Louis Board of Health, published a paper entitled *The chief local factors in the causation of disease and death* (Luedeking 1884), in which he wrote the following:

[In St. Louis, in 1883, the population density of 9.8 persons to the acre] is indeed a low density compared with that of most metropolitan cities: that of London, for instance, is given at 52.5 to the acre in 1883. And yet we find the annual rate of mortality per thousand in London in 1883 to have been but 20.4, while that of St. Louis was 21.35. With such a variance existing in the relative densities, it must needs force itself upon our conviction that inherent faults in our sanitation must be the cause.

In this paper Luedeking compares crude death rates between cities and finds that mortality in St. Louis is slightly higher than in London, even though population density is substantially lower in the former city. He then implicitly uses previous knowledge to attribute the unexpected similarity in mortality, given very different population densities, to deficient sanitation in St. Louis. This paragraph is illustrative of a process in which the application of causal inference to the improvement of population health is attempted: observing an unexpected difference (or a surprising similarity), identifying a cause based on observed data and expert knowledge, and recommending a public health action.

This provides an interesting example of a pragmatic concept of cause in epidemiology. Today, health authorities would probably avoid such strong causal statements. However, it seems unfair to neglect that improving sanitation in St. Louis would very likely decrease mortality substantially at the time.

A cause can be defined as a person or thing that acts, happens, or exists in such a way that some specific thing happens as a result; the producer of an effect (Dictionary.com 2011). On the one hand, this definition reflects the notion that causation is an essential component of the human understanding and interaction with the world. On the other hand, although this seems like a straightforward definition, which is probably in agreement with many if not most individuals' concept of cause, it raises a number of questions: Does the cause always produce the effect? Are other causes involved in producing the effect? If the cause was removed would the effect be produced? Formal discussions of these and other questions have been the focus of philosophical and scientific approaches to causation and the appropriate notion of cause for a certain discipline is influenced by the kind of causal knowledge that the discipline aims at producing.

While theories on causation and causal inference have been abundantly discussed in the philosophical literature, an operational concept of causation is essential to conduct scientific research. In fact, science has developed experimentation as a useful approach to dealing with the complexity of causal inference. In etiologic epidemiology we are interested in understanding the mechanisms of disease causation and we aim at identifying targets for intervention in order to be ultimately able to reduce the burden and consequences of disease in the population.

In epidemiologic research, however, the multifactorial etiology of human disease, the non-modifiable nature of a number of health-related factors, and mainly the vastly unethical nature of experimentation in human subjects brought about the need to design and conduct studies that are knowingly imperfect approximations to the experimental ideal. In fact, in etiologic studies of human disease we are faced with a number of problems that threaten causal inference and whose avoidance and discussion are at the core of epidemiologic research.

In practical terms, stating that causality is the best explanation for an observed association is equivalent to ruling out, with reasonable confidence, alternative explanations such as reverse causation, selection bias, information bias, confounding and chance. The formalization and discussion of these alternative explanations has become in fact so important in epidemiologic research that it was pointed out that these methodologic issues became the main focus of epidemiology textbooks, at the expense of little attention devoted to the discussion of such fundamental issues as theories of causation or hypothesis formulation (Krieger 1994). Indeed, there has been a shift in recent years towards framing the thinking and teaching of epidemiologic methods into a more solid theoretical basis for causal inference (Rothman et al 2008).

Even though causal inference is such a central issue in epidemiology, and perhaps because of that, different views on causation have proliferated in the epidemiologic literature. A systematic review of scientific publications (Parascandola & Weed 2001) has identified several different explicit or implicit definitions of cause within the epidemiological literature, which the authors classified in the following categories:

- production: causes are seen as part of the production of disease;
- necessary causes: causes are conditions without which the effect cannot occur;
- sufficient/component causes: one sufficient cause guarantees that the effect will occur, and each sufficient cause is made up of component causes, none of which is enough to produce the effect;
- probabilistic causes: causes are seen as conditions which increase the probability of an effect, regardless of whether or not they are necessary or sufficient;
- counterfactual causes: the presence of a cause, compared with its absence, makes a difference in the occurrence of the outcome, while all else is held constant.

While no single model can aspire to provide the answer to causal questions in epidemiology, inferring causation from observed data in human populations is a complex task which extends beyond the discussion of systematic or random errors, some of which may be dealt with through statistical methods.

The aim of this chapter is to provide a brief overview of selected frameworks frequently used to assist causal inference in epidemiology. Although there are many interesting approaches to causation in the epidemiologic literature, the ones referred below were chosen for historical significance or because of their increasing relevance in epidemiologic research. An additional interesting aspect of the approaches chosen is that they originate from different areas of knowledge, from philosophy (the sufficient and component causes model and the counterfactual model) to medicine/biology (Hill's considerations) and computer science (causal diagrams).

2. Frameworks for causal inference

2.1 Bradford Hill's considerations regarding causation

During the first half of the 20th century it became increasingly clear that monocausal theories of human disease were virtually useless to explain chronic conditions (Broadbent 2009). Models that were previously applied to explain the distribution of disease proved useful, to a large extent, to prevent or treat communicable conditions. However, they were clearly insufficient to uncover the multifactorial etiology of complex chronic diseases and therefore inadequate to identify targets for chronic disease prevention. The increasing interest in understanding the etiology of non-communicable diseases brought about the challenge of re-thinking the process of causal inference from observed data.

In 1965, in his famous paper entitled *The environment and disease: association or causation?*, Sir Austin Bradford Hill recognized the fundamental problem of deriving a causal interpretation from observed associations between exposure and disease (Hill 1965). In this widely known paper, his aim was to provide guidance regarding the process that goes from finding an association between an exposure and a disease to deciding that causation is the most likely explanation for that association. His approach clearly intends a detachment from the philosophical discussion of causation. Rather than proposing a theoretical model for causal inference, he puts forward a set of empirical aspects of associations that should be examined to guide the judgment of causality, namely:

a. **Strength**: this consideration is based on the premise that the stronger an association is the less likely it is that there is some alternative unknown explanation rather than causation;
b. **Consistency**: this refers to the replication of the findings in different methodological, geographical and time settings;
c. **Specificity**: this refers to the high probability that an exposure is causally linked to some outcomes more than to others;
d. **Temporality**: this means that the putative cause must precede the effect and is probably the only indisputable criterion for causality;
e. **Biologic gradient**: this refers to the existence of a dose-response relation by which increased dose of exposure is related with increased expression of the outcome;
f. **Plausibility**: this refers to the agreement of the examined association with existing biological knowledge;
g. **Coherence**: this argues for the importance that the association is not conflicting with scientific knowledge on the disease;

h. **Experiment**: this refers to the possibility of eliciting the outcome by experimentally introducing exposure or, in human populations, an alternative such as the possibility of preventing the outcome by removing the exposure;
i. **Analogy**: this refers to the existence of similar outcomes with exposures of the same kind.

It is noteworthy that the ranking of these considerations was intentional. As acknowledged by Hill, none of these items is necessary for deciding that an association translates a causal relation (except for temporality), and the whole set is not sufficient to prove causation. Therefore, the author himself clearly states that this should not be used as a checklist for causal inference, though it has thereafter frequently served that purpose. Such widespread misuse has probably exposed the limitations of this set of considerations and they have often been dismissed as having little utility in causality assessment. However, it should be noted that one of the major contributions of Hill's paper is probably not only the list of viewpoints but also his reflection that, in the presence of an association, the fundamental question that the practice of epidemiology attempts at answering is: "is there any other of explaining the set of facts before us, is there any other answer equally, or more, likely than cause and effect?". In fact, the key notion is that, if a more likely explanation for the observed association exists, it will probably emerge from the analysis of one or more of Hill's considerations. Another important contribution of this paper is the clear statement that significance testing is useful to quantify the magnitude of the role of chance but adds nothing to the purpose of deciding whether or not an association is causal.

Aiming at analyzing the role of the infection with the human papilloma virus as a potential necessary cause for cervical cancer, Bosch et al underwent the massive process of reviewing available evidence and formally assessing the concordance of observed data with the considerations published by Hill, as well as those subsequently adopted by the International Agency for Research on Cancer (Bosch et al 2002). In this extensive review, by combining those considerations with the sufficient and component causes model, the authors conclude that the role of the infection is consistent with that of a necessary cause for cancer. Although compelling evidence of a causal relation had been available for a long time, their work takes a formal approach to ruling out alternative explanations and is additionally relevant in showing the role of Hill's important considerations in current causal inference.

2.2 Sufficient and component causes model

Aiming at bringing together a philosophical view of cause and the practice of epidemiology, Kenneth Rothman proposed an application of a sufficient and component causes model to epidemiology (Rothman 1976). Central to this model are the notions that each person is susceptible to multiple diseases and that each disease is a multifactorial outcome that results from the co-occurrence of several factors. The minimum set of causes enough to elicit disease is called a **sufficient cause**. Since it is reasonable to assume that not all individuals develop the disease through the same causal process, different sufficient causes are possible for the same disease, each with a different combination of factors (Figure 1, sufficient causes I to IV). Each of the factors that build up one or more of the sufficient causes is called a **component cause** (Fig. 1, CC_1 to CC_7). One of the interesting features of this model is that it enables the representation of sets of component causes that are assumed to intervene in disease causation but have not yet been identified (component causes U in Figure 1).

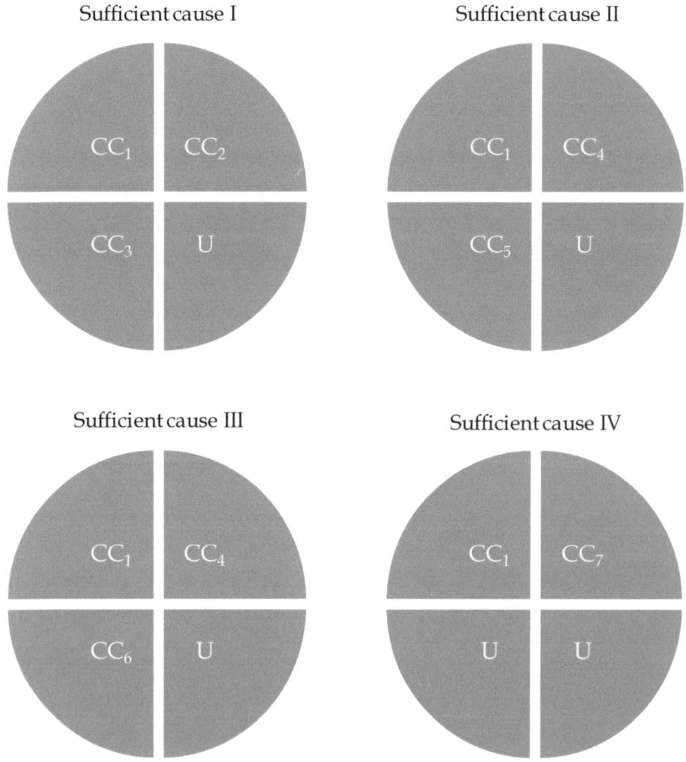

Fig. 1. Hypothetical examples of four sufficient causes for a disease. CC_1 to CC_7 - known component causes; U - unknown component cause(s)

In order to have a causal interpretation, component causes must be defined relative to a clearly defined contrast, i.e. a reference state with which the index state is compared. Since the underlying reality from which causes emerge may have various patent or latent dimensions, each of which may be seen as a continuum, component causes should be defined in relation to a number of attributes. These attributes are essential to conceptualize the presence of each component cause relative to the above-mentioned reference state. To clarify this, we may consider an example where we are studying the occurrence of an event such as venous thromboembolism in women as a possible adverse reaction to the use of a particular, clearly identified hormonal preparation. To define the use of that specific medication as a component cause, we should specify attributes such as **dose** (What mass of drug per day does the component cause refer to? Is the dose defined in relation to body size? Is the cumulative amount of life exposure a relevant attribute?), **duration** (How much exposure time should be considered in the index state? How is intermittent use of the drug relevant to the cause? Is there a particularly decisive biological timing of exposure, such as a specified gynecological age?), **induction period** (Which is the relevant time interval between the occurrence of the first component cause in the specific sufficient cause(s) of thromboembolism in which the hormone preparation is included and the completion of that sufficient cause?), and **reversibility** (Is it reasonable to assume a transient effect of hormone preparations on thromboembolism? Can the elimination of that exposure be considered complete, i.e. is a woman who never used the preparation in the same circumstances relative to the presence of the component cause as a woman who has never used it?). Although these examples of attributes are by no means exhaustive, they illustrate a part of the complexity in the decision of what constitutes a component cause. At the same time they elucidate on the need for its definition as clearly as possible when discussing causation.

Additionally, component causes may be **necessary** for the occurrence of disease if they are present in every possible sufficient cause (such as CC_1). Disease occurs in an individual when one of the sufficient causes is completed, i.e. all its component causes are present. The period throughout which component causes accumulate to finally produce clinical disease is called the **latent period**.

It should be noted that different component and therefore sufficient causes have different frequencies in the population. The notion of risk at the individual level can therefore be translated into whether or not a sufficient cause is completed. At the group level risk becomes the proportion of people in whom a sufficient cause is completed. An implication of this reasoning to observed data is that the strength of association of a component cause with the occurrence of disease is directly dependent on the frequency of the other causes with which it shares a sufficient cause.

It also results from this model that if one component cause may be identified and prevented, all cases of disease that result from the sufficient cause or causes in which that component cause is present will be avoided. This is in accordance with the intuitive notion that identifying and subsequently eliminating a necessary cause will eradicate disease since it will impair the completion of all sufficient causes. In terms of measures of impact, this model implies that the etiologic fraction of a component cause is the proportion of disease that is attributable to the sufficient causes that contain that component.

This model provides a clear conceptual meaning for effect modification or biological interaction: two component causes can be said to interact synergistically simply if there is one sufficient cause that contains both of them. There is full synergism if they are only involved in producing the disease through the sufficient cause in which they are both present, i.e., there is no other sufficient cause in which one of them is present rather than the one in which they interact (complete synergism between CC_2 and CC_3 but partial synergism between CC_4 and CC_5). One of the interesting features of this model is that it clearly distinguishes the concept of interaction - a biological concept which can be represented under this framework - from the concept of confounding - a phenomenon which is introduced by the observer and has no biological role in disease causation.

Although the sufficient and component causes model has been used mainly as a conceptual framework for causal thinking, namely for teaching purposes, an interesting application to data from the European Prospective Investigation into Cancer and Nutrition has been published (Hoffmann et al 2006). The authors identified all possible combinations in a set of known component causes of myocardial infarction (smoking, hypertension, obesity and lack of exercise). Every possible combination was considered to be part of a set of sufficient causes and the population attributable fraction regarding that combination of factors was taken as a measure of the proportion of disease attributable to that class of sufficient causes in the population. The authors argue that beyond its theoretical contribution, by allowing for the modeling of sufficient causes without necessarily knowing all of the component causes, the model may be used to guide public health interventions.

2.3 Counterfactual model

According to counterfactual theories in philosophy, causation may be reflected upon by hypothesizing what would have occurred had the conditions been different from the actual conditions observed. In terms of counterfactual conditionals, the meaning of a cause A can be defined in the form "If A had not occurred, C would not have occurred" (Menzies 2009). Although it had been long explored in the philosophical literature, the application of the counterfactual model, or potential outcomes model, to epidemiologic research is recent (Greenland & Robins 1986).

According to the counterfactual approach, when assessing whether an exposure causes an outcome, most of the time we are interested, even if not explicitly stated, in comparing the occurrence of the outcome when the exposure is present with its occurrence if the exposure was absent and all other factors remained equal (Maldonado & Greenland 2002). If we could compare these outcomes and they were different, we would conclude that there was a causal relation between the exposure and the outcome. In other words, the counterfactual ideal contrasts the occurrence of the outcome in the actual exposure status (the observed, **factual** outcome) with the occurrence of outcome in the **same** individual or population had the exposure not been present (the unobserved, **counterfactual** outcome).The counterfactual or potential outcomes model formalizes this contrast in terms of epidemiologic research.

At the individual level, subjects may be classified according to four susceptibility types under the model, defined according to the combination of both potential outcomes (factual and counterfactual). Even though we can only observe factual outcomes, each individual can theoretically be classified according to two responses: the occurrence of the outcome had he been exposed and the occurrence of the outcome had he not been exposed. Table 1 shows the occurrence of the outcome according to each susceptibility type. If we consider an adverse outcome, susceptibility type 1 designates individuals who will develop the outcome whether or not they are exposed – they are **doomed**. Type 2 groups individuals who will develop the outcome if they are exposed but not if they are unexposed - **causative exposure**; among these, the exposure has a causal effect on the outcome. Individuals in whom the outcome will occur if the exposure is absent but not if the exposure is present are grouped in type 3 - **preventive exposure**. Finally, subjects are called **immune** (type 4) if they will not develop the outcome during the observation period whether or not they are exposed. It should then be noted that in types 1 and 4 factual and counterfactual outcomes are the same, i.e., the exposure has no effect on the occurrence of the outcome. The presence of the exposure relative to its absence affects only types 2 and 3.

Counterfactual susceptibility type	Occurrence of outcome if exposed	Occurrence of outcome if not exposed
Type 1 – doomed	1	1
Type 2 – exposure causal	1	0
Type 3 – exposure preventive	0	1
Type 4 – immune	0	0

Table 1. Counterfactual susceptibility types classified according to the occurrence of outcome in factual/counterfactual exposure conditions. Legend – 1: present, 0: absent

Although we can admit the theoretical existence of a counterfactual contrast, for each individual we can observe only one outcome while the other remains, by definition, unobserved. Therefore, we cannot classify an individual into his susceptibility type. Since potential outcomes include a response that would have been observed in an exposure experience that did not actually take place, if individual A is exposed and the outcome occurs we can classify him as type 1 or 2 but we will not be able to distinguish between these two types. Therefore, we will not be able to differentiate between an individual who would have developed the outcome whether or not he had been exposed and one who developed the outcome because of the exposure. This non-identifiability issue arises from the fact that the same observed association (occurrence of the outcome given exposure) may originate from both causal (type 2) and noncausal (type 1) relations. In the same way, if the outcome is not observed among an exposed individual B, that information does not allow for the distinction between an individual in whom the exposure was preventive and one who was immune to the outcome (types 3 and 4, respectively).

Greenland & Robins add that the observation that an exposed individual develops the outcome while an unexposed does not develop the outcome has no causal interpretation unless the assumption that these two individuals belong to the same susceptibility type is added to the observed data. This assumption implies that individuals are exchangeable, i.e. that if individual A had been unexposed and individual B had been exposed the same overall result would have been observed. Confounding becomes then equivalent to a lack of exchangeability and therefore may be defined in terms of comparability. Because counterfactual parameters are by definition unobservable, the exchangeability assumption is not verifiable. In practical terms this means that the comparability between exposed and unexposed subjects (i.e. the magnitude of confounding) cannot be measured directly from observed data.

Although this model is applicable to the individual, the unobserved nature of counterfactuals impairs causal inference at the individual level. Therefore, in epidemiology, we are frequently interested in estimating average effects in a population of an exposure in the occurrence of a disease. In a population, the counterfactual reasoning translates into comparing the probability of the occurrence of the outcome if the entire population had one exposure distribution (Figure 2, A1) with the probability of occurrence if the entire population had an alternative exposure distribution (A0). A causal effect would be present if these counterfactual probabilities were different (Maldonado & Greenland 2002).

It should be emphasized that under the counterfactual approach, an effect measure compares the frequency of the outcome under **two** exposure distributions, but in **one** target population during **one** etiologic time period. Since the true causal effect is by its counterfactual definition never observable (because the two exposure distributions cannot occur simultaneously in the same target population), causal inference has to rely on the contrast between the actual frequency of the outcome in the observed target population (A1) and the actual frequency of the outcome in a population which is a **substitute** for the counterfactual disease frequency in the target population with regard to the exposure under study (B0). The more similar the substitute is to the target population the more likely it is that the true causal contrast ($risk_{A1}/risk_{A0}$) is reflected in the estimated contrast ($risk_{A1}/risk_{B0}$). Bias in etiologic studies may be seen as resulting from the existence of relevant differences between the substitute and the target.

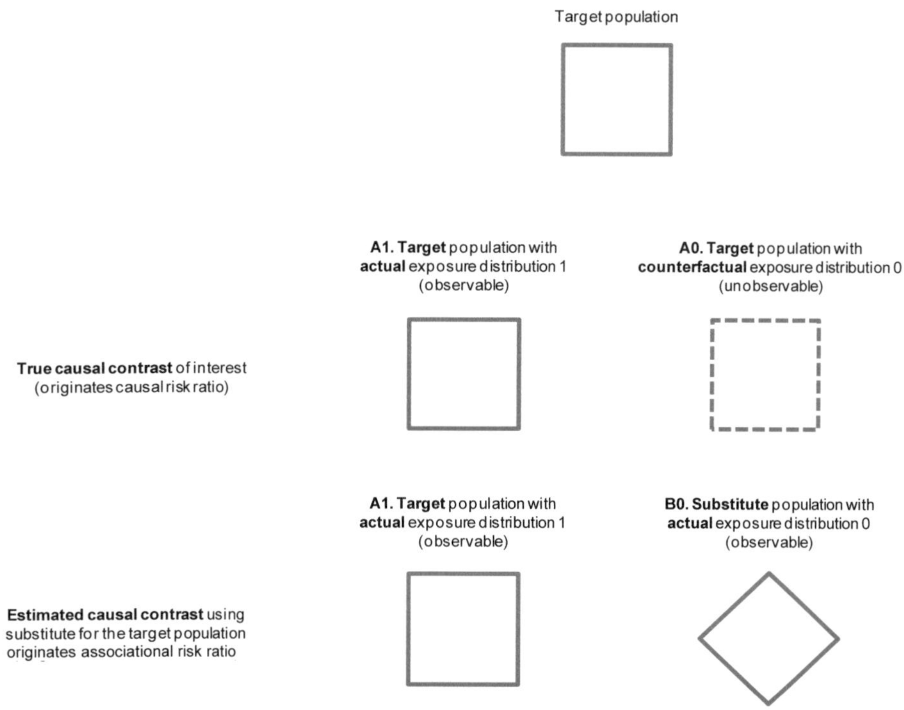

Fig. 2. Ideal causal (counterfactual) contrast and estimated causal contrast.

In the counterfactual framework, randomization can be seen as a means of obtaining the observed contrast as close as possible to the counterfactual ideal. If we assume perfect randomization and no random error, both groups (exposed to the index intervention and unexposed) are as similar as possible with regard to measured and unmeasured factors. As a consequence, the probability of developing the outcome among the control group equals the probability of developing the outcome in the intervention group had the latter not received the intervention (counterfactual). In this circumstance, groups are considered exchangeable and the causal risk ratio is accurately estimated by the associational risk ratio.

An application of the counterfactual framework to discuss selection criteria and generalizability of safety conclusions in randomized controlled trials has been recently published (Weisberg et al 2009). For a number of reasons, in trials of pharmacological interventions it is usual to exclude individuals with increased probability of drop-out or adverse events. This option is chosen at the expense of generalizability regarding the safety of the intervention, since selection probability is dependent on the baseline risk of adverse event. In their work, Weisberg *et al* argue that trials usually screen out individuals at high risk of an adverse event by measuring indicators of such risk. They make the point that those indicators are also predictive of the probability of experiencing adverse events in the **absence** of treatment (i.e. under placebo) since they are measured before the intervention starts. The authors assume that these indicators remain better predictors of the probability of adverse event under placebo than if treatment is introduced. As a result of those strict selection criteria, individuals most likely to have an adverse event if placed in the placebo arm of the trial have higher probability of being excluded. In counterfactual terms, this means that there is an underrepresentation of individuals for whom the intervention would be preventive, i.e. who would have the adverse event if under placebo but not if they received the active treatment.

Table 2 presents the hypothetical results proposed by the authors for a trial where the outcome is an adverse event. Two scenarios are posed: one in which all counterfactual susceptibility types regarding the adverse event under study have the same selection probability, which corresponds to their prevalence in the target population, and another in which there is selective undersampling of individuals who would have had the event under placebo, i.e. doomed and preventive susceptibility types. In this example, the authors use counterfactual susceptibility types to illustrate that the ratio of the risks of adverse event between the two arms may be biased and a conclusion of a causal effect may be derived when the observed association is due only to selection criteria which originate a dependence between counterfactual susceptibility types and the probability of entering the trial.

Under non-differential selection criteria					
Counterfactual susceptibility type	Proportion in the population	Selection probability	Number of participants in each arm	Adverse events under active treatment	Adverse events under placebo
Doomed	6%	100%	15	15	15
Causal	4%	100%	10	10	0
Preventive	4%	100%	10	0	10
Immune	86%	100%	215	0	0
			Risk of adverse event	*10.0%*	*10.0%*
Under differential selection criteria					
Counterfactual susceptibility type	Proportion in the population	Selection probability	Number of participants in each arm	Adverse events under active treatment	Adverse events under placebo
Doomed	6%	20%	3	3	3
Causal	4%	80%	8	8	0
Preventive	4%	20%	2	0	2
Immune	86%	80%	172	0	0
			Risk of adverse event	*5.9%*	*2.7%*

Table 2. Selection probability for a hypothetical randomized trial according to counterfactual susceptibility types (adapted from Weisberg 2009).

This is an interesting example of the use of counterfactual thinking for illustrating selection bias. Although one may assume, contrarily to the authors, that individuals who are at greater risk of developing adverse events under treatment (doomed and causal rather that doomed and preventive) are underrepresented, the issue of different selection probabilities given different susceptibility types would remain relevant.

More often than not, experimental studies are not feasible and causal inference relies on observational data. In non-randomized studies, confounding emerges if the chosen substitute does not accurately represent the target population under the counterfactual condition, i.e. if the two groups of contrasting exposure distributions that are compared with respect to the occurrence of the outcome are not exchangeable. Such inadequate substitute may originate relevant differences between the observed (associational) risk ratio and the true (causal) risk ratio.

Today, there is growing use of the counterfactual model of causation in epidemiologic research. The application of the counterfactual framework to epidemiologic research has been subject to discussion (Dawid 2002; Elwert & Winship 2002; Kaufman & Kaufman 2002; Shafer 2002). In practice, it should be noted that this framework does not aim at clarifying mechanisms of disease causation and that there is a potential for impossible counterfactuals, which are not amenable to intervention and have therefore limited interest in public health. Nevertheless, the model provides, for individuals or populations, a causal interpretation to measures of association. More importantly, the counterfactual ideal is relevant in the design and analysis of etiologic studies since it provides a framework for choosing the target population as well as an appropriate substitute for that target. It is also an important approach to clarify threats to validity.

2.4 Causal diagrams

One of the most intuitive ways of representing and communicating hypothetical causal relations between epidemiological variables is to visually depict the paths believed to relate them, namely exposure, outcome and possible confounders. For a long time the use of such visual tools to assist causal inference was informal and lacked theoretical support. The development of computer science and the corresponding need for improvement of the quality of the decision process on the basis of the relations between previously defined and empirical data from complex systems led to the development of a solid theoretical basis for the use of graphical models (Pearl 1995).

This body of work allowed for the formal application of causal diagrams outside the artificial intelligence domain to a number of areas where causal inference relies on the combination of causal assumptions with observational data. Causal diagrams have been increasingly used in epidemiology and have proved to be a helpful approach to conceptualize research questions and analytical issues (Greenland et al 1999). Indeed, one of the most interesting features of these diagrams is that, by depicting qualitative and nonparametric assumptions of causal mechanisms linking variables in a dataset and knowing a number of mathematical rules, it is possible to characterize the nature of common systematic errors in causal inference, as well as to guide study design.

Causal diagrams used in epidemiology are known as **directed acyclic graphs** (DAGs). The relations between variables in a DAG are translated in a set of formal rules known as ***d*-separation rules** (where *d* means "directional"), which are used to judge whether variables are associated (*d*-connected) or independent (*d*-separated) (Pearl 2009). In a DAG, variables are named **nodes** and are linked by arrows called **edges**. Since a variable cannot be, at the same instant, a cause and a consequence of another variable there are no cycles in DAGs. In the following example, E and O are nodes connected by an edge. In DAG terminology E is a parent or ancestor of O, and O is a child or descendant of E.

E→O

A **path** is a sequence of edges that connect two variables regardless of the direction of the edges, such as the following path that links variables A and O. This path is called **unblocked** because there are no head to head arrows colliding along the path:

A→X→E→O

If two edges meet head to head the node where they meet is called a **collider**. In the following example, where Y is a collider, the path between A and Y is unblocked (A and Y are *d*-connected) but the path between A and O is blocked by Y (A and O are *d*-separated):

A→X→E→Y←O

Any one of these nodes (or variables) may be **conditioned on** or, in other words, it may be set at a specific value. In classic epidemiologic language, this is most of the times equivalent to adjustment for or stratification according to X. If a **non-collider** such as X is conditioned on, as shown by the square symbol around it, the path between A and Y becomes **blocked** and A and Y become *d*-separated:

A→$\boxed{X}$→E→Y←O

If, however, a **collider** such as Y is conditioned on, the path between A and O becomes **unblocked** and A and O become *d*-connected:

A→X→E→$\boxed{Y}$←O

Pearl provided also a very clear example of the meaning of conditioning on a collider. Suppose that there are two reasons for a car not starting: not having fuel and having a dead battery, according to the following diagram:

Dead battery → Car does not start ← No fuel

These causes are marginally independent, i.e., having information on one of them tells us nothing about the other (they are *d*-separated). Indeed, knowing that the battery is dead does not improve our prediction of whether or not there is fuel. However, if the collider is conditioned on, i.e., if we known that the car does not start, knowing that the battery is not dead tells us that there must be no fuel. Dead battery and no fuel, which were marginally independent, become dependent (*d*-connected) by conditioning on their common effect. If the descendant of a collider such as Z is conditioned on, the path between A and O also becomes unblocked:

A→X→E→Y←O
↓
$\boxed{Z}$

A DAG is causal only if it includes the common causes of any two nodes represented (Markov condition). In the previous case, if there is a variable X which is a common cause of E and O it must be depicted in the diagram. This condition simplifies the diagram since it implies that any variable which is not a common cause of two or more variables in the DAG does not need to be depicted in the graph.

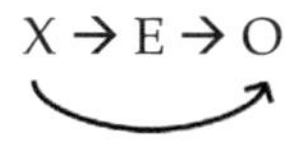

In the previous diagram the path that connects E to O through X (E←X→O) is called a **backdoor path**. If the common cause of E and O is conditioned on, that backdoor path will be closed. Consequently, if X is the only common cause of E and O, after adjustment for X, the statistical association found between E and O will be a result of the true causal effect of E on O, which is equivalent to eliminating confounding.

Using the above-mentioned rules, and assuming no random error, statistical associations between variables can be found in the three following causal diagram scenarios:

1. They are cause (E) and effect (O):

E→O

2. They share common causes (X) that have not been conditioned on (open backdoor path):

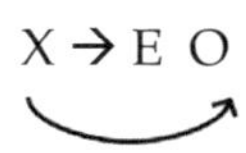

3. They share common effects (Y) that have been conditioned on:

E→Y←O

While the first alternative depicts a **true causal effect** of E on O, the second scenario is the graphical representation of **confounding** and the third translates **selection bias**.

A very interesting example of the application of causal diagrams to judge the appropriateness of conditioning on available variables has been presented to explain the so-called "birth weight paradox" (Hernandez-Diaz et al 2006). In perinatal epidemiology, birth weight is a routinely collected variable because of its ability to predict adverse outcomes during infancy. Probably as a result of its importance and wide availability, birth weight is frequently an adjustment or stratification variable in the analysis of the effects of several other exposures on infant mortality.

From the comparison of the associations found among low birth weight infants with those found in normal weight infants emerged what was called the birth weight paradox: the associations between known adverse exposures such as maternal smoking and infant mortality was weaker among low birth weight infants than among normal weight children. In other words, although it was known that smoking caused low birth weight and increased infant mortality, it was estimated that the effect of smoking on mortality was greater in normal weight infants. As a consequence, it was hypothesized that maternal smoking could be protective against infant mortality in low birth weight children.

To explain this apparent paradox, Hernandez-Diaz *et al* proposed several DAGs depicting *a priori* assumptions about the causal relations between variables. They proposed that even using a simple set of causal assumptions it may be shown that bias may arise from adjustment to birth weight. Convincing evidence exists that there are common causes of low birth weight and mortality (U), such as birth defects and malnutrition. In those circumstances, the most simplistic DAG that could be drawn would be the following:

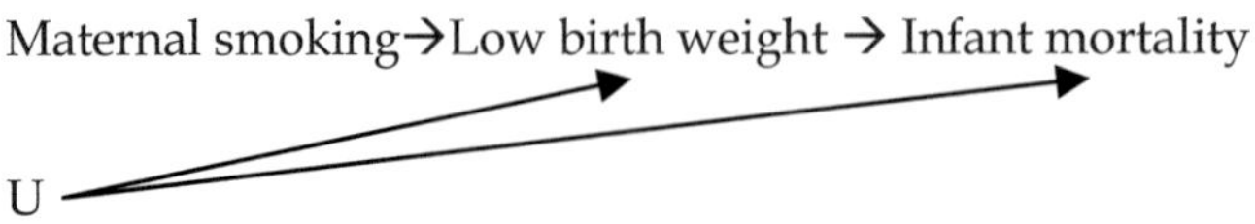

Low birth weight is a collider in this graph, since it is a common effect of smoking as well as of other causes (U). Conditioning on birth weight will create a spurious dependence between maternal smoking and the other low birth causes. Indeed, if we know that a child had low birth weight and that the mother never smoked, then it is more likely that the child had low birth weight because of another (probably more serious) cause than maternal smoking, such as a birth defect. That other cause will probably be a stronger determinant of infant mortality than smoking.

Therefore, in low birth weight infants, smoking may appear protective of infant mortality only because, after birth weight stratification, it indicates lower probability of other causes of low birth weight and therefore of infant mortality. This bias will emerge even if the "true" causal DAG includes an effect of low birth weight on infant mortality and/or an effect of maternal smoking on mortality not mediated by birth weight, as shown in the following diagram:

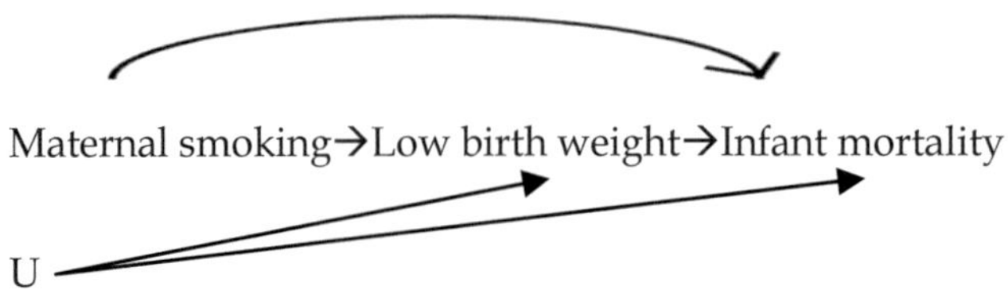

This interesting example of the introduction of selection bias in the analysis of data illustrates the usefulness of causal diagrams in distinguishing between variables that measure common causes and those which measure common effects. In fact, one of the points made by the authors of the example referred above is that the choice of variables to include in regression modeling should not be driven by their availability or biological relevance alone, but after a hypothesis has been formulated on what their role in the causal pathway might be.

Another important example of a decision in data analysis where causal diagrams may be of importance is the analysis of change, which is of great importance with the increasing abundance of prospectively collected data. Imagine we are studying the physiological increase in bone strength (measured through bone mineral density) throughout adolescence. We are interested in assessing whether adiposity in early adolescence (measured as body fat mass) has an effect on the extent of bone strength increase between early and late adolescence. Suppose that we have a dataset with the following variables:

- Bone mineral density in early adolescence (BMD_{early})
- Bone mineral density increase from early to late adolescence (BMD_{change})
- Total body fat mass in early adolescence (Fat_{early})

There is a body of evidence indicating that total body fat has an overall positive effect on bone strength at the same age. Additionally, there is also evidence that baseline bone density has an effect on the change in bone strength throughout the following years. Our causal DAG could be the following:

$Fat_{early} \rightarrow BMD_{early} \rightarrow BMD_{change}$

What we want to know is if there might be an effect of fat on BMD change that is independent of bone mineral density in early adolescence, as depicted in the following diagram:

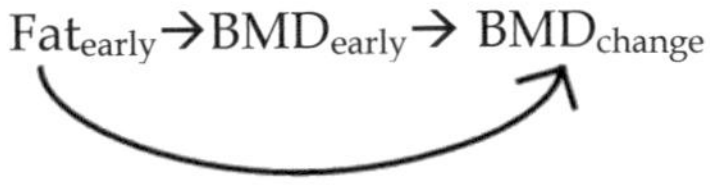

One of the questions we frequently have when facing this kind of research problems is whether or not we should adjust for baseline characteristics, in this case for BMD in early adolescence. Using different examples, the point has been made that it is very likely that there are unmeasured common causes of variables shown in the previous diagram (Glymour et al 2005; VanderWeele 2009). According to rules previously presented, any common causes of two variables in a DAG have to be depicted. That means that the previous DAG is probably not a good representation of the true causal structure, and that the following diagram could be more consistent with previous expert knowledge:

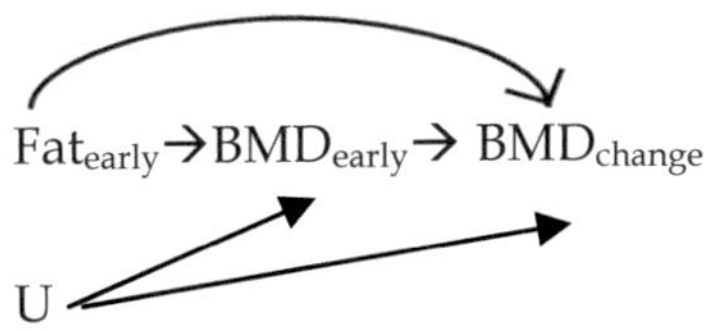

This addition of unmeasured common causes to the diagram turns BMD_{early} into a collider, which means that adjusting for (or conditioning on) that variable creates a spurious association between those common causes and adiposity, which were marginally independent before adjustment. This means that an adjusted estimate may be biased, since we may be in truth measuring the association between those unmeasured common causes and bone strength change and estimating it as the true effect of adiposity on bone strength change.

If we consider that one of those unmeasured common causes may be lean body mass, we may see conditioning on a collider similarly to the car example: if an adolescent has low body fat and high bone strength, that may be due to increase lean mass, which has documented positive effect on bone properties. Adjusting for baseline BMD (a collider) could therefore originate biased effect estimates. Only by identifying and measuring all common causes of any two variables in the diagram would we be able to adjust for them, blocking all backdoor paths and thus eliminating confounding.

As seen from the examples above, by applying a small set of formal mathematical rules these diagrams provide a tool for identifying sources of bias in study design or in the analysis of results, thus providing an interesting framework for causal inference. DAGs have the additional advantage of clearly depicting assumptions about the causal structure of data, thus improving clarity in the communication of hypothesized causal relations between variables. Since they are nonparametric qualitative models which do not by themselves provide information on the magnitude of effects, DAGs may be used to assess to which extent previous assumptions are compatible with observed data.

Causal diagrams should not be expected to provide the answer to causal questions. DAGs are useful exactly because we will most probably never know the "true" DAG for most causal mechanisms. These diagrams provide a common framework for clarifying causal assumptions and guiding study design and data analysis in such a way that it is not contradictory with those assumptions.

3. Conclusion

Epidemiologic research is primarily driven by the observation of difference, which in human populations virtually never corresponds to an ideal contrast. Epidemiologists then try to explain that difference and to identify the factors that can be acted upon to improve population health.

The development and widespread use of statistical modeling techniques has dramatically improved our ability to efficiently quantify statistical associations between variables. It has allowed us to model relations between enormous numbers of variables. In the context of etiologic research, the magnitude and even the statistical significance of the associations estimated have been used as evidence for causation, while a more formal causality assessment has frequently gone undiscussed.

In order to quantify the role of different types of findings in the appraisal of causality, an interesting experience conducted among 159 epidemiologists, where each subject was shown computer-simulated summaries of evidence of the relation between an exposure and an outcome (Holman et al 2001). In this study, the factors with the strongest influence in causal attribution by epidemiologists were statistical significance and refutation of alternative explanations, followed by strength of association and coherence.

The frameworks presented strengthen the point that etiologic research aims at disclosing causal relations rather than co-occurring characteristics. Assumptions regarding causation are present in virtually all domains of scientific research. In areas where controlled experiments are admissible, the observation of difference may frequently be taken as evidence for causation and the theory underlying causal thinking remains implicit. However, causal inference in epidemiology can seldom be a result of such ideal experiments. The observational nature of most epidemiologic research is probably the main reason for the search for frameworks to guide causal inference in the study of the etiology of human disease.

None of the models presented can be expected to uncover the complexity of disease causation. Nevertheless, these frameworks are important contributions for the design and analysis of epidemiological studies, as well as for integrating observed data and prior knowledge with the purpose of judging whether or not a true causal effect is the best explanation for differences observed.

4. Acknowledgment

Project grant FCT-PTDC/SAU-ESA/108407/2008 and individual grant SFRH/BD/40656/2007 from the Portuguese Foundation for Science and Technology are gratefully acknowledged.

5. References

Bosch FX, Lorincz A, Munoz N, Meijer CJ, Shah KV. (2002). The causal relation between human papillomavirus and cervical cancer. J Clin Pathol 55:244-65

Broadbent A. (2009). Causation and models of disease in epidemiology. Stud Hist Philos Biol Biomed Sci 40:302-11

Dawid AP. (2002). Counterfactuals: help or hindrance? Int J Epidemiol 31:429-30; discussion 35-8

Dictionary.com (2011). cause. (n.d.). Dictionary.com Unabridged. Retrieved September 23, 2011, from Dictionary.com website: http://dictionary.reference.com/browse/cause.

Elwert F, Winship C. (2002). Population versus individual level causal effects. Int J Epidemiol 31:432-4; discussion 5-8

Glymour MM, Weuve J, Berkman LF, Kawachi I, Robins JM. (2005). When is baseline adjustment useful in analyses of change? An example with education and cognitive change. Am J Epidemiol 162:267-78

Greenland S, Pearl J, Robins JM. (1999). Causal diagrams for epidemiologic research. Epidemiology 10:37-48

Greenland S, Robins JM. (1986). Identifiability, exchangeability, and epidemiological confounding. Int J Epidemiol 15:413-9

Hernandez-Diaz S, Schisterman EF, Hernan MA. (2006). The birth weight "paradox" uncovered? Am J Epidemiol 164:1115-20

Hill AB. (1965). The environment and disease: association or causation? Proc R Soc Med 58:295-300

Hoffmann K, Heidemann C, Weikert C, Schulze MB, Boeing H. (2006). Estimating the proportion of disease due to classes of sufficient causes. Am J Epidemiol 163:76-83

Holman CD, Arnold-Reed DE, de Klerk N, McComb C, English DR. (2001). A psychometric experiment in causal inference to estimate evidential weights used by epidemiologists. Epidemiology 12:246-55

Kaufman JS, Kaufman S. (2002). Estimating causal effects. Int J Epidemiol 31:431-2; discussion 5-8

Krieger N. (1994). Epidemiology and the web of causation: has anyone seen the spider? Soc Sci Med 39:887-903

Luedeking R. (1884). The Chief Local Factors in the Causation of Disease and Death. Public Health Pap Rep 10:329-31

Maldonado G, Greenland S. 2002. Estimating causal effects. Int J Epidemiol 31:422-9

Menzies P. (2009). "Counterfactual Theories of Causation", The Stanford Encyclopedia of Philosophy (Fall 2009 Edition), Edward N. Zalta (ed.), URL = <http://plato.stanford.edu/archives/fall2009/entries/causation-counterfactual/>

Parascandola M, Weed DL. (2001). Causation in epidemiology. J Epidemiol Community Health 55:905-12

Pearl J. (1995). Causal diagrams for empirical research. Biometrika 82:669-710

Pearl J. (2009). Causality: Models, Reasoning and Inference: Cambridge University Press; 2 edition.

Rothman K, Greenland S, Lash T. (2008). Modern Epidemiology: Lippincott Williams & Wilkins. Philadelphia, 2008.

Rothman KJ. (1976). Causes. Am J Epidemiol 104:587-92

Shafer G. (2002). Estimating causal effects. Int J Epidemiol 31:434-5; discussion 5-8
VanderWeele TJ. (2009). Marginal structural models for the estimation of direct and indirect effects. Epidemiology 20:18-26.
Weisberg HI, Hayden VC, Pontes VP. (2009). Selection criteria and generalizability within the counterfactual framework: explaining the paradox of antidepressant-induced suicidality? Clin Trials 6:109-18.

3

Causal Diagrams and Three Pairs of Biases

Eyal Shahar and Doron J. Shahar
University of Arizona
USA

1. Introduction

An association between variables is an idea whose meaning is usually grasped intuitively. In most minds, the statement "Variables *D* and *E* are associated" does not call for an explanation. Far less clear is the meaning of causation on which volumes have been written by both philosophers and scientists. Courses in epidemiology teach students to recite the mantra 'association is not causation', which is true of course—the words are not synonyms—but the two ideas are connected, and one may be developed from the other.

Considering association to be a basic idea, we define causation as a special type of association between two time-point variables: an association *that is directed forward in time*. It is often depicted by a single-headed arrow pointing toward a later time. If *E* is antecedent to *D*, then $E \rightarrow D$ denotes "Variable *E* is a cause of variable *D*". If *F* follows *E* and is antecedent to *D*, then $E \rightarrow F \rightarrow D$ denotes "Variable *E* is a cause of variable *D* via an intermediary variable *F*". All branches of science, from particle physics to cancer epidemiology, share a single theme: the study of causation.

The effect of *E* on *D* is defined as the strength of the causation between *E* and *D*. We can estimate the magnitude of that effect (which may be null or negligible) by studying the association between the two variables. In some cases, estimating the marginal ('crude') association between *E* and *D* would suffice; no further action is needed. Often, however, other variables should be taken into account. A causal diagram—a set of variables and arrows (Pearl, 1995)—clearly explains what should be done to estimate a particular effect. Moreover, causal diagrams help to clarify a long-standing confusion about the taxonomy of biases (Sackett, 1979; Grimes & Schulz, 2002). In fact, almost any claim of bias can be depicted in a diagram.

If causal diagrams are such a powerful tool, can't science be turned into a computerized algorithm of discovery? Unfortunately, no. To estimate the effect $E \rightarrow D$, we have to display background causal theories in the form of other arrows; those arrows are often the subject of heated exchanges about sources of bias. No computer program can replace the human debate, and no verdict should be issued either. It is always possible that some critical variables were displayed incorrectly, or not displayed at all. Moreover, scientists often struggle with an inevitable trade-off between bias, variance, and effort. For example, reducing bias costs extra variance and reducing variance costs extra bias. No algorithm can strike a balance between the two. It is a human decision.

2. Effect modification

The effect *E*→*D* might depend on the value of another cause of *D*, say *Q* (*Q*→*D*). For instance, the harmful effect of heparin injection (*E*) on bleeding (*D*) could depend on aspirin use (*Q*): heparin might have a stronger effect on bleeding in the presence of aspirin in the blood than in its absence. This phenomenon is called effect modification; *Q* is called an effect modifier (Shahar & Shahar, 2010a). Effect modification of *E*→*D* by *Q* requires *Q* to have at least one value (say, *Q*=1), such that the effect *E*→*D* when *Q*=1 differs from that effect when *Q*=*q*≠1. If *Q* takes more than two values, the effect *E*→*D* might be unique to each value of *Q*. In the general case of multiple modifiers, every combination of their values might dictate a unique effect. For instance, the effect of heparin on bleeding could vary according to the combined values of aspirin use (yes, no), sex (male, female), genotype (A, B, C), and weight (continuous). The simple idea of effect modification opens the door to endless variations.

So far we have considered *E*→*D* to be the effect of interest and *Q* (*Q*→*D*) to be the modifier. But the causal situation of *E* and *Q* is symmetrical: *E*→*D*←*Q*. The variable *Q* does not have some special property of a modifier which *E* is lacking. Indeed, we may consider *Q*→*D* to be the effect of interest and *E* to be the modifier. Effect modification is therefore a reciprocal phenomenon (Shahar & Shahar, 2010a): given two causes, *E* and *Q*, of some outcome, *E* modifies *Q*'s effect if and only if *Q* modifies *E*'s effect.

To depict a theory of effect modification of *E*→*D* by *Q*, we will place the lower case *q* above the arrow *E*→*D*. That intuitive notation indicates that the effect behind the arrow depends on the value of *Q*. Given reciprocity, we should also place the lower case *e* above the arrow *Q*→*D*. An arrow with no letter denotes a theory of no effect modification; *E* has the same effect on *D* for every value of any other cause of *D*.

Whether modified or not, an effect has to be estimated on some scale: usually a difference scale (e.g., probability difference) or a ratio scale (e.g., probability ratio). Therefore, the magnitude of any effect depends on the chosen scale. For instance, a probability difference of one percentage point could mean a two-fold probability if computed from 2% and 1%, or a three-fold probability if computed from 1.5% and 0.5%. Likewise, the magnitude—and sometimes direction—of effect modification are scale dependent. Which scale is preferred, if either, is beyond the scope of this chapter.

Whenever effect-modification is 'small enough' on a given scale, it may be ignored, even if it is not sharply null. This practice is analogous to ignoring a 'small enough' effect in a causal diagram: when the effect *E*→*D* is assumed to be too small to be of interest, we may omit the arrow altogether. Similarly, when effect modification by *Q* is assumed to be negligible, we may omit the letter *q* above the arrow *E*→*D*. Except for precise theoretical considerations, the prevailing dichotomy between 'null' and 'not null', or between 'modified' and 'not modified', is not warranted in science, because 'small enough' is not more interesting than exactly null or exactly unmodifed.

3. Confounding bias

Let *E*→*D* be the effect of interest, which may be strong, weak, or even precisely null. The marginal ('crude') association between *E* and *D* (of whatever magnitude) is due, in part, to the effect *E*→*D* (Figure 1). Unfortunately, however, that arrow is not the only contributor to the marginal association.

Figure 1 also shows a variable *C*, which is antecedent to *E* (and therefore antecedent to *D* as well). By definition *C*→*E* and *C*→*D*, regardless of the magnitude of these effects. Recalling that causation is a forward association in time, the structure *E*←*C*→*D* does not depict causation between *E* and *D* because the path of arrows from *E* to *D* requires backward movement in time. Starting at *E*, we first travel back to *C*, which is antecedent to *E*, and then travel forward to *D*. Nonetheless, this path contributes to the marginal association between *E* and *D*, so long as the effects *C*→*E* and *C*→*D* are not precisely null.

Such a variable *C*—a common cause of *E* and *D*—is called a confounder. The path *E*←*C*→*D* is called a confounding path. Note that a confounder is a cause of *D* *not only via E*. The structure *C*→*E*→D, for example, does not depict a confounder even though *C* is cause of *E* (directly) and a cause of *D* (via *E*). It does not contribute to the marginal association between *E* and *D*.

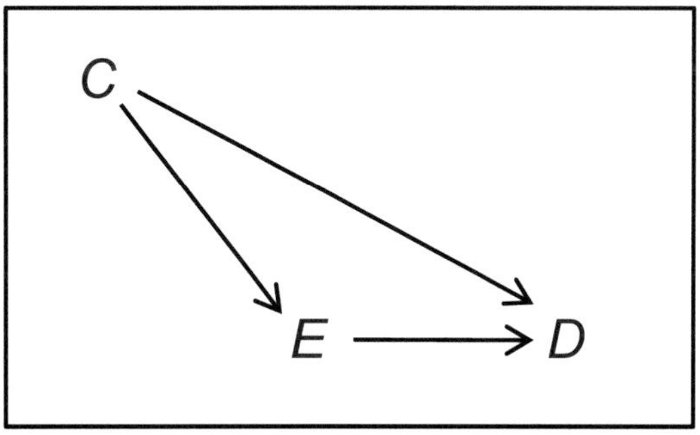

Fig. 1. Two sources of the marginal association between *E* and *D*: *E*→*D* (the effect of interest) and *E*←*C*→*D* (a confounding path)

Evidently, if we try to estimate the effect of *E* on *D* by their marginal association, some bias will be present—confounding bias (Figure 1). That association reflects not only the magnitude of the effect of interest (*E*→*D*), but also the magnitude of a confounding path (*E*←*C*→*D*). Again, the contribution of each source can range from very large to null. When the contribution of a confounding path is 'small enough', confounding bias is still present but may be ignored.

Assume, for example, that *C* is body fat at time 1; *E* is serum glucose at time 2; *D* is blood pressure at time 3; and the effect of interest is *serum glucose→blood pressure*. The marginal association between serum glucose and blood pressure is driven, at least in part, by the path *serum glucose←body fat→blood pressure*. Therefore, some confounding bias is present—assuming that neither effect of body fat is precisely null.

The magnitude of confounding bias depends on the strength of the effects *C*→*E* and *C*→*D*. The weaker the effects of the confounder—the smaller is the bias. If one of these effects is precisely null, confounding bias does not exist at all. The distribution of the values of the confounder also plays a role: For example, a 100:0 distribution of some binary confounder will not generate bias (Section 3.1). Finally, the direction of the effects *C*→*E* and *C*→*D* determines the direction of the bias. Confounding bias could lead to any kind of distortion in an attempt to find the effect *E*→*D*: over-estimation, under-estimation, or even missing the direction of the effect.

The last statement should not be interpreted as a claim about the relation between any estimate and the true effect ('the causal parameter'). That relation remains unknown, and an estimate from a biased study could happen to be closer to the unknown parameter than an estimate from an unbiased study. Claims about bias should therefore point the finger at the *method* that has generated an estimate ('the estimator'), not at the estimate itself. The term 'bias' alludes to a discrepancy between the theoretical result of a study at infinity and the causal parameter. Some writers consider "at infinity" as infinite replications of the study. We prefer to consider it as an infinite-size version of the study.

3.1 Deconfounding

Most, if not all, of the methods to eliminate confounding bias are based on conditioning, which means (in its simplest form) restriction to one value of a variable. Conditioning (denoted by a box) dissociates a "variable"—now just a value—from both its causes and its effects, because a *value* is not associated with any other variable. For example, rather than estimating the marginal association between *E* and *D*, we would estimate a conditional association—the association between *E* and *D* when the confounder *C* is restricted to a single value. Since the confounding path has been blocked (Figure 2, Diagram A), the only source of the conditional association is the effect *E*→*D*.

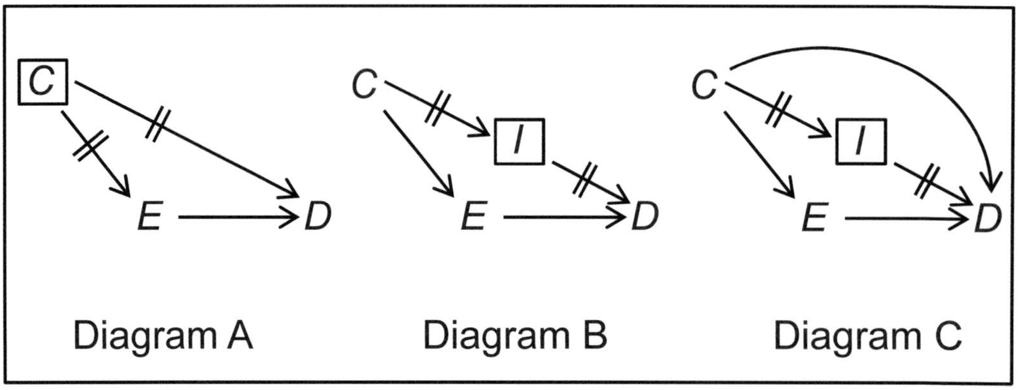

Fig. 2. Conditioning (denoted by a box) dissociates a variable from its causes and its effects (denoted by two lines over incoming and outgoing arrows). After conditioning, confounding bias is eliminated (Diagrams A and B) and is either reduced or increased (Diagram C)

It is not always necessary to deconfound by conditioning on the confounder. A confounding path may sometimes be blocked by conditioning on an intermediary variable (*I*) along the path (Figure 2, Diagram B). That would not suffice, however, if the effect of the confounder is not exclusively mediated by the intermediary (Figure 2, Diagram C). In that case, conditioning on the intermediary might reduce, but not eliminate, confounding bias because one confounding path is still open (*E*←*C*→*D*). Whether bias will be reduced at all depends on the two paths by which *C* affects *D* (*C*→*I*→*D* and *C*→*D*). If both of them deliver causation of *D* in the same direction, confounding bias will be reduced. Otherwise, the bias will actually increase, because the association of *C* with *D* will be strengthened, rather than weakened, after conditioning on *I*. Similar arguments apply to conditioning on an intermediary variable between C and *E* (C→*I*→*E*).

3.2 Deconfounding by restriction, stratification, or regression

Conditioning may be achieved by restricting the sample to people who share a single value of the confounder—for example, recruiting only women into the study. Alternatively, conditioning may be achieved by stratification of the sample on the values of the confounder. If the confounder, *C*, is a categorical variable with *k* values, stratification will generate *k* estimates of the effect *E*→*D*, one per each value (stratum) of *C*. Assuming no effect modification between *E* and *C*, all of the estimates may be replaced with a single weighted average, which is a deconfounded estimator of the effect *E*→*D*.

To remove confounding by several categorical variables, we may stratify on all of them simultaneously and compute a weighted average of as many estimates as we get (again, assuming no effect modification). Of course, as the number of strata increases, the number of stratum-specific observations decreases and at some point the method will fail: reduction of confounding bias will cost too large of a variance. The method will also fail when we have to condition on continuous variables where stratification is practically impossible. In those cases, regression analysis usually substitutes for a simple weighted average. The variables are added to the right hand side of a regression model.

3.3 Deconfounding by randomization

A confounding path (*E*←*C*→*D*) may be eliminated by another method, besides conditioning on the confounder *C*, or on some intermediary on the path. Suppose that *E* has a cause, *R*, which is not a confounder, and that *R* and the confounder *C* are effect modifiers with respect to *E* (Figure 3, Diagram A). Suppose further that the effect *C*→*E* is null for some value of *R*, say, *R*=1. If we restrict the sample to *R*=1 (condition on *R*), the confounder *C* will not be associated with *E*, and the confounding path will no longer exist (Figure 3, Diagram B).

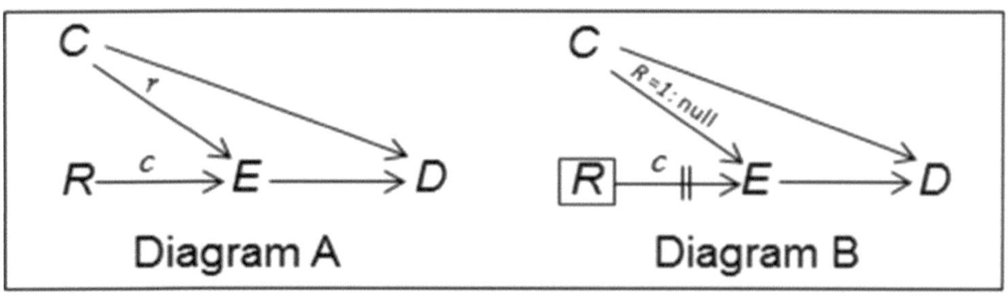

Fig. 3. Deconfounding by conditioning on *R*, a modifier of the effect *C*→*E* (Diagram A), assuming that the effect *C*→*E* is null when *R*=1 (Diagram B)

That method operates in a randomized trial (Figure 4). The first cause on the horizontal path is the randomization mechanism (*R*), which takes a value for each possible mechanism (e.g., a coin toss, a computer program), as well as one value for 'not randomized'. *R* is a cause of the treatment offered, $E_{OFFERED}$, because the probability of offering some treatment in a randomized study differs from that probability in a non-randomized study. $E_{OFFERED}$, in turn, is a cause of E_{TAKEN}—the treatment actually taken by a patient—and E_{TAKEN} is a cause of *D*.

Both *E*-variables have other causes, too, some of which are also causes of *D* not via *E* (Figure 4). When the effect of interest is $E_{OFFERED}$→*D*, *C*-type variables are confounders. When the effect of interest is E_{TAKEN}→D, both C-type variables and Q-type variables are confounders. (Q-type variables are causes of E_{TAKEN} not via $E_{OFFERED}$.) Notice that R is a cause of both E-variables, but it is not a confounder.

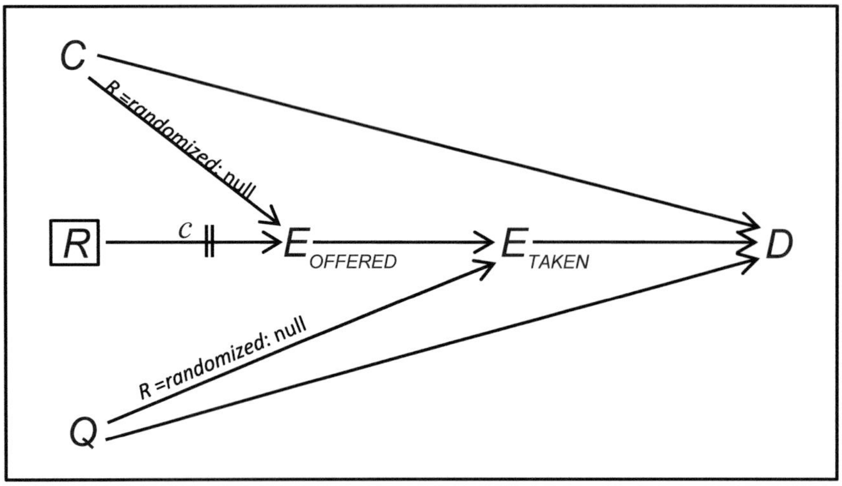

Fig. 4. Deconfounding by randomization (R), a modifier of the effects C→$E_{OFFERED}$ and Q→E_{TAKEN}, assuming that these effects are null when R=*randomized* (by some mechanism)

Randomization in a trial implies conditioning on the variable R (Figure 4). To estimate the effect of $E_{OFFERED}$ on D, we invoke a theory of effect modification and assume that C-type variables have a null effect on $E_{OFFERED}$ when randomization is executed (R=*randomization mechanism*), in contrast to a non-null effect otherwise (R=*not randomized*). It is not that difficult, however, to propose C-type variables that have a non-null effect on $E_{OFFERED}$ even within a randomized trial (Shahar & Shahar, 2009).

Although the effect of offering a treatment ($E_{OFFERED}$→E_{TAKEN}→D) is of interest to the physician, the patient is far more interested in the effect of taking a treatment (E_{TAKEN}→D). To estimate the latter effect, we may invoke, again, a theory of effect modification: the effect of *both* C-type variables and Q-type variables on E_{TAKEN} is null when R=*randomization mechanism*, and non-null when R=*not randomized* (Figure 4).

Scientists readily assume a null effect of C→$E_{OFFERED}$ in a randomized trial, but are often reluctant to assume a null effect of Q→E_{TAKEN}. Therefore, they would estimate the effect of $E_{OFFERED}$, but not of E_{TAKEN}. At least two reasons underlie that diverging behaviour: First, only C-type variables operate as confounders for $E_{OFFERED}$→D, whereas both C-type variables and Q-type variables operate as confounders for E_{TAKEN}→D. Second, E_{TAKEN} is further away from R than $E_{OFFERED}$, and therefore, effect modification by R might be weaker.

3.4 Matching: Attempting to deconfound efficiently

There are two common forms of matching: 1) matching the confounder distribution in the categories of E (a matched cohort study); 2) matching the confounder distribution in the categories of D (a matched case-control study). Both methods try to remove confounding bias more efficiently—reduce the variance—than would have been achieved otherwise with a given sample size. In both cases, however, the saving of variance is not guaranteed and is not free.

Deconfounding with matching relies, in part, on a phenomenon called colliding (Section 4). We, therefore, defer the explanation until the end of the next section.

4. Colliding bias

Let *E*→*D* be the effect of interest, and let *C* be a shared effect of *E* and *D* (Figure 5, Diagram A). The structure *E*→*C*←*D* does not depict causation between *E* and *D*, because the path of arrows from *E* to *D* via *C* requires backward movement in time. Starting at *E*, we first travel forward to *C*, and then travel *backward* to *D*, which is antecedent to *C*.

Furthermore, that path—unlike a confounding path—does *not* contribute to the marginal association between *E* and *D*, because a common effect (a future variable) does not induce an association between its causes (past variables). The path *E*→*C*←*D* is an innocent bystander; it does not deliver any bias.

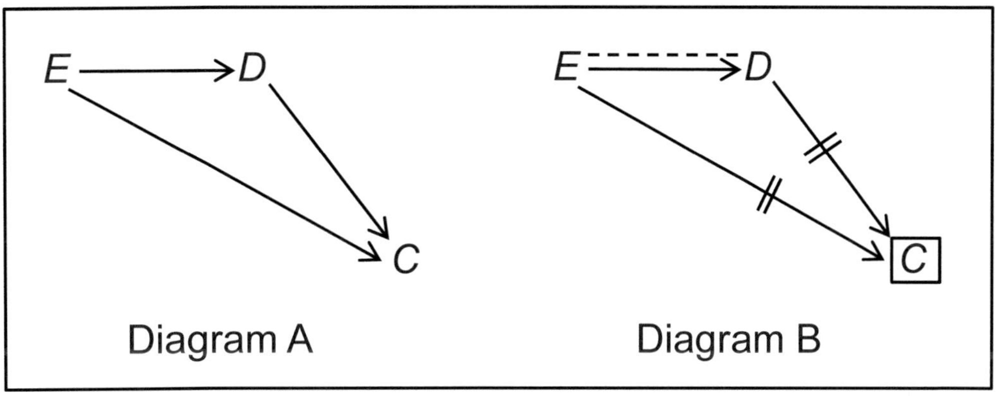

Fig. 5. The path *E*→*C*←*D* does not contribute to the marginal association between *E* and *D* (Diagram A). But conditioning on *C* (Diagram B) often contributes to the conditional association between the colliding variables *E* and *D* (denoted by a dashed line)

Since the arrowheads in *E*→*C* and *D*→*C* 'collide' at *C*, the variables *E* and *D* are called 'colliding variables'; *C* itself is called 'a collider on the path *E*→*C*←*D*'. Note that a collider, just like a confounder, is a path-specific term. A variable may be a collider on one path and not a collider on another. For example, if *C* is a cause of another variable, *F* (*C*→*F*), then *C* is not a collider on the paths *E*→*C*→*F* and *E*→*D*→*C*→*F* even though it is still a collider on the path *E*→*C*←*D*.

As we have seen, conditioning on a confounder removes confounding bias. In contrast, conditioning on a collider sometimes *adds* bias. After conditioning on *C* (Figure 5, Diagram B), the colliding variables *E* and *D* will be associated not only due to the effect *E*→*D*, but also due to a newly-formed association between them (*E*---*D*). Consequently, the estimator contains a new type of bias—colliding bias. How much bias will be added, and whether bias will be added at all, depends on several factors: the value to which *C* is restricted; effect-modification between *E* and *D* on the probability ratio scale; and the type of post-conditioning analysis (a weighted average, regression, or none). Unlike confounding bias, some rules that govern colliding bias depend on the scale and analysis by which effects are estimated.

Why does conditioning on a collider sometimes create an association between the colliding variables? (And why does a confounder create an association between its effects?) Formal proofs are available, but we will just provide intuitive explanations. Considering confounders first: Suppose that sex is a cause of both aspirin use and estrogen use (*aspirin use*←*sex*→*estrogen use*), such that the probability of taking each drug is higher in females than in males. If we know that Jordan takes aspirin, we may guess that baby Jordan was a girl, and therefore, we may also guess that "she" takes estrogen, too. The ability to guess estrogen use from aspirin use reflects a marginal association between the two variables.

Conditioning on a collider is a little more complicated. Suppose that vital status is an effect of two causes, aspirin use and statin use (*aspirin use*→*vital status*←*statin use*), such that the probability of *vital status=alive* is higher for users of either drug. If we know, for example, that Taylor did not take aspirin, that knowledge alone does not allow an informed guess about whether Taylor took a statin drug. There is no marginal association between the colliding variables. Nonetheless, an association will be created after conditioning on vital status. For example, if we *also* know that Taylor is alive (*vital status=alive*), we may now guess that Taylor took a statin drug.

Confounding bias is part of the causal structure over which we have no control. We can remove the bias, but we cannot make the arrows disappear. Colliding bias, however, is not part of causal reality. We create the bias by conditioning—a human decision that may be avoided. If that's not feasible or possible, the bias can sometimes be removed by conditioning on other variables, as explained later.

4.1 Types and structures of colliding bias

Confounding bias takes a single causal structure: *E*←*C*→*D*. Colliding bias takes many forms, because the colliding variables are not always the cause-and-effect of interest. We describe, next, two types and several structures of colliding bias, and methods to avoid or remove it.

4.1.1 Sampling colliding bias

In one of the early examples of colliding bias, *E* was cholecystitis, *D* was diabetes, *C* was hospitalization status, and the effect of interest was *cholecystitis* →*diabetes*. Both cholecystitis and diabetes are assumed to be causes of hospitalization. Colliding bias was inadvertently added by restricting the studies to hospitalized patients—that is, conditioning on hospitalization status (Berkson, 1946). As a result, the conditional association between cholecystitis and diabetes was driven, at least in part, by a non-causal component. The bias could have been avoided by ignoring hospitalization status in the sampling protocol.

The classical structure of colliding bias may be elaborated by adding an intermediary variable, *I*, between *E* and *C* (Figure 6, Diagram A). Although the pair of colliding variables is *I* and *D*—not *E* and *D*—colliding bias is still present, because the new association between *I* and *D* contributes to the association between *E* and *D* via the new path *E*→*I*---*D*. (Think of a dashed line on a path as an open bridge that transmits associations from side to side in the absence of an arrow, or in addition to an arrow.)

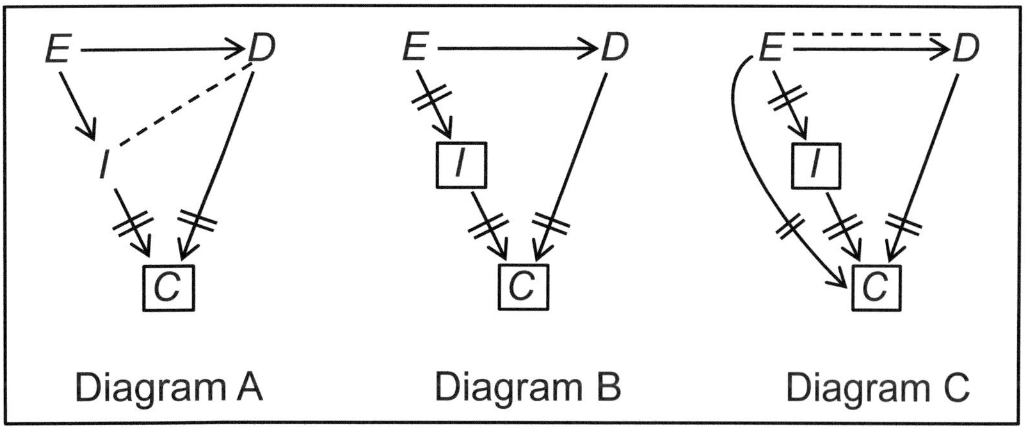

Fig. 6. Colliding bias that is transmitted via an intermediary *I* (Diagram A) can be eliminated by conditioning on *I* (Diagram B), unless *E* affects *C* not only through *I* (Diagram C)

A case-control study is prone to this structure of colliding bias. Let *C* be a binary variable that indicates whether a person is selected into a study (*C*=1) or not (*C*=0). In a case-control study, the effect *D*→*C* is typically strong, because people with the disease are much more likely to be sampled than their disease-free counterparts. Since only sampled people (*C*=1) are actually studied, conditioning on *C* is inevitable.

All that it takes to turn *C* into a collider is an effect *E*→*C*. Such an effect may be introduced, inadvertently, by a sampling decision. For example, if the effect of interest is *weight* (*E*)→*hip fracture* (*D*), and *weight* (*E*)→*diabetes* (*I*), selecting diabetic patients as controls (*I*→*C*) will create the structure in Figure 6 (Diagram A). That unfortunate sampling decision will add a path of colliding bias: *weight* (*E*)→*diabetes* (*I*)---*hip fracture* (*D*).

As explained before, prevention is the best remedy: do not sample controls on the basis of diabetes status. Simply ignore the variable during selection. If the bias is already present, it may be removed by conditioning on diabetes status, the intermediary variable (Figure 6, Diagram B). That additional conditioning dissociates *I* from both *E* (denoted by two lines over the arrow) and *D* (denoted by the deletion of the dashed line)—thereby eliminating the path of colliding bias. If the effect of *E* on *C* is not exclusively mediated by *I*, the solution will fail (Figure 6, Diagram C).

Colliding bias in a case-control study could take another form (Figure 7, Diagram A). Here, the colliding variable, *Z*, is a cause of *E*—not an effect of *E*. After inevitable conditioning on *C* (selection status), the newly formed path *E*←*Z*---*D* contributes to the conditional association between *E* and *D*. This structure will operate, for example, in a case-control study of the effect of assisted living (*E*) on injury (*D*), if health insurance (*Z*) affects assisted living status and insured people are preferentially selected as controls. Again, the bias can be avoided by ignoring insurance status during control selection, or removed by conditioning on this variable (Figure 7, Diagram B).

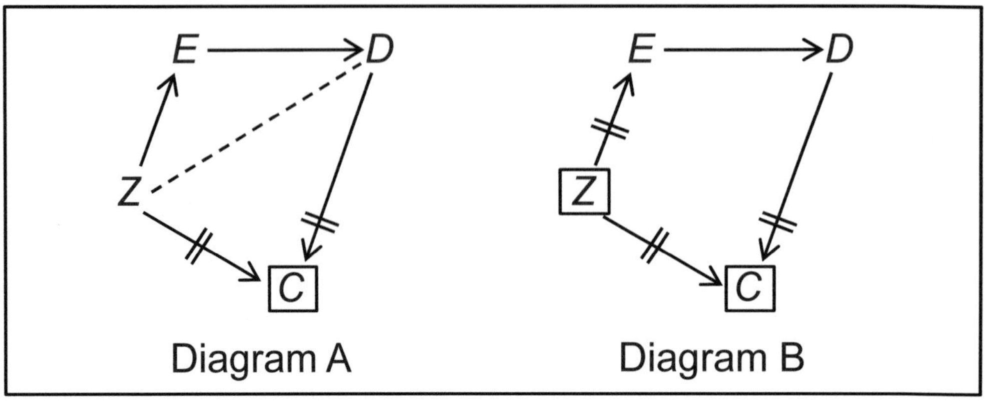

Fig. 7. Colliding bias in a case-control study where *Z*, a cause of *E*, also affects selection (Diagram A). The bias can be removed by conditioning on *Z* (Diagram B).

Disease status in a cohort study follows selection into the cohort and cannot be a cause of selection status. Nonetheless, another type of collider could create sampling colliding bias. Let *C* indicate whether a cohort member is observed at the end of the study (*C*=1) or not (*C*=0). Since the final sample is restricted to *C*=1, conditioning on *C* is built into the design.

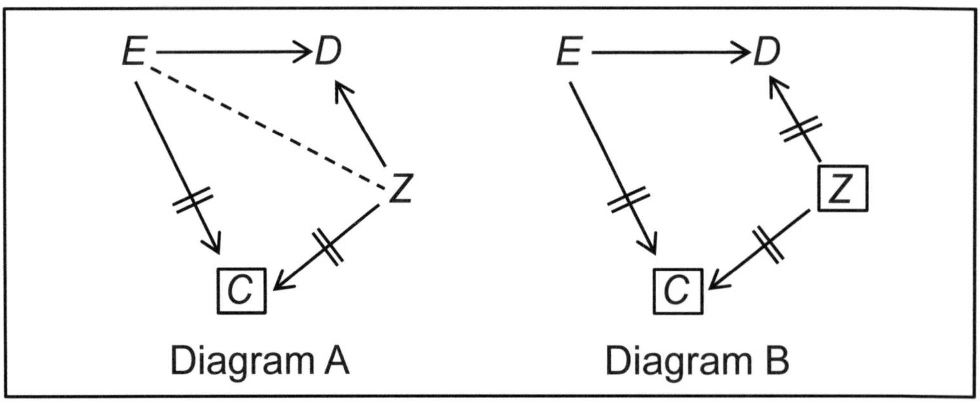

Fig. 8. Colliding bias in a cohort study where *E* affects 'censoring status' (*C*) and *Z* is a common cause of *C* and *D* (Diagram A). The bias can be removed by conditioning on *Z* (Diagram B).

Colliding bias would be present if *E*→*C* and some cause of the disease, *Z*, is also a cause of *C* (Figure 8, Diagram A). For example, in a cohort study of health education (*E*) and lung function (*D*), health education (*E*) is a cause of loss to follow-up (perhaps via interest in continued participation), and *Z* might be 'place of residence'—a cause of lung function (*D*), say, via amount of pollutants in the lungs, and also a cause of loss to follow-up (*C*). Again, the bias can be removed by conditioning on *Z*, which would block the path *E*---*Z*→*D* (Figure 8, Diagram B). Notice that colliding bias will also be created if *E* and *C* are associated due to a common cause, rather than *E*→*C*.

4.1.2 Analytical colliding bias

Colliding bias might arise during data analysis by a deliberate decision to condition on a variable. Whether colliding bias will be added depends on the causal structure and the group of variables that is chosen for conditioning (in addition to previously mentioned factors).

Figure 9 (Diagram A) shows a 'crown-like' structure for a study of the effect of *E* on *D*. Two paths connect *E* with *D*: The path we wish to estimate (*E*→*D*), and a path with two colliders, *C1* and *C2*, neither of which is an effect of *E* or *D* (*E*←*X*→*C1*←*Y*→*C2*←*Z*→*D*). Since there are no confounders, the marginal association between *E* and *D* is an unbiased estimator of the effect *E*→*D*. No deconfounding is needed.

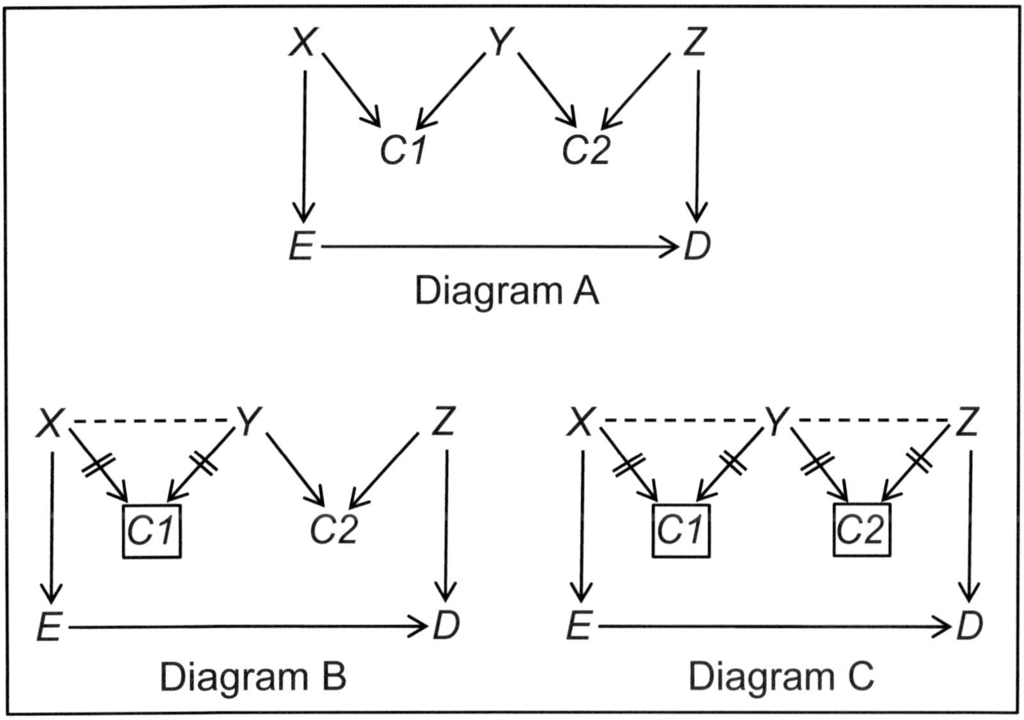

Fig. 9. The effect *E*→*D* can be estimated by their marginal association (Diagram A). Unnecessary conditioning on the collider *C1* does not add bias (Diagram B), but unnecessary conditioning on both *C1* and *C2* opens a new path and adds colliding bias (Diagram C)

Unnecessary conditioning on *C1* (Figure 9, Diagram B) will create an association between the colliding variables *X* and *Y*, but will not add colliding bias because *C2*, the other collider, blocks the new path (*E*←*X*---*Y*→*C2*←*Z*→*D*). Conditioning on *C2* alone will not add bias either. And in all cases, conditioning on a collider on a path between *E* and *D*—or even on several colliders—will not add colliding bias so long as at least one collider on that path remains intact. Colliding bias will arise only when we condition on *every* collider on a path (Figure 9, Diagram C).

But why would anyone condition on *C1* and *C2* in the first place?

The answer is simple. Worried about confounding bias, many scientists choose covariates (variables for conditioning) by informal verbal arguments about 'potential confounders', or by statistical procedures such as stepwise regression. A common method is the 'change-in-estimate' rule, according to which conditioning on a variable is needed, if the estimated association changes after conditioning. All of these methods fail to distinguish between confounders and colliders. Therefore, they are just as likely to add colliding bias as they are to remove confounding bias. To remove confounding in a rationalized way, variables should be displayed in a causal diagram and conditioning should follow the rules of open and blocked paths.

A variable could play the role of both a confounder and a collider for a given effect. Figure 10 (Diagram A) shows three confounders—*X*, *Y*, and *C1*—for the effect *E*→*D*, one of which (*C1*) is also a collider on the path *E*←*X*→*C1*←*Y*→*C2*←*Z*→*D*, and on the shorter path *E*←*X*→*C1*←*Y*→*C2*→*D*.

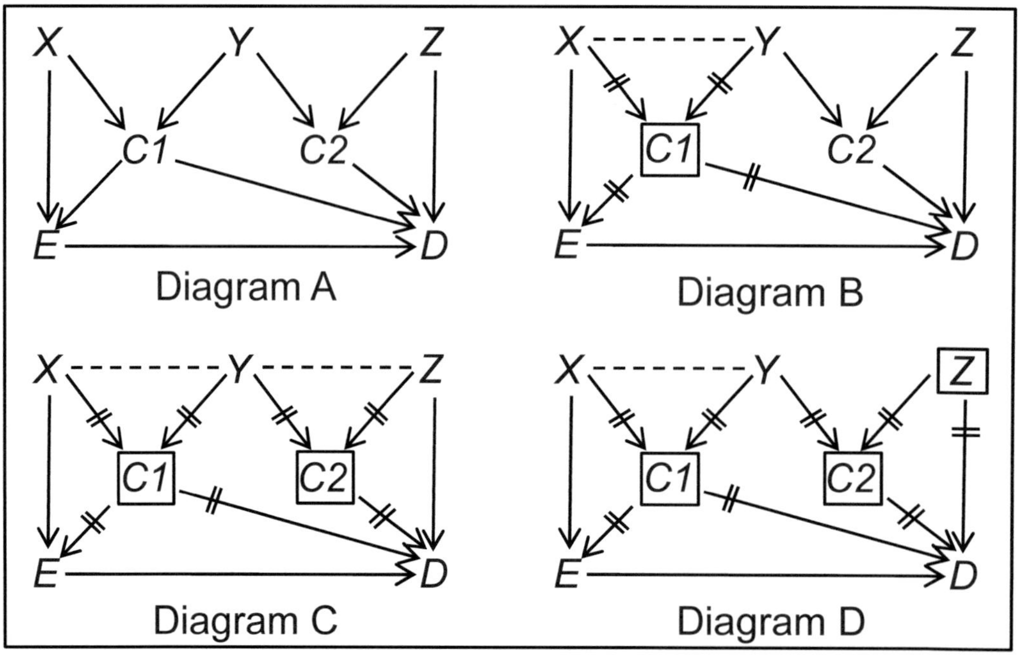

Fig. 10. Confounding by *X*, *Y*, and *C1* (Diagram A) is eliminated by conditioning on *C1* but colliding bias is added (Diagram B). Conditioning on both *C1* and *C2* still creates colliding bias (Diagram C), whereas conditioning on *C1*, *C2*, and *Z* eliminates confounding bias without adding colliding bias (Diagram D)

Conditioning on *C1* is essential for deconfounding, and will also block the confounding paths of both *X* and *Y*. At the same time, however, colliding bias will be added by the new path *E*←*X*---*Y*→*C2*→*D* (Figure 10, Diagram B).

The new bias may be removed by conditioning on any intermediary on the new path: *X*, *Y*, or *C2*. Suppose, however, that neither *X* nor *Y* was measured, and the only practical way to block the path is to condition on *C2*. But *C2* is also a collider, and conditioning on this variable will now add colliding bias via the 'п-shaped' path: *E*←*X*---*Y*---*Z*→*D* (Figure 10, Diagram C). What is the final remedy? Condition on *Z* as well (Figure 10, Diagram D).

The lesson of Figure 10 is illuminating. Confounding bias due to three confounders (*C1*, *X*, and *Y*) that could have been removed by conditioning on two of them—{*C1*, *X*} or {*C1*, *Y*}—was eventually removed by conditioning on three variables: a variable that is both a confounder and a collider (*C1*); a collider that also resides on a confounding path (*C2*); and a variable that is neither a confounder nor a collider (*Z*). None of the commonly used methods for covariate selection, other than the rules of a causal diagram, can unequivocally show that the substitution above is valid for that causal structure.

4.1.3 Some other structures of colliding bias

There are many other structures of colliding bias, three of which are shown in Figure 11. Let *I* be an intermediary between *E* and *D* (*E*→*I*→*D*), and let *C* be a common effect of *E* and *I* (*E*→*C*←*I*). Unnecessary conditioning on *C* contributes to the association between *E* and *I* (Diagram A). As a result, two components make up the conditional association between *E* and *D*: *E*→*I*→*D* (the effect of interest) and *E*---*I*→*D* (colliding bias). No simple remedy is available.

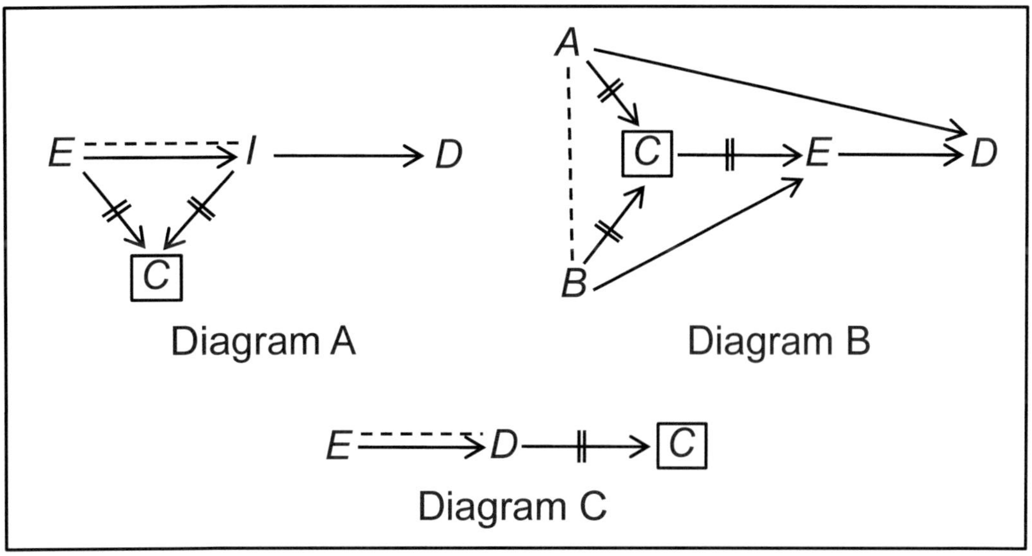

Fig. 11. Three structures of colliding bias: unnecessary conditioning (Diagram A); conditioning on an intermediary on a confounding path (Diagram B); conditioning on an effect of *D* when *E* and *D* collide at *C*, but *E* affects *C* only through *D* (Diagram C)

In Diagram B of Figure 11 the collider, *C*, is a cause of *E* and a common effect of a confounder (*A*) and a cause of *E* which is not a confounder (*B*). Conditioning on the collider adds bias through the path *E*←*B*---*A*→*D*, which can be removed by conditioning on *B* or *A*. (In fact, conditioning on *A* alone would remove confounding bias without adding colliding bias.)

A special type of colliding bias is shown in Diagram C of Figure 11. The structure is simple: *D* is a cause of *C*, and *E* is also a cause of *C* (albeit only via *D*). Therefore, *D* and *E* collide at *C* (unless *E*→*D*→C is a precisely null effect). We may call this structure 'uni-path' colliding bias, to distinguish it from colliding via separate paths ('bi-path' colliding bias). Note that if *E* affects *C* not only through *D* (*E*→*C*), the structure is, again, 'bi-path' colliding bias. (There is no additional 'uni-path' bias.)

The causal structure in Diagram C of Figure 11 depicts a classical case-control study in which controls are sampled from disease-free people at a fixed follow-up time (the 'cumulative' design). As we have seen, disease status (*D*) affects selection status (*C*), and conditioning on C is inevitable because only sampled people are studied. Does every case-control study contain some uni-path colliding bias, unless the effect *E*→*D* is precisely null?

The answer depends on the measure of effect. If the effect is estimated by a probability ratio or a probability difference, colliding bias is indeed present (Figure 11, Diagram C). But if the effect is estimated by an odds ratio, the dashed line *E---D* is *not* created (proof omitted). Therefore, odds ratios should be computed from a case-control study, unless the bias in probability measures is small. When the sampling fraction of controls is known, probability measures can be computed with no colliding bias, but the causal diagram is different.

The same structure (Figure 11, Diagram C) also describes a cross-sectional study in which the disease of interest (*D*) affects vital status (*C*). Since only alive people are typically studied, conditioning on C is built into the design, and some uni-path colliding bias is present. Consider, for instance, a cross-sectional study of the effect of genotype (*E*) on myocardial infarction (*D*), which, in turn, affects vital status (*C*). Unless the effect *genotype (E)*→*myocardial infarction status (D)*→ *vital status (C)* is precisely null, some colliding bias is present—whenever probability ratios are estimated. What is the remedy (when the bias isn't small)? Estimate the odds ratio, as in a case-control study.

It is interesting to compare the structure *E*→*D*→*C* with the structure *C*→*E*→*D*, which was mentioned before (Section 3): Changing the role of *C* from an effect of *E* and *D* to a cause of *E* and *D* turns *C* from a 'uni-path collider' into a 'pseudo-confounder'. But conditioning on a 'pseudo-confounder'—unlike conditioning on a 'uni-path collider'— will *not* add bias, regardless of which measure of effect is computed. It will, however, unnecessarily increase the variance of the estimated effect.

4.2 Beneficial colliding

In Section 3.4, we mentioned that deconfounding with matching relies, in part, on colliding. In fact, to match means to create a collider by sampling, and to condition on that variable. Interestingly, what has been called colliding bias so far, will prove helpful in the context of deconfounding.

Figure 12 (Diagram A) shows the causal structure of a matched cohort. The effect of interest is *E*→*D*; *Z* is a confounder on which we match; and *C* denotes selection status. Matching the distribution of *Z* in the categories of *E* means that both *E* and *Z* affect selection status (*C*). Recall that conditioning on *C* is a feature of every study, because only selected people are studied.

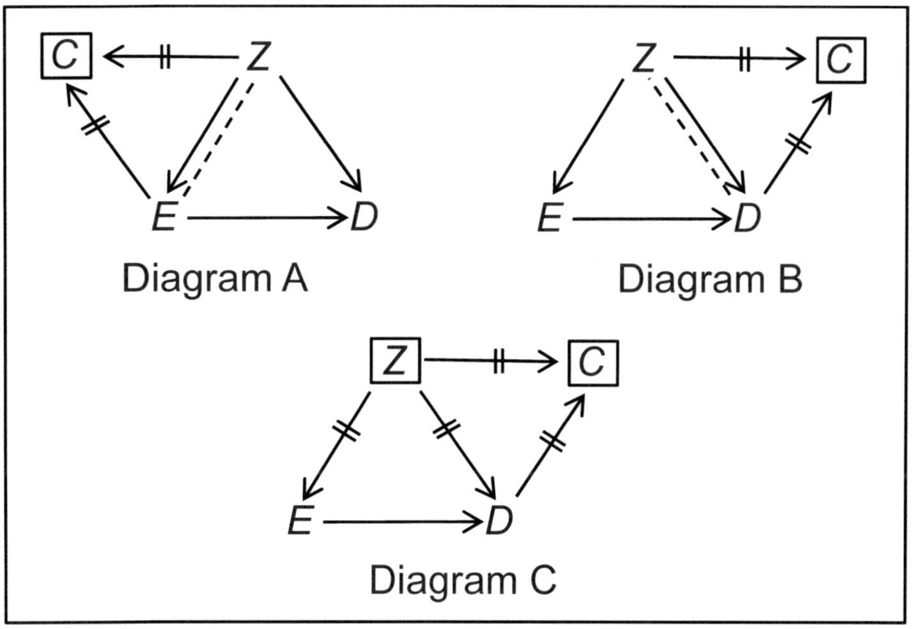

Fig. 12. The causal structures of a matched cohort (Diagram A) and a matched case-control study (Diagram B). In a matched case-control study, matching adds colliding bias (Diagram B), which is eliminated by conditioning on the confounder (Diagram C)

At first glance, it seems that the situation is worse because colliding bias (*E*---*Z*→*D*) has been added to confounding bias (*E*←*Z*→*D*). Not so. Although matching has contributed to the association between *E* and *Z*, that addition *counteracted* the contribution of *Z*→*E*—nullifying the overall association between the two variables. Indeed, as we know *E* and *Z* are not associated after matching. Since the 'associational sum' of *Z*→*E* and *Z*---*E* is null, bias has been removed.

Thinking back for a moment, we have seen three methods to dissociate a confounder Z from *E*: conditioning on Z (or on an intermediary on the path), which prevents an arrow from creating an association; conditioning on a modifier such that the effect *Z*→*E* is null (randomization); and conditioning on a collider, which nullifies the 'associational sum' of *Z*→*E* and *Z*---*E* (matching in a cohort).

The situation is a little more complicated in a matched case-control study, where we match controls to cases on Z (Figure 12, Diagram B). Analogous to a matched cohort, matching contributes to the association between Z and *D*, and the two variables are no longer associated: the 'associational sum' is null. But in this case the overall null association is composed from *three* paths, not two: *Z*→*D*; *Z*---*D*; and *Z*→*E*→*D*. Therefore, the 'sum' of *Z*→*D* and *Z*---*D* alone is *not* null, which means that colliding bias has indeed been mixed with confounding bias (unless the effect *Z*→*E*→*D* is precisely null). To deconfound, we must therefore condition on the confounder Z as well (Figure 12, Diagram C).

If so, why should we invest effort in matching controls to cases and then condition on Z, rather than condition on Z in an unmatched design? The answer comes from the domain of variance.

The estimator from a matched case-control study is often more efficient: the variance is smaller than the variance we would have computed from an unmatched study of equal size.

To match or not to match controls to cases (with deconfounding in mind) is a trade-off between effort and variance, not between bias and variance. Unfortunately, however, the extra effort does not guarantee the saving of variance—neither in a case-control study nor in a cohort study. In fact, the variance in a matched design might sometimes be larger than the variance in an unmatched design of the same size.

5. Colliding bias and confounding bias: A pair

Table 1 contrasts colliding bias with confounding bias. As can be seen, many characteristics of colliding bias can be obtained from those of confounding bias by inserting an opposite idea: "effect" instead of "cause"; "closed" instead of "open"; "value" instead of "distribution"; "not conditioning" instead of "conditioning", and so on. Indeed, colliding bias and confounding bias make up a pair of antithetical biases.

	Confounding bias	**Colliding bias**
Main feature	Common (shared) cause of two variables	Common (shared) effect of two variables
Causal structures	Single: $E \leftarrow C \rightarrow D$	Several. For example: $E \rightarrow C \leftarrow D$ ('bi-path') $E \rightarrow C \leftarrow L \rightarrow D$ ('bi-path') $E \rightarrow D \rightarrow C$ ('uni-path')
Type of path	Associational (open)	Blocked (closed)
Presence of bias	Not conditioning on one of the confounders (of the relevant association)	Conditioning on all of the colliders (on the relevant path)
Magnitude of bias depends on:	1. the distribution of C 2. the magnitude of C's effects on E and D	1. the value of C 2. the magnitude of effect modification between the causes of C ('bi-path' bias) 3. the magnitude of E's effect on C ('uni-path' bias) 4. the measure of effect ('uni-path' bias)
Removal of bias (primary method)	Conditioning on all of the confounders (of the relevant association)	Not conditioning on at least one collider (on each relevant path)
Removal of bias (secondary method)	Conditioning on an effect of the confounder (on the confounding path), rather than conditioning on the confounder	Conditioning on a cause of a collider (on the colliding path), in addition to conditioning on the collider

Table 1. Antithetical characteristics of confounding bias and colliding bias

6. Effect-modification bias

As we saw in Section 2, the effect *E*→*D* could be uniform for any value of any other cause of *D* (Figure 13, Diagram A), or could vary across the values of another cause (Figure 13, Diagram B), two other causes (Figure 13, Diagram C), or any number of causes. The reciprocal phenomenon of a varying effect was called effect modification (Section 2).

If only one binary modifier exists (*Q*=0; *Q*=1), the effect *E*→*D* is described by two causal parameters: one parameter when *Q*=0, and another when *Q*=1. If we erroneously assume a single causal parameter (Figure 13, Diagram A), our estimator is obviously biased. A theoretical result of the study at infinity will not deliver two parameters. Since the bias arose from failure to estimate a modified effect (Shahar, 2007), it is called 'effect-modification bias'.

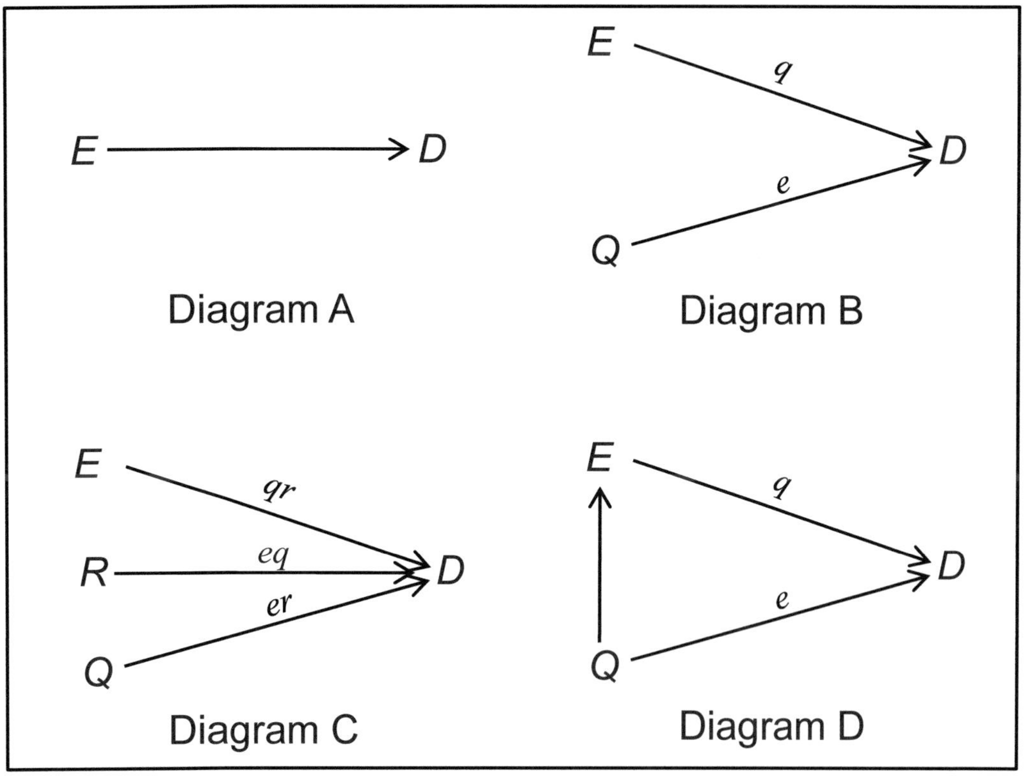

Fig. 13. Unmodified effect *E*→*D* (Diagram A); *Q* modifies the effect *E*→*D* (Diagram B); Both *Q* and *R* modify the effect *E*→*D* (Diagram C); *Q*, a common cause of *E* and *D*, modifies the effect *E*→*D* (Diagram D).

Effect-modification bias will also be present if several variables modify the effect *E*→*D*, yet only some of them are considered as modifiers (Shahar & Shahar, 2010a). In the simplest example, both *Q* and *R* are modifiers (Figure 13, Diagram C), but we assume that the effect of *E* on *D* varies only according to the value of *Q* (Figure 13, Diagram B). If *E*, *Q*, and *R* are all binary variables, we mistakenly estimate two causal parameters for the effect *E*→*D* (*Q*=0; *Q*=1), instead of four (*Q*=0 and *R*=0; *Q*=0 and *R*=1; *Q*=1 and *R*=0; *Q*=1 and *R*=1). In general, some bias will be present whenever there are *k* distinct parameters for some modified effect and we estimate only *j* ($j<k$).

Effect-modification bias often arises whenever a modifier, *Q*, happen to be a cause of *E*—a structure that resembles confounding (Figure 13, Diagram D). If *Q* is treated as a covariate for "adjustment" (e.g., by regression), effect modification bias is present.

6.1 Magnitude of the bias

To illustrate quantitative aspects of effect-modification bias, we first consider two causes (*E* and *Q*), both of which are binary, reciprocal modifiers; there are no other modifiers (Figure 13, Diagram B). We confine the discussion to probability ratios, because the arguments below do not hold for every measure of effect.

Suppose that the causal parameters for *E*→*D* are a probability ratio of 2.5 when *Q*=0 and 3.5 when *Q*=1. If we erroneously assume that *Q* is not a modifier, our single estimator at infinity will produce a value that is a weighted average of 2.5 and 3.5—a biased estimator of both numbers. The weights are a function of the effect *Q*→*D* and the distribution of *Q* in the study. In general, the magnitude of the bias is inversely related to the weight: the larger the weight for some value of a missed modifier, the smaller is the bias for that value. For instance, if the weights for 2.5 and 3.5 were 0.1 and 0.9, respectively, the biased average (3.4) is closer to 3.5 than to 2.5. Of course, the magnitude of the bias also depends on the magnitude of effect modification between E and *Q*. For example, if the causal parameters were 2.6 and 2.7, effect modification bias will be minimal for both *Q*=0 and *Q*=1, regardless of the weights in our biased estimator.

We consider, next, three causes (*E*, *Q*, and *R*) and similar basic assumptions: binary variables and no other modifiers (Figure 13, Diagram C). The effect of interest, *E*→*D*, is estimated again by probability ratios.

E	Q	R	Pr (D=1)	E→D 4 causal parameters (probabaility ratios)	E→D 2 estimators (probability ratios)
0	0	0	0.1		
1	0	0	0.2	2	2
0	0	1	0.2		
1	0	1	0.4	2	2
0	1	0	0.3		
1	1	0	0.6	2	$2 \le p \le 3$
0	1	1	0.3		
1	1	1	0.9	3	$2 \le p \le 3$

Table 2. Effect-modification bias when *Q* and *R* modify the effect *E*→*D*, yet only *Q* is assumed to be a modifier

Assuming an infinite-size study, Table 2 shows the probability of *D*=1 for every combination of the values of *E*, *Q*, and *R*, as well as four causal parameters. Although three of the four parameters are identical, effect modification by *Q* and *R* is evident because one parameter is different (*E*→*D* when *Q*=1 and *R*=1). If we erroneously assume that only *Q* is a modifier (Figure 13, Diagram B), only two estimators exist: one estimator for *Q*=0 and another for *Q*=1. Each estimator assumes that the value of *R* makes no difference—for example, the effect *E*→*D* when *Q*=1 and *R*=1 is assumed to be identical to the effect *E*→*D* when *Q*=1 and *R*=0 (Table 2, right column). Given our false assumption, how much bias is present?

As before, ignoring the modifier *R* means taking a weighted average of two causal parameters (over *R*=0 and *R*=1). When *Q*=0, that's a weighted average of 2 and 2, and no bias is present, regardless of the weights (Table 2). When *Q*=1, however, the probability ratio (*p*) in an infinite-size study is a weighted average of 2 and 3, which is constrained in the interval [2, 3]. The exact value of *p* depends on the weights. Again, the larger the weight for some value of *R*, the smaller is the bias for that value.

6.2 Is there effect-modification bias?

Figure 14 shows that *E* affects *D* by two paths: one path via an intermediary variable *I* and another 'direct' path. The diagram also shows another cause, *Q*, and effect modification between *E* and *Q*, but the symbol of effect modification is displayed only on the 'direct' arrows (*E*→D, *Q*→*D*). Suppose we assume that *Q* is not a modifier and we estimate the effect of *E* on *D*, ignoring *Q*. Is there effect-modification bias?

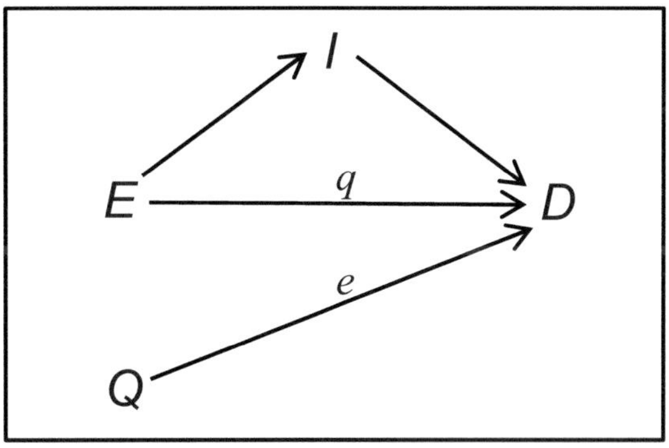

Fig. 14. The direct effect *E*→*D* is modified by *Q*, but the indirect effect (via *I*) is not

To answer the question, we should first state which effect of *E* is of interest: the indirect effect via *I*, the 'direct' effect, or the total effect? Of these, only two are modified by *Q*: the 'direct' effect and the total effect (because the modified 'direct' effect contributes to the total). Nonetheless, there is no modification of *E*→*I*→*D*: the effect of *E* via this path is uniform for all values of *Q*. Consequently, effect-modification bias is present if we estimate the total effect or the 'direct' effect, but is absent if we estimate the indirect effect.

Figure 14 shows that the effect *Q*→*D* is different for at least one value of *E*, yet the effect *E*→*I*→*D* does not vary according to the value of *Q*. Does it mean that reciprocity of effect modification does not hold? No. Reciprocity still holds for the *total* effect of each cause.

To summarize, effect modification between two or more causes of *D* implies effect modification of *at least* one path between each variable and *D*, and effect modification of the variable's total effect (ignoring theoretical, precise cancellations). It does not imply effect modification of *every* path by which a variable affects *D*. By the same token, a claim of effect-modification bias should specify the relevant path(s).

We conclude this section with an interesting question: What are the consequences of assuming effect modification when it is absent? For example, what happens if we mistakenly assume that a binary variable, *Q* (*Q*→*D*) modifies the effect *E*→*D* and unnecessarily substitute two estimators for one?

As far as effect-modification bias is concerned, no harm was done: both estimators are unbiased. But they are inefficient. Assuming no other reason to condition on *Q* (and no colliding bias), the variance has increased with no return in reduced bias or reduced effort. Other times, some effect-modification bias may be traded for variance: we may ignore a modified effect and accept a small bias—in return for reduced variance.

7. Causal-pathway bias

Figure 15 shows three paths by which *E* affects *D*: one path via *I*; another via *J*; and a third, direct arrow. The 'direct' path, which was mentioned in Section 6.2, is not a direct effect, but simply serves as summary notation for all other paths of causation.

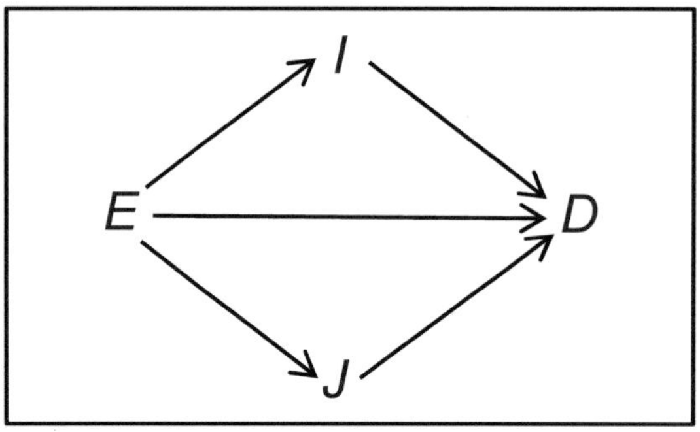

Fig. 15. *E* affects *D* via *I*; via *J*; and via all other paths (denoted by a direct arrow)

We may wish to estimate several kinds of effects of *E* on *D* (Table 3): the total effect (first row); the effect by all paths except via *J* (second row); the effect by all paths except via *I* (third row); and the 'direct' effect (last row).

Path(s) of interest	Examples of causal-pathway bias
E→I→D E→D E→J→D	Conditioning on *I*, *J*, or both
E→I→D E→D	Conditioning on *I*, not conditioning on *J*, or both
E→D E→J→D	Conditioning on *J*, not conditioning on *I*, or both
E→D	Not conditioning on *I* and *J*

Table 3. Path(s) of interest and examples of causal-pathway bias

Causal-pathway bias will operate whenever there is a mismatch between the path(s) we actually estimate and the path(s) we wish to estimate. The mismatch might result from excluding a path of interest, or from including a path that is not of interest. A path will be excluded if it is blocked (for example, by conditioning on an intermediary); a path will be included if it remains intact.

The right column of Table 3 shows examples of causal-pathway bias. For instance, the bias will be present if we are interested in the total effect of E on D (first row) and we mistakenly condition on I. Likewise, the bias will be present if we are interested in the 'direct' path (last row), and we fail to condition on both I and J. The magnitude of causal-pathway bias depends the magnitude (and direction) of the effect via the path(s) that are mistakenly blocked, or remain open. (In principle, multiple mistakes could add up to no or little bias.)

7.1 The placebo effect

The attempt to block the so-called placebo effect is a classical example of an attempt to remove causal-pathway bias. Figure 16 (Diagram A) shows some elements of a randomized trial (Section 3.3) along with the 'placebo path' between $E_{OFFERED}$ and D.

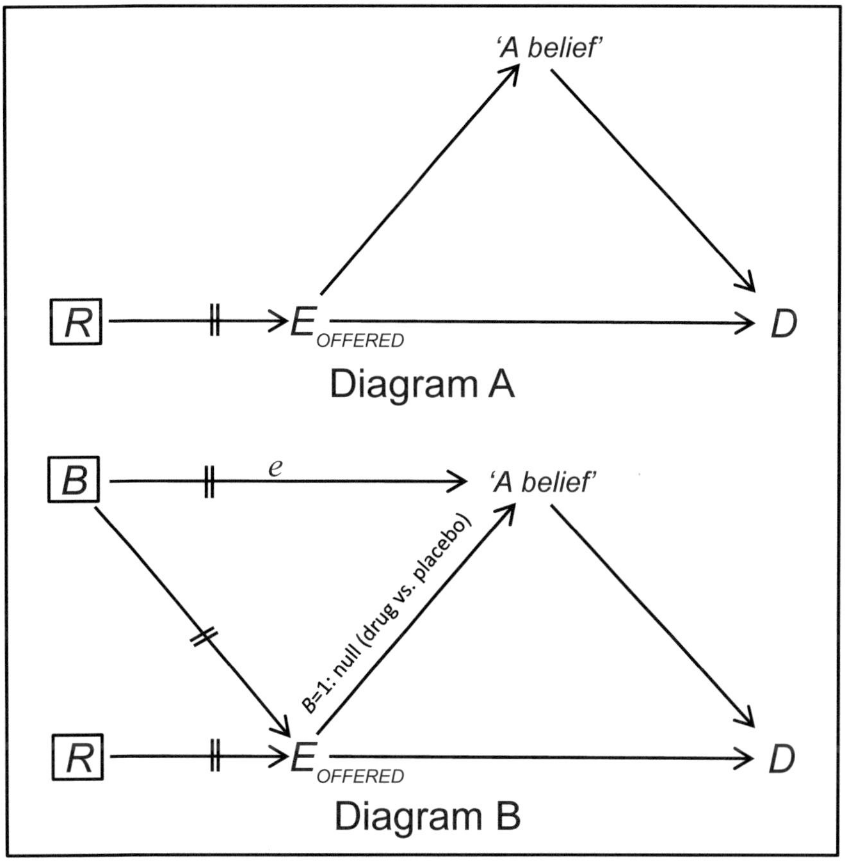

Fig. 16. The placebo path in a randomized trial (Diagram A); Removal of causal-pathway bias when we estimate the 'direct' effect $E_{OFFERED} \rightarrow D$ (Diagram B)

In a simple case, $E_{OFFERED}$ takes three values: offering of a drug, offering a placebo pill, or offering neither. What a patient believes to have taken is assumed to affect the outcome, *D* (if he also believes that taking the drug will help more than taking placebo, or more than taking nothing). That is the placebo effect, which may be negligible for some outcomes and strong for others. If the placebo effect is not precisely null, $E_{OFFERED}$ affects *D* not only 'directly', but also via the 'belief' variable (Figure 16, Diagram A).

We may therefore consider at least two kinds of effects of $E_{OFFERED}$: the total effect and the 'direct' effect. Since the variable takes three values, there are three causal contrasts: drug vs. placebo; drug vs. nothing; and placebo vs. nothing.

Randomized trials typically try to estimate the 'direct' effect of $E_{OFFERED}$ for the contrast between offering a drug and offering placebo. Assuming that the placebo effect is not negligible, the placebo path should be blocked to remove causal-pathway bias. As we saw before, a path may be blocked by a number of methods, one of which is built on the idea of effect modification. That method is chosen in a double-blinded randomized trial (Figure 16, Diagram B).

The variable *B* indicates whether blinding is part of the protocol (*B*=1) or not (*B*=0). To block the placebo path, we assume that *B* modifies the effect $E_{OFFERED}$→*A belief*, such that the effect is null when blinding is executed (and not null in non-blinded studies). Of course, our theory of a null effect, given blinding, might not be true. For example, the presence or absence of side effects might cause patients to believe that they know what they took.

If we wish to estimate the total effect of $E_{OFFERED}$, we should consider, again, effect-modification between *B* and *E*. Notice that when *B*=1 (blinding), the 'direct' path is also the total effect, because the placebo path should not exist. But when *B*=0 (no blinding), the total effect is the sum of the 'direct' path and the placebo path. Therefore, a blinded trial contains causal-pathway bias for the total effect in the absence of blinding.

Which of the two types of total effect is of greater interest: with blinding or without? Regulators care about the first type (total effect='direct' path), and they are interested only in the contrast between offering a drug and offering a placebo pill. Physicians and patients care about the second type (total effect='direct' path + placebo path) and about the contrast between offering a drug and not offering it. There are two reasons for the latter preference. First, physicians don't usually blind their patients to the treatment they offer them, so the placebo path is part of the effect in daily medical practice. Second, physicians don't usually choose between offering a drug and offering placebo, but between offering and not offering a drug. From that point of view, a placebo-controlled, blinded trial contains causal-pathway bias, whereas an open trial of a drug vs. no drug does not. As its name implies, the bias is tied to the causal path(s) of interest.

7.2 'Over-adjustment'

Perhaps the most common type of causal-pathway bias arises from conditioning on an intermediary between *E* and *D*—when the total effect is of interest (Table 3, first row). For example, we wish to estimate the *total* effect of estrogen use (*E*) at time 1 on coronary heart disease (*D*) at time 2, yet we condition on the blood concentration of estrogen (*I*) at an interim time. If the effect *E*→*I*→*D* is not precisely null, some causal-pathway bias is present because a path of interest has been blocked. If instead, we wish to estimate the effect of estrogen use on coronary heart disease *not* via the blood concentration of estrogen, failure to condition on that variable will lead to causal-pathway bias.

Causal-pathway bias due to conditioning on an intermediary is often called 'over-adjustment', a poorly standardized term (Schisterman et al., 2009). Other kinds of mistaken conditioning may also be called 'over-adjustment': conditioning that increases the variance with no return; conditioning that creates colliding bias; and 'adjustment' that leads to effect-modification bias. Sometimes, 'over-adjustment' from one point of view may be justified as an intentional trade-off between two types of bias.

7.3 Relation to other biases

Trying to remove causal-pathway bias, we might sometimes remove, and sometimes add, other biases. Figure 17 shows four examples. In Diagrams A, B, and C, the effect of interest is the 'direct' path $E \rightarrow D$. In Diagram D, it is the horizontal path $E \rightarrow J \rightarrow D$. Therefore, in all four examples we condition on the intermediary, I, to remove causal-pathway bias.

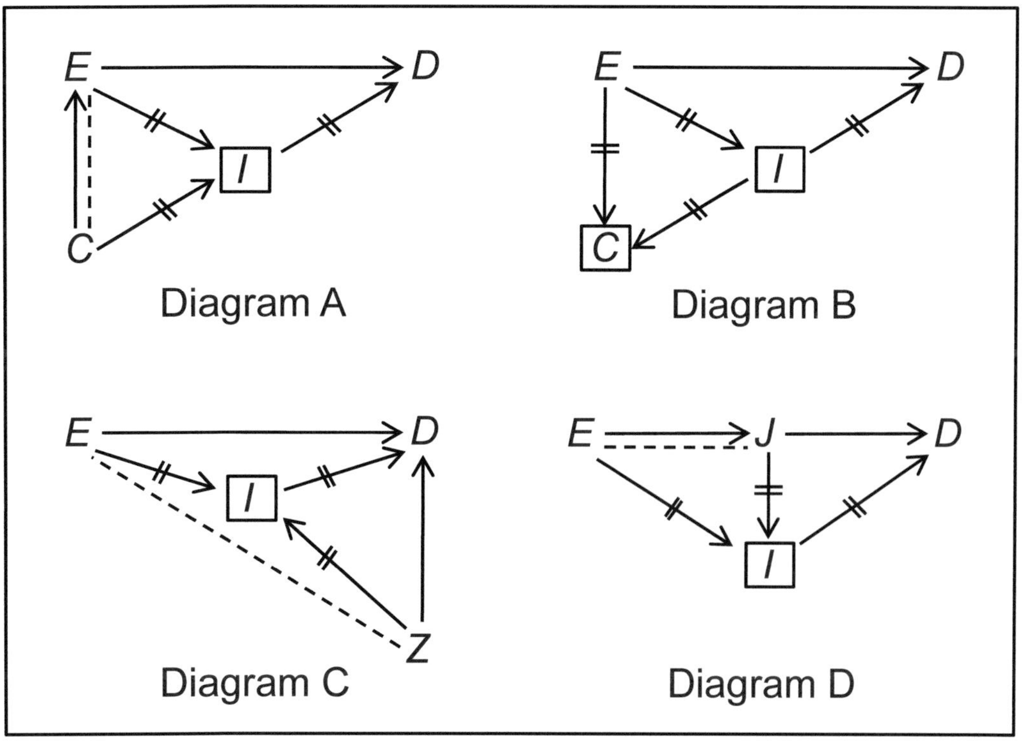

Fig. 17. Consequences of removing causal-pathway bias: confounding bias removed (Diagram A); colliding bias removed (Diagram B); colliding bias added (Diagrams C and D)

In Diagram A, removal of causal-pathway bias has also removed confounding bias, whereas in Diagram B, removal of causal-pathway bias has also removed colliding bias (due to conditioning on C). On the other hand, in Diagrams C and D the attempt to remove causal-pathway bias has resulted in colliding bias.

8. Causal-pathway bias and effect-modification bias: A pair

Table 4 contrasts causal-pathway bias with effect-modification bias. As can be seen, the two may be considered a second pair of antithetical biases.

	Effect-modification bias	**Causal-pathway bias**
Main feature	Failure to consider modification of an effect	Failure to consider path(s) of an effect
Causal structure	Multiple causes with modification. For example, $E \rightarrow D$ $Q \rightarrow D$ $R \rightarrow D$	A single cause with multiple paths. For example, $E \rightarrow D$ $E \rightarrow I \rightarrow D$ $E \rightarrow J \rightarrow D$
Type of path(s)	Modified causation	Causation
Presence of bias	1. Not conditioning (mistakenly) on a modifier 2. Conditioning on a modifier and (mistakenly) taking a weighted average across its values	1. Not conditioning (mistakenly) on an intermediary 2. Conditioning (mistakenly) on an intermediary, regardless of whether a weighted average is taken
Magnitude of bias depends on:	Magnitude of effect modification	Magnitude of effect
Removal of bias	Conditioning on modifiers	Conditioning (or not conditioning) on intermediaries

Table 4. Antithetical characteristics of effect-modification bias and causal-pathway bias

9. Information bias

A value of a variable is an unknown value of a property of an object, such as a person's height. When estimating the effect $E \rightarrow D$, we do not know, and cannot know, the values of E and D. Their true values remain missing forever, and so are the values of modifiers, confounders, colliders, and intermediaries on a path. All that we can do in science is to replace each variable of interest with another variable that is assumed to provide the missing information (Shahar, 2009). That inevitable substitution may be called imputation, because imputation in statistics means replacing a missing value (Shahar & Shahar, 2010c). To distinguish between a variable of interest and its imputed version, we'll denote the latter by the subscript I—for 'imputed'. Note that E_I, D_I and all other imputed variables exist *at the moment at which the estimated effect is computed*, not sooner (Shahar & Shahar, 2009).

Information bias is present whenever the association we estimate—using imputed variables—differs from the association we wish to estimate. The bias arises because imputed variables are not exact copies of the variables they replace.

9.1 Imputation by 'measurement'

Figure 18 shows a simple example where E_I, D_I, and C_I, are effects of the variables E, D, and C, respectively. The 'direct' path between a variable and its imputation usually indicates 'measurement'. As explained elsewhere, however, that single arrow abbreviates a far more elaborated causal structure (Shahar & Shahar, 2010c).

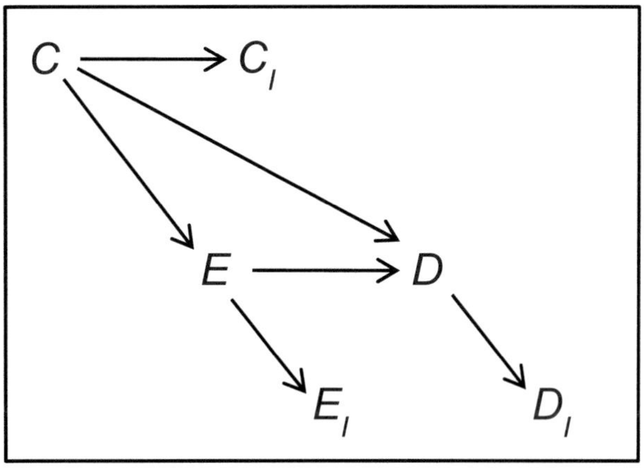

Fig. 18. Information bias is present if the association between E_I and D_I after conditioning on C_I differs from the association between *E* and *D* after conditioning on *C*

Since *C* is a confounder, conditioning on *C* is required, and the effect of interest should be estimated by the conditional association between *E* and *D*. In practice, however, we estimate the association between E_I and D_I (not *E* and *D*), after conditioning on C_I (not C). If the value produced by the estimator at infinity differs from the causal parameter, information bias is present. Unbeknown to us, information bias might be large, small, or even absent, depending on the similarity between imputed variables and the variables they replace.

An imputed version of a variable differs from the original variable in part due to indeterministic causation (Popper, 1988; Shahar & Shahar, 2011) and in part due to other causes of the former, such as measurement method (not shown in Figure 18). Choosing a standardized measurement of some variable, say *E*, means conditioning on the variable 'measurement method'. We assume effect modification between *E* and 'measurement method', such that the value of E_I better resembles the value of *E* when one particular method is used.

9.2 Imputation using a derived variable

Whenever imputation by 'measurement' is not feasible or possible, the values of an imputed variable, say A_I, may be obtained from other variables, say X_I and Y_I, in a two-step process: First, we assume that the values of some derived variable, denoted *D*, which are created from the values of *X* and *Y*, provide information on the unknown values of *A*. Second, we obtain information on the unknown values of *D*. Assuming that the first step was valid, the variable D_I (the imputed version of *D*) is entitled to be called A_I. If the first step is not valid, the imputation is useless (Section 10.1).

But why would the values of one variable, say *X*, provide information on the values of another, say *A*, when *X* is not a measurement of *A*?

The answer is simple: because the two variables are associated by some mechanisms: *X* is a cause of *A*; *A* is a cause of *X*; *X* and *A* share a common cause; or we condition on all colliders on a path between X and A. As we saw, a non-null association means that the value of one variable provides information on the value of another.

Imputing the values of A using a derived variable, D, requires more than non-null associations between A and the makers of D. We must also choose a function that will specify how the values of D are related to its makers (Shahar & Shahar, 2010c). If D is derived from just one variable, X, the function may be as simple as "If $X=x$, then $D=x$". Obviously, if D is derived from two variables or more, the function would be more complicated.

Figure 19 shows an example. The unknown values of body surface area (A) are imputed from height (X) and weight (Y), which are assumed to be associated with body surface area (A) due to a gene (G)—a common cause of all three variables. As before, the values of X_I and Y_I are obtained by 'measurements' ($X \rightarrow X_I$ and $Y \rightarrow Y_I$).

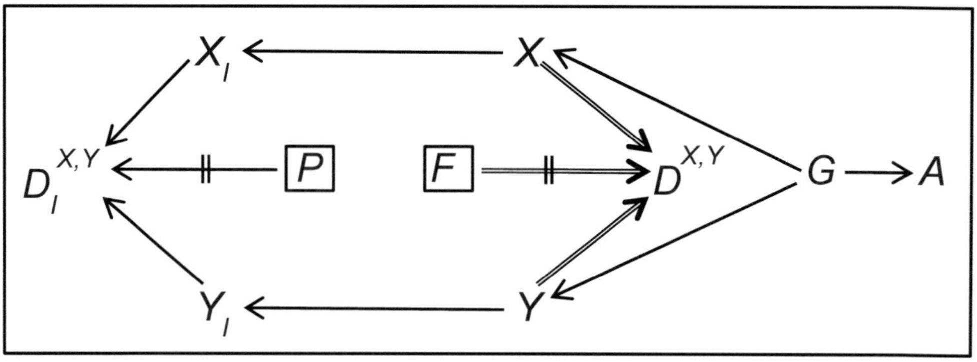

Fig. 19. The values of $D_I^{X,Y}$ substitute for the unknown values of body surface area (A), relying on the unknown values of height (X) and weight (Y)

Notice some new notation in Figure 19. First, the derived variable was labelled $D^{X,Y}$ to indicate its makers. Second, the choice of one derivation function means conditioning on the universe of all functions (denoted by F). Third, the arrows into $D^{X,Y}$ were drawn in the mathematical notation of 'imply', because theoretical derivation of the unknown values of $D^{X,Y}$ from the unknown values of X and Y is not causation (Shahar & Shahar, 2011). Imputation, in contrast, is a causal process that includes a choice of some computation program (denoted by P). For example, the values of X_I and Y_I are keyed onto a calculator, and the value of $D_I^{X,Y}$ appears on the display.

About half a dozen functions have been proposed for the imputation of body surface area from height and weight, most of which take the form $f(X,Y)=kX^mY^n$. Indeed, the biggest challenge of imputation by a derived variable is often the choice of the function. That choice may be based on mathematical constraints, other theories, or an empirical method.

Imputation through a derived variable is also used when the values of a variable, A, were measured in some people, but not in others—a problem of missing data in the traditional sense. In that case the function is chosen, in part, by empirical means. For example, we may fit a linear regression model of A_I (as obtained by 'measurement') on X_I,Y_I, and Z_I to the non-missing part of the sample, and then use the regression equation to impute the missing values: $A_I=D_I^{X,Y,Z}=\beta_0+\beta_1X_I+\beta_2Y_I+\beta_3Z_I$. Eventually, some of the unknown values of A are imputed by 'measurement' and some by a derived variable.

9.3 Invalid imputations

A derived variable, *D*, cannot substitute for *A* when its makers have null associations with *A*. But there are several other situations in which imputation by derivation is invalid. First, we should not impute the cause of interest from the effect of interest and vice versa. Obviously, the derivation itself creates an association between the imputed versions of the two variables.

Second, we should not impute an effect of the cause of interest using a variable that is not associated with that cause (ignoring some exceptions of precisely null effects). For example, *Q* should not be used to impute *D* if the structure is $E \rightarrow D \leftarrow Q$, because the association between *E* and *Q* is null (*D* is a collider), regardless of the magnitude of the effect $E \rightarrow D$.

Third, a variable should not be used in an imputation if conditioning on this variable is required to estimate the effect of interest. A variable cannot play a dual role in a single estimator (e.g., appear twice in linear regression): either it is used for imputation or it is used for conditioning (Shahar & Shahar, 2010c). (Conditioning, as we saw, might be needed to remove some other bias.)

Figure 20 (Diagram A) shows an example of imputation when conditioning is required to estimate the effect $E \rightarrow Y$. The values of D_I^C (imputation from C) replace the unknown values of *E*, the cause of interest (Diagram A). But conditioning on *C* is required to block the confounding path. Unless that path can be blocked by some other means (Diagram B), the imputation is invalid (Diagram A).

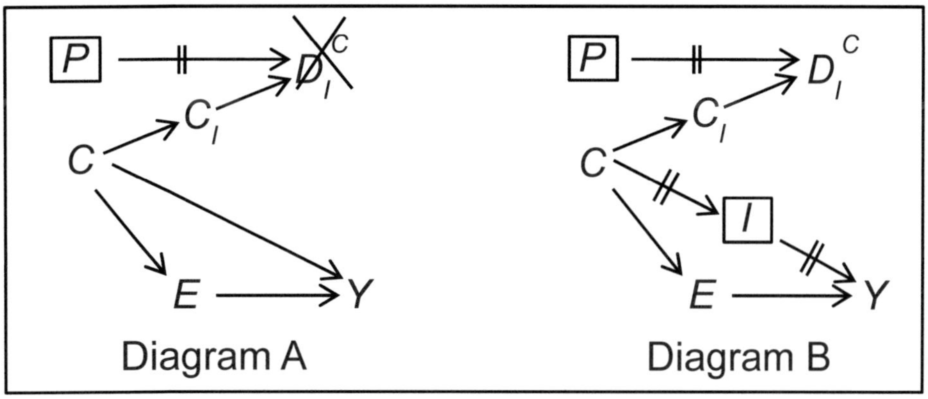

Fig. 20. The values of D_I^C substitute for the unknown values of *E*. The imputation is not valid (Diagram A), unless the confounding path due to C can be blocked without conditioning on C (Diagram B).

Consider, for instance, a study of the effect, at infancy, of exposure to respiratory viruses (*E*) on airway obstruction 10 years later (*Y*). That exposure may be imputed by the binary variable 'day-care attendance' (C), assuming that the causal parameter for the effect *day-care attendance* (C)→*exposure to respiratory viruses* (*E*) is not null. The imputation is, of course, imprecise because a binary variable substitutes for a continuous property ('viral load'). But it is *a priori* invalid if day-care attendance is a confounder (*exposure to respiratory viruses* (E)←*day-care attendance* (C)→*airway obstruction* (Y)), and conditioning on that variable is needed. Nonetheless, if the magnitude of the confounding path is small, the imputation may be justified as a trade-off: small confounding bias is tolerated in return for reduced effort (which would have been invested in imputing 'viral load' by other means).

9.4 Undesired paths between imputed variables

Sometimes, the cause of interest (E) affects the imputed version of the effect of interest (D_I) not only via the path $E \rightarrow D \rightarrow D_I$, but also via other paths (e.g., $E \rightarrow M \rightarrow D_I$), a phenomenon called 'differential measurement error' (Figure 21, Diagram A). For example, estrogen use (E), as a cause of endometrial cancer (D), is also a cause of vaginal bleeding (M) which, in turn, is a cause of endometrial cancer diagnosis. Other times, the effect of interest (D) is a cause of the imputed version of the cause of interest (E_I), as shown in Figure 21, Diagram B. For example, cancer status in a case-control study might affect reported exposure to smoking (the so-called recall bias). It is also possible that E_I and D_I will share some cause besides E (Figure 21, Diagram C). All of these structures make an undesired contribution to the association between E_I and D_I, thereby adding information bias.

Again, the bias may sometimes be removed or reduced by conditioning. For example, conditioning on M will block the path $E \rightarrow M \rightarrow D_I$ (Figure 21, Diagram A), whereas conditioning on Z will block the path $E_I \leftarrow Z \rightarrow D_I$ (Figure 21, Diagram C). Of course, in practice we condition on M_I and Z_I (not shown), not on M and Z.

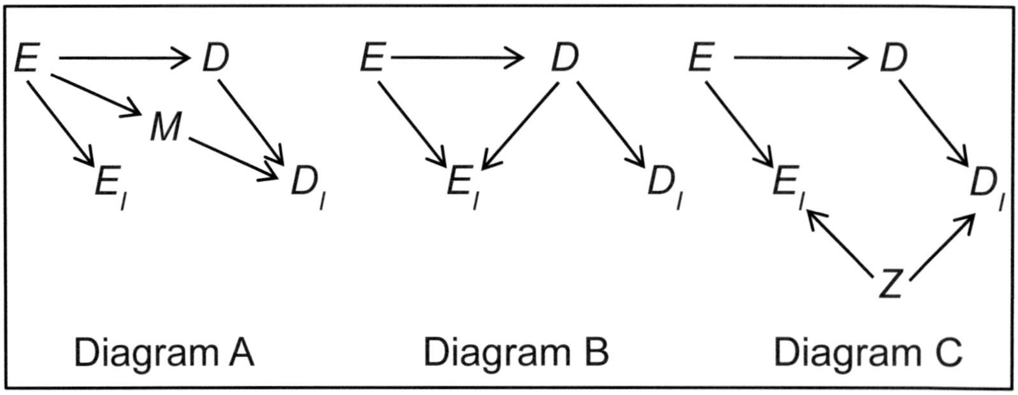

Fig. 21. Several causal structures that contribute to information bias

9.5 Relation to other biases

Information bias hampers attempts to remove all four, previously described biases: confounding bias, colliding bias, effect-modification bias, and causal-pathway bias. When any of them is present, information bias takes its toll by leaving residual bias behind. For example, if C is a confounder, conditioning on C_I—when it differs from C—will not fully remove confounding bias. Even if no other bias is present, information bias could still be present because the association between E_I and D_I might not be identical to the effect of E on D, as is evident from the structure $E_I \leftarrow E \rightarrow D \rightarrow D_I$.

10. Thought bias

Antecedent to all causal inquiry is the question of variable existence. Is there indeed a property of an object that is a cause and effect of other variables, or do we erroneously think so? Does variable *A* exist in the natural world, or did we just make up a name? Physicians, perhaps more than many scientists, have long recognized the question, as they occasionally debate the existence of a medical syndrome (Bohr, 1995; Gale, 2005; Grundy, 2006).

If we think that *A* exists—and it does not—bias must be present in any study in which *A* plays a key role: thought bias (Shahar & Shahar, 2010c). Unlike previously described biases, thought bias arises not because the estimator produces a value that differs from the causal parameter, but because there is no causal parameter to begin with. If such an *A* is thought to be a cause or an effect of interest, there is no effect to estimate. And if it is thought to be responsible for some bias, there is no bias to remove. A variable that does not exist cannot account for confounding bias, colliding bias, effect-modification bias, causal-pathway bias, or information bias. Obviously, thought bias should be considered before any other bias. Sadly, it has been missed by many scientists—within, and outside of, epidemiology.

In its trivial form, thought bias exists whenever a made-up name, say *Kwatcha*, is claimed to be a property of an object. But most of the time the bias takes one of two other forms: derived variables and constructs.

10.1 Thought bias type 1: Derived variables

In Section 9.2 we explained how the unknown values of a variable, *A*, may be imputed from two other variables, *X* and *Y*, using a derived variable $D^{X,Y}$. The unknown values of $D^{X,Y}$ substituted for the unknown values of *A*, and $D_I^{X,Y}$—the imputed version of $D^{X,Y}$—was entitled to be called A_I.

Quite often, however, it is mistakenly assumed that $D^{X,Y}$ itself—a variable that belongs to the abstract world of mathematical ideas—is a cause or an effect of other variables. For example, it is assumed that body-mass index, waist-to-hip ratio, the difference between cognitive function at two times, and hypertension status are all causal variables in the natural world. That assumption should be rejected for numerous reasons, as explained elsewhere (Shahar & Shahar, 2010b; Shahar & Shahar 2010c). Theoretical derivations—no matter which function and how many variables line up behind them—are not properties of objects. They are mathematical entities. They are not part of the causal structure of the universe, and therefore, they have neither causes nor effects.

The origin of the entrenched mistake may be traced to several sources (Shahar & Shahar 2010c): First, in statistics there is no difference between natural variables (properties of objects) and derived variables (mathematical entities). Second, it is easy to confuse *the using of a function* to estimate the effect of some variable with the claim that *some (unknown) output of a function* has an effect. Third, derived variables play an essential role in medical practice and elsewhere. We have to derive 'hypertension status' from blood pressure in order to 'diagnose' patients and treat them. Of course, that does not mean that 'hypertension status'—a theoretical derivation from the unknown blood pressure—is a property of any patient. Finally, an *empirical* version of a theoretical derivation is a property of an object. For instance, *classification* of a patient as hypertensive or normotensive, based on measured blood pressure, might have all kinds of effects. It is easy to miss the distinction between the non-existent effects of D and the possible effects of an empirical version of D.

10.2 Thought bias type 2: Constructs

We all hold some rough ideas that may be called constructs: athleticism, attractiveness, assertiveness, intelligence, fitness—to name a few examples. But just like derived variables, constructs belong to the world of abstract ideas. They are not properties of any human being, and therefore, they have neither a clear set of causes nor any effects. Thought bias arises whenever we 'impute' the non-existing values of a construct, and try to estimate its non-existing effects (Shahar & Shahar, 2010c).

Note that 'constructs in the mind' are properties of a person, which may have causes and may have effects. For example, although 'assertiveness' and 'attractiveness' are not properties of any woman, 'perceived assertiveness' and 'perceived attractiveness'—mental state variables—are properties of the *perceiver*. Therefore, they may have all kinds of causes and effects. That subtle distinction between constructs and 'constructs in the mind' is as easy to miss as the distinction between a theoretical derivation and its empirical version.

11. Thought bias and information bias: A pair

Table 5 contrasts thought bias with information bias—a third pair of antithetical biases. Notice that we can depict the presence of information bias in a causal diagram (A_I and A are separate variables), but not its removal. In contrast, we can depict the removal of thought bias, but not its presence (Shahar & Shahar, 2010c).

	Information bias	**Thought bias**
Main feature	A_I has the wrong values	A is the wrong variable
Causal structure	Surrogate path for the causal path of interest	Non-existent causal path of interest
Reason for bias	A exists, but its values in the natural world are unknown	A does not exist; it has no values in the natural world
Presence of bias	Using A_I when its values differ from A's values	Using A_I when A does not exist
Removal of bias	A_I actually provides perfect information on A	A_I is assumed to provide worthless information on A
Relation to other biases	Succedent	Antecedent
Causal diagram	Can depict its presence, but not its removal	Can depict its removal, but not its presence

Table 5. Antithetical characteristics of information bias and thought bias

12. Conclusion

It is difficult to overstate the relevance of causal diagrams to epidemiology and to other branches of science. A causal diagram serves as a universal language that decodes causal theories; exposes half-baked theories; and reveals the uncertainty of scientific assertions.

Most important, causal diagrams can depict different types of bias, and can show how to avoid, remove, or reduce them. We can only wonder why they continue to be ignored by most scientists, and why they rarely show up in scientific publications. Perhaps the benefits cited above are viewed as threats. For example, how can I know that my diagram is correct and no confounder is missing?

Well, I cannot know, and no one can know, either. All causal knowledge is inference from premises that are never known to be true. (And they are never even 'reasonable'.) Science is no more than the interplay between three ordered components: The first is a set of axioms (Shahar & Shahar, 2011); the second is a set of explicit (and fallible) theories (Shahar, 2011); and the third is empirical work (estimation). No rhetoric can change that fact.

Of the six types of bias that were described here, only three have been emphasized in epidemiology and elsewhere: confounding bias, colliding bias (under the historical misnomer 'selection bias'), and information bias. Effect-modification bias has often been ignored, especially by authors who develop the math of 'sufficient causes' and 'counterfactuals' (i.e., determinism). Causal-pathway bias has been recognized (e.g., blinded, placebo-controlled trials), although it was not formally named. Causal diagrams not only reduce the taxonomy of biases to six types, but they also eliminate the need for long-winded explanations of dozens of biases, many of which are just multiple historical names for a single causal structure.

Is there any type of bias that cannot be depicted in a causal diagram (besides thought bias), or was not described here?

Three candidates come to mind: various forms of missing data problems (in the traditional sense of the term); publication bias; and model misspecification. Missing data problems can be displayed in a causal diagram (Shortreed & Forbes, 2010; Daniel et al., 2011), and they usually belong to the category of information bias. To the extent that 'publication bias' refers to a meta-analysis, the problem is, again, of missing data. Model misspecification is a non-standardized term, which is sometimes used to indicate the omission of covariates, and sometimes used to indicate misrepresentation of the true dose-response function. Nonetheless, if the term 'bias' refers to the theoretical value in an infinite-size study, a statistical model is not part of the estimator. In a bias-free, infinite-size study, the causal parameter may be directly obtained from true probabilities, with no need to imagine any model.

Our organization of six biases in three antithetical pairs is not the only possible grouping. For example, confounding bias and causal-pathway bias are anchored in the causal structure that we wish to study, whereas other biases arise because we try to study that structure. Colliding bias and effect-modification bias may be distinguished from other biases as the cost that we sometimes pay for injecting math into causal reality. (No, nature is not a mathematician.)

The grouping of biases one way or another might have appealing features, but the take-home message of this chapter is different: Next time that you estimate an effect, be sure to decode your causal theories by variables and arrows. Do not hide them behind the text. And if you cannot fully decode your theories, maybe they are not quite ready for empirical work.

13. Acknowledgment

We thank InTech for the invitation to write this chapter, and the reviewer—for the suggestion to describe all three pairs of biases.

14. References

Berkson, J. (1946). Limitations of the application of fourfold table analysis to hospital data. *Biometrics*, 2:47-53

Bohr, T.W. (1995). Fibromyalgia syndrome and myofascial pain syndrome. Do they exist? *Neurologic Clinics*, 13: 365-384

Daniel, R.M, Kenward, M.G., Cousens, S.N. & De Stavola, B.L. (2011). Using causal diagrams to guide analysis in missing data problems. *Statistical Methods in Medical Research*, published online 9 March 2011 [DOI: 10.1177/0962280210394469]

Gale, E.A. (2005). The myth of the metabolic syndrome. *Diabetologia*, 48: 1679-1683

Grimes, D.A & Schulz, K.F. (2002). Bias and causal associations in observational research. *Lancet*, 359: 248–252

Grundy, S.M. (2006). Does the metabolic syndrome exist? *Diabetes Care*, 29: 1689-1692

Pearl, J. (1995). Causal diagrams for empirical research. *Biometrika*, 82: 669–688

Popper, K.R. (1988). *The open universe: an argument for indeterminism*. London, Routledge

Sackett, D.L. (1979). Bias in analytic research. *Journal of Chronic Diseases*, 32: 51-63

Schisterman, E.F., Cole, S.R. & Platt, R.W. (2009). Overadjustment bias and unnecessary adjustment in epidemiologic studies. *Epidemiology*, 20: 488–495

Shahar, E. (2007). Estimating causal parameters without target populations. *Journal of Evaluation in Clinical Practice*, 13: 814-816

Shahar, E. (2009). Causal diagrams for encoding and evaluation of information bias. *Journal of Evaluation in Clinical Practice*, 15: 436-440

Shahar, E. (2011). A method to detect an unknown confounder : something from nothing ? *Journal of Evaluation in Clinical Practice*, published online 13 Mar, 2011 [DOI: 10.1111/j.1365-2753.2011.01652.x]

Shahar, E. & Shahar, D.J. (2009). On the causal structure of information bias and confounding bias in randomized trials. *Journal of Evaluation in Clinical Practice*, 15: 1214-1216

Shahar, E. & Shahar, D.J. (2010a). On the definition of effect modification. *Epidemiology*, 21: 587

Shahar, E & Shahar, D.J. (2010b). Causal diagrams and change variables. *Journal of Evaluation in Clinical Practice*, published online 12 Sep, 2010 [DOI: 10.1111/j.1365-2753.2010.01540.x]

Shahar, E. & Shahar, D.J. (2010c). Causal diagrams, information bias, and thought bias. *Pragmatic and Observational Research*, 1: 33–47

Shahar, E. & Shahar, D.J. (2011). Marginal structural models: much ado about (almost) nothing. *Journal of Evaluation in Clinical Practice*, published online 24 Aug, 2011 [DOI:10.1111/j.1365-2753.2011.01757.x]

Shortreed, S.M & Forbes, A.B. (2010). Missing data in the exposure of interest and marginal structural models: A simulation study based on the Framingham Heart Study. *Statistics in Medicine*, 29: 431—443

4

Qualitative Research in Epidemiology

Susana Silva and Sílvia Fraga
University of Porto Medical School,
Institute of Public Health of the University of Porto
Portugal

1. Introduction

By using integrated knowledge from natural sciences with insights from population sciences and the humanities and social sciences, qualitative research has been gaining a greater influence both in the development of epidemiology (Daly et al., 2007; Lloyd, 2000; Long & Eskin, 1995) and in the organization and delivery of healthcare (Shuval et al., 2011). In spite of the growing acceptance of qualitative methods in health sciences, most biomedical scientists have tended to devalue the contributions of interpretative research methods (Albert et al., 2008).

Traditional epidemiology is dominated by a positivist perspective, which means that social reality is seen as stable and therefore the best way to analyze it is through the rigorous application of a limited range of quantitative techniques (Popay, 2003). By contrast, qualitative research and interpretative methods have been dismissed as subjective, soft and unscientific (Green & Britten, 1998) or second class science (Shuval et al., 2011), and their findings have been deemed thin, trite, and banal (Lambert & McKevitt, 2002).

The following quotation from a reviewer's comment on an original qualitative paper submitted for publication in 2010 by Susana Silva and colleagues illustrates the perception of this methodology as an "entertaining" and "enjoyable" mode of inquiry. The reviewer, who recognized his/her "ignorance" in the field of qualitative methods, reported that "this article [is] very entertaining to read. (…) I do not feel competent to assess the scientific strengths and weaknesses of the study presented in the article. (…) There may be aspects of the study design, and the representativeness of the findings that could be addressed, which I cannot comment on due to my ignorance in these disciplines. Nevertheless, the readers (…) might as well enjoy reading this paper". While this sympathetic response from a reviewer can be drawn on the emotive quality of quotations included in the article, the excerpts are not self-validating and require analysis (Daly et al., 2007: 44).

This thought partly reflects the training and academic background of epidemiologists, where some dichotomies still characterize the methodological debate, such as medical science versus social science and positivism versus interactionism/constructionism (Baum, 1995). Black (1994) argued that epidemiologists were unaware of qualitative methods and some took pride in their ignorance in the nineties, but nowadays epidemiologists are starting to recognize the potential of qualitative research and they are becoming more familiar with these methods. The *Journal of Clinical Epidemiology*, for example, published a comment on the strength of evidence in qualitative research, arguing that qualitative studies are able to illuminate the "black box" of complex interventions (Jones, 2007), as was demonstrated by Campbell and colleagues (2000) in the analysis of the design and execution of randomized trials. In fact, the use of an iterative phased approach that harnesses qualitative and quantitative methods should lead to improvement in study design, execution and generalizability of results (Campbell et al., 2000).

The findings of the Economic and Social Research Council International Benchmarking Review of the field of health and medical research within United Kingdom sociology, published in 2010, identified the separation between a quantitative (epidemiological) and qualitative (interpretive) work as important reason contributing to its weaknesses. According to this report, there is an increasing demand for the qualitative skills of health and medical sociologists, but sometimes they have to accept marginal roles in large health and medical research teams, as the lack of strong quantitative skills renders them unable to take principal investigator roles, making it harder for them to obtain opportunities to collaborate on international projects (Economic and Social Research Council, 2010: 14). Furthermore, the decreased likelihood of funding opportunities for qualitative research remains a potential obstacle to its growth, although contributing to qualitative research has historically been at the forefront of new research agendas (Muntaner and Gómez, 2003).

Such a framework impacts on scientific journals at two interrelated levels. First, in some cases editors' and reviewers' skills are inadequate to appraise qualitative studies, and this might result either in their rejection or in the publication of papers of poor quality (Daly et al., 2007). Second, while leading medical and healthcare journals apply for qualitative research papers and develop criteria for their evaluation, the proportion of original qualitative research articles in medical journals is low (Shuval et al., 2011).

Journals' policies impact on the publication of qualitative research, through the appearance of specific guidelines for authors and editorials/methodological papers on the subject, irrespective of the journals' impact factor (Shuval et al., 2011). Since 1997 the *British Medical Journal* (BMJ) has been establishing guidelines for qualitative articles (Greenhalgh & Taylor, 1997), and in 2001 the *Lancet* published criteria for qualitative inquiry (Malterud, 2001). The *British Medical Journal* (BMJ) and the *Journal of the American Medical Association* (JAMA) have accepted qualitative research papers since 1990, and the *Lancet* published the first qualitative articles in the second half of the nineties (Yamazaki et al., 2009). In *The New England Journal of Medicine* it became possible to find articles based on a qualitative and interpretative perspective only after 2010 (Kesselheim et al., 2010). Currently we have found more than 60000 publications in Medline using qualitative methods.

In the last 20 years, the publishing of original qualitative research papers by leading medical and healthcare journals, as well as the foundation of journals like *Qualitative Health Research* (1991) and the *International Journal of Qualitative Studies on Health and Well-Being* (2006), specially devoted to the discussion of theoretical and empirical issues on qualitative research in health, have been contributing to shape the way biomedical scientists and practitioners look at qualitative methods. At the same time, flexible research methods and socio-environmental approaches have been used by public health researchers in order to answer complex questions embedded in social, political and economic factors (Baum, 1995).

Popay (2003) synthetized the contributions of qualitative research to epidemiology in two contrasting models:

- The enhancement model, which perceives qualitative research as adding a little extra to the knowledge provided by traditional epidemiological research through explaining unexpected results, generating hypotheses to be tested by quantitative epidemiological research, and helping to develop measures of social phenomena.
- The epistemological model, which presupposes an equal relationship between qualitative and quantitative approaches, recognizing the possibility of challenge and tension between them, expressed on the following specific contributions of qualitative methods to epidemiological research: addressing different kinds of questions; shifting the balance between the researcher and the researched; and adding conceptual and theoretical depth to knowledge.

The first perspective - the enhancement model - is most common when conceiving the relationship between qualitative research and epidemiology. However, the publication of explicit criteria to construct a hierarchy of evidence-for-practice for assessing qualitative empirical studies in the *Journal of Clinical Epidemiology* may serve as a basis to strengthen the epistemological model, in the sense that these criteria, based on the study type and its features and limitations, would both assist in transparency in peer review and help practitioners identify the research which provides the strongest basis for action (Daly et al., 2007).

The objective of this chapter is to discuss the contributions of qualitative methods to the development of epidemiological research, arguing that qualitative and quantitative methodologies are complementary approaches to answer different research questions. This discussion is informed by the authors' research experience in the context of reproductive and genetic technologies and the social determinants of health in adolescents. Our aim is to focus on the following four main topics related to the role and scope of qualitative methods used in epidemiology:

- To address the main techniques of data collection and analysis, and to critically appraise their appropriateness to study designs.
- To discuss the representativeness of the findings and their internal validity (the study investigates what it is meant to investigate) and external validity (in what contexts the findings can be applied).
- To examine how mixed-method research, using qualitative and quantitative approaches, can contribute to deepen traditional epidemiological research.
- To explore the challenges and embodied practices that emerge from undertaking qualitative research.

2. Data collection and analysis

More than describing the principles and approaches of the main techniques used to collect and to analyse qualitative data (see Green & Thorogood, 2009, Part I), this section aims to show how qualitative research makes sense in the epidemiological way of doing and thinking. Qualitative data provide answers to specific research questions in epidemiological studies, by focusing on the understanding of meanings, beliefs, and attitudes from the point of view of the social actors (Lloyd, 2000; Mays & Pope, 1995), allowing in depth analysis of human behaviour. Qualitative methods are useful for studies with the following broad objectives (Alderson, 2001: 5-6):

- To explore and map out a little known field and to give voice to habitually silenced and excluded groups.
- To provide detailed findings on people's views and experiences and to understand how they make sense of their beliefs, values, rules and behaviours with a flexibility which standardized quantitative enquiries cannot cater for.
- To discuss new questions and emerging theories or conclusions through data collection, working reflexively.
- To reveal and analyse complexity, difference, ambiguity, contradiction and gradual changes which are hard to capture in more static quantitative measures.

2.1 Qualitative interviews

The interview is the most commonly used technique for producing data in qualitative health research. While the interview is generally seen as an informal and spontaneous dialogue, there are two main differences between them: first, the interviewees are the protagonists and the interviewers must listen very carefully and encourage him/her to speak; second, the guide of the interview aims to obtain data to answer the research questions.

Qualitative interviews have been categorised as structured, unstructured, semi-structured, and in-depth:

- In a structured interview, the interviewer follows a previously defined set of questions in a specific order. The interview often produces data to be submitted to quantitative analysis.
- Unstructured interviews are more or less equivalent to guided open conversations about the field in which the interviewer is gathering information. It is usually conducted in conjunction with the collection of observational data in the context of ethnographic studies.
- The semi-structured interview lies between the above mentioned categories. There is an interview guide with a set of predetermined open-ended questions, but several questions may emerge during the interview. It is the most commonly used strategy to obtain data for qualitative health research, and it requires from the interviewer a great knowledge of the subject that is being studied.
- An in-depth interview generally starts with open and thematically oriented questions. A few specific and effective questions for eliciting the necessary information may be asked, even if they differ from the planned itinerary, as they follow the interviewee's knowledge and interest.

The qualitative interviews, especially in-depth interviews, require several skills from the interviewer, who must be trained, both in the objectives of the research, and in the social and technical norms of interviewing, namely regarding the following aspects:

- Methods for recording interview data, such as audiotape recording, videotape recording and note taking. To maintain high quality in the audiotape recording, the most frequently used method, the interviewer should take into account the following factors: the avoidance of excessive background noise; checking the batteries; placing the recorder in a suitable position; testing the recorder before using it; having a back-up recorder ready to be used; asking for specific consent for tape-recording prior to an interview. Recorded data need to be carefully guarded and eventually destroyed after completion of the transcription or analyses.

- Processes for transcribing data. Although this process remains relatively unexplored, the accuracy of transcribed data is difficult to appraise, because transcribers must make judgments when capturing the spoken word in text form. Thus, to ensure accuracy during interpretation, most experienced researchers listen to the audiotape while reading the transcriptions (DiCicco-Bloom & Crabtree, 2006).
- Strategies and procedures for working with interpreters on cross-language qualitative interviews, and their influence on the data generation process and on the validity of the data, in a context where an "interpreter-facilitated" approach seems to be an effective alternative to more commonly used and more laborious and expensive translation practices (Williamson et al., 2011).

Researchers face two main issues concerning sampling procedures when conducting qualitative interviews - the method of sampling and the number of participants:

- The strategies used to recruit the participants depend on the objectives of the study. In some situations, like a small number of potential participants or in exceptional cases, sampling decisions have to be made opportunistically (opportunistic or convenience sampling). However, most qualitative investigations rely on purposive (or purposeful) and theoretical sampling, which means that they select participants who are likely to generate appropriate and useful data to address the research question, grounded on an iterative process in order to maximise the depth and richness of the information. While purposive sampling selects participants with different characteristics which are relevant to the study to cover as wide a range as possible, theoretical sampling aims to fill in gaps discovered at earlier stages or to expand the range of participants linked to an issue which has come to be seen as important in order to illustrate and test emerging theories.
- The sample size is generally determined by data saturation, which means that recruitment continues until no new categories or themes emerge from the interview data. Awareness of the saturation point requires a reflexive attitude and experience of at least two researchers. In sum, qualitative studies aim to obtain a theoretical representative sample, regardless of its size.

In epidemiology, qualitative interviews have been used to collect data that quantitative methods are unable to discover. For instance, smoking is becoming more frequent among adolescents (Fraga et al., 2006) despite the many prevention campaigns which targeted them. These results were obtained from the baseline of an epidemiological cohort of adolescents and led us to conclude that tobacco epidemics did not seem to be under control. These adolescents were the target of many campaigns in schools and through the media at the time of the interview. Therefore the authors wanted to understand how the information about tobacco and smoking was absorbed by adolescents. With the purpose of understanding this trend, Fraga and colleagues conducted 30 semi-structured qualitative interviews with adolescents in order to assess how they perceived smoking behaviour, concluding that adolescents were aware of the serious health implications of smoking, but they only referred to it as a long-term effect in adulthood and no consequences during adolescence were reported (Fraga et al., 2011a).

As Baum stated, "while the causal link between tobacco and lung cancer may be explained by experimental and quasi-experimental methods, the power of tobacco companies and their advertising strategies, the reasons people continue to smoke despite strong evidence about the health risks it entails and the social meanings of smoking (...) require qualitative research inquiry" (Baum, 1995: 464). However, the collaboration between epidemiology and qualitative research in the substance use field is a difficult one, partly because qualitative research often adds issues of context and meaning that challenges the traditional epidemiological data of interest (Reisinger, 2004).

Silva and Machado (2010) explored similar issues in the case of unsuccessful in vitro fertilization programmes. Eleven semi-structured qualitative interviews (four heterosexual couples and seven women) were conducted with Portuguese in vitro fertilization patients in order to analyse the social meanings of the failure of these treatments and the strategies deployed by the patients in the reconstruction of expectations toward them despite evidence about the limitations, risks and uncertainties they entail. The authors concluded that the uncertainties and risks of in vitro fertilization procedures and their implications in the mobilization and in the actions of different social and/or professional groups should be central topics in debates on medicine and bioethics in a broader sense and in the local ethics of clinical research and doctor-patients relationships. Furthermore, these debates should incorporate the experiences of women and men who try to have a biological child by using these techniques and should produce reflection about the social, cultural, technical and medical changes that are necessary to make these technologies increasingly successful. These are important considerations underlying patient-friendly medicine because they could minimize the negative feelings that many patients might have, especially women - for example, that they themselves are to blame for an unsuccessful in vitro fertilization treatment cycle.

Another example of the contributions of qualitative research might be the findings in a paper about the public perceptions of genome-based knowledge and bio-information technologies. Semi-structured qualitative interviews performed with 31 inmates in three prisons for male adults in the north of Portugal between May and September 2009 were useful in the understanding of Portuguese prisoners' awareness of the new gold standard for individual identification - DNA profiling or DNA fingerprinting. Individuals currently imprisoned seemed to grasp the advantage of keeping a convicted person's DNA profile on the national forensic DNA database as a protective measure to prevent being "rounded up" by the police when a crime has occurred and the released prisoner fits the (non-DNA based) search criteria for suspects. Moreover, the prisoners argued in favour of a universal DNA database - something that civil liberty advocates would strongly disagree with (Machado et al., 2011).

While single interviews allow the researcher to deeply explore social and personal issues, interviewing couples may offer a potentially strong basis to understand the processes by which the social relationships and gender identities are deployed to construct meanings and to provide significance to personal experiences in health, illness, and medicine. For example, the emergence of a new type of "hermaphrodite patient" (Ploeg, 2001) – the couple – in the case of in vitro fertilization treatments challenges epidemiology to analyse issues related with this new unit of analysis (Kenny et al., 2006).

With the purpose of understanding how ovarian stimulation makes sense within the context of heterosexual couples' relationships, for example, Silva and Machado conducted 15 semi-structured interviews with Portuguese patients who have undergone in vitro fertilization programmes performed with eggs collected in stimulated cycles. The authors concluded that the cultural assumptions underlying women's duties regarding maternity reinforce a moral framework in which the pain and the complications associated with ovarian stimulation were naturalized, normalized and accepted. Furthermore, this paper shown how men can be incorporated into roles that are supportive of women's social well-being and reproductive health by means of two essential devices: increasing cross-gender interactions, emotions, co-operation and men's involvement in the injection of hormones into his partner's body; the re-construction and the challenging of the discourses and practices surrounding the vulnerable and 'inappropriate' women and strong men, so that women do not blame themselves for the reproductive failings of heterosexual couples (Silva & Machado, 2011b).

There are also group interviews, where the interviewer simultaneously gathers data from several participants. Besides assessing individual participant's perspectives about a certain issue, the researcher obtains information on strategies of interaction between participants, allowing the understanding of how knowledge is produced in daily life. However, the public nature of the process prevents a deep exploration of individual matters. Some examples of group interviews include consensus panel, focus group, natural group or community interview.

The focus group is the most commonly used strategy in qualitative health research. The choice of this technique is related both with the researcher's working preferences and study objectives. A focus group is a small group of 6 to 12 people who are invited to jointly discuss a particular theme, under the guidance of a moderator. Sometimes there is a co-moderator or note-taker that assists the moderator. The co-moderator takes some written notes about the emerging themes and participants' interactions during the session and ensures that tape recorders are working. Moderators must be very familiar with the interview guide and the objectives of the study and must have a strong background in the issue that is under discussion. The role of a moderator is to establish a relaxed atmosphere, to enable all participants to tell their stories and to listen very carefully. The physical setting is particularly important for the success of this technique. It should be quiet and comfortable, without any disturbance.

2.2 Documental analysis

Documental analysis refers to the use of a wide range of existing written and/or visual sources related to a topic. In qualitative health research, the main documentary sources are mass media outputs, such as newspapers or magazines, public documents, research articles, personal and work diaries, and photographs or video recordings (Green & Thorogood, 2009: 173 ss.).

While existing documents are one of the most accessible and widely available sources that can be used in epidemiological studies, health researchers cannot take them for granted as reliable sources of information. All formal procedures must be described very carefully in order to answer a research question. The use of standardized and well documented procedures as in a systematic literature review contributes to increase reproducibility and transparency of the qualitative findings from documental analysis.

The analysis of the portfolio of risks presented in the Portuguese law of assisted reproductive technologies (Law n.º 32/2006, July 26th) and in consent forms that must be signed by the beneficiaries of these techniques is an illustration of documental analysis (Silva & Machado, 2011a). This study aimed to understand how medical practitioners and legal framers attribute meanings to the benefits and risks involved in assisted reproductive technologies. The authors concluded that these assessments reproduce existing relations and practices, particularly the social power of medicine and technology, the dominant perceptions about women´s and men's bodies and the geneticization of genealogy. However, they also generate new ways of thinking and talking about individual and institutional management of expectations, risks and responsibilities imbued with hope and trust, whereby some citizens' rights may be weakened. New rights based on genetic information, such as the right to genetic identity, the right to genetic inheritance, the right to know one's genetic history, and the right not to inherit genetic problems that can be scientifically detected and eliminated, demand both a "healthier" genetic society and changes in the social definition of identity, affiliation and citizenship. At the same time, individual and institutional responsibilities are now based on co-production of medicine, law and social order to guarantee the success and acceptability of assisted reproductive technologies, benefiting from the creation of new social actors and new scientific fields to regulate them, such as biolaw, bioethics, and The National Council of Medically Assisted Reproduction.

Another example that demonstrates the utility of this technique is related to the use and storage of genetic information in forensic DNA databases (Machado & Silva, 2009). The authors aimed to explore the practices of informed consent in the context of DNA sample collection for forensic processing in Portugal, and they concluded that these practices need to incorporate responses to risks and also uncertainties posed by collecting DNA samples and DNA profiling.

Drawing on three different documentary sources - the Portuguese law of assisted reproductive technologies (Law n.º 32/2006, July 26th) and the Portuguese law concerning the DNA profile database for civil and criminal identification purposes (Law n.º 5/2008, February 12th); information available on the websites of two non-public centres for reproductive medicine that recruit egg donors and/or semen donors in Portugal; and news articles published in the press about the intentions to create the first public egg and sperm bank in this country - Silva and Machado (2009a) analyzed the discourses on donation of biological material in two distinct contexts: the medical context of gamete (eggs and sperm) donation; and volunteers for donation of DNA material for the forensic national DNA database. Framing these narratives in rhetorical devices of gift, altruism, informed consent and social responsibility, the authors concluded that several parallelisms between donor characteristics (e.g., gender, age, professional status, clinical and gynaecological history, and altruistic motivations) and the dominant social, cultural and political order were established, creating multiple inequalities in terms of citizens' interactions with biotechnology. The fulfilment of the apparent possibility that any citizen could become a biological material donor depends on the existence of some requirements, grounded on biological and genetic factors, but overall socio-cultural, economic, moral and emotional criteria. The inequalities and genetic (in)security are naturalised through two discursive patterns: the reduction or suppression of risks associated to biotechnology by emphasising the rhetoric of gamete quality and the safety of genetic databases and by reaffirming the dominant conception of DNA as an objective measure of individual identity; and purification, a discursive mechanism which stresses individual responsibility in the donation of biological material in order to achieve collective well-being - procreation and security, a task assisted by biotechnology.

2.3 Observation

In qualitative health research observational methods provide direct access to what people do, as well as to what they say and think. Observation has been categorised as participant and non-participant, depending on the involvement of the researcher with the activities and people under scrutiny. Participant observation refers to the cases when the researcher takes part in the activities and directly interacts with participants. Thus, it requires reflexivity from the researcher, as well as the use of "epidemiological imagination" (Ashton, 1994), that is, the ability to make links based on new strategies to collect and analyse data. Ethnographic observation is commonly used to study health beliefs of groups or communities and to understand health care organization. It is especially effective in the analysis of the meanings and functions of physical places and the study of social interactions.

Béhague and Gonçalves (2008), for example, show how ethnographic analyses reveal multiple pathways of influence and causality when interpreting epidemiological results on the determinants of mental morbidity and age of sexual initiation, obtained in the 1982 birth cohort from Pelotas, Southern Brazil. The authors concluded that the following set of mediating factors generally related to particular experiences of specific subgroups account for the epidemiological results: the awareness and experience of inequities; the role of violence in everyday life; traumatic life events; social isolation and emotional introversion; and approaches towards psychological maturation. These factors "are likely to vary depending on the specificity of socio-political and economic contexts. As such, to be adequately tailored to each setting, public health strategies need to be based on a more detailed, in-depth and context-specific understanding of the *reasons* accounting for the salience of statistical associations" (Béhague and Gonçalves, 2008: 8).

The authors of this chapter will use ethnographic observation within an on-going project aiming to address the negotiation of expectations, rights and duties of parents of very preterm babies in the context of Neonatal Intensive Care Units (project "Parenting roles and knowledge in neonatal intensive care units", PTDC/CS-ECS/120750/2010). This technique will be used to describe the configuration of the physical spaces; to analyse the organization of care; and to understand the interactions between mothers and fathers, parents and babies, and parents and staff. In this study, the researcher will not be in a familiar setting, which facilitates the achievement of an analytic distance. The analysis of the co-constitution of parenting (both mothering and fathering) and medical technologies, and biomedical and embodied knowledge in the context of Neonatal Intensive Care Units has been grounded on qualitative studies of the experiences and views of parents of children born prematurely on the following main domains: informed consent practices and perceptions of risk (Alderson et al., 2006); information and communication needs (De Rouck & Leys, 2009); meanings of acceptable quality of future life (of offspring) and legitimacy of end-of-life decisions (Vermeulen, 2004); and breastfeeding (Renfrew et al., 2010).

2.4 Analysis and interpretation

To organize, classify and compare data is the first step in the process of analyzing qualitative material. Computer-assisted qualitative data analysis software, such as NVivo Research Software®, NUD*IST, ATLAS.ti or Ethnograph, are available to assist in data management and they can draft content analysis through coding and systematic retrieval of data. Although these tools have seen an overall improvement since 2000 (Yamazaki et al., 2009), they neither spontaneously classify nor compare data.

Qualitative data analysis ideally occurs concurrently with data collection. During this iterative process, the investigators generate an emerging understanding about research questions with two main objectives: first, this preliminary analysis leads to the identification of issues where data need to be further enriched; second, it informs the sampling process, in the sense that researchers are aware of the point in the data collection in which no new categories/themes emerge - data saturation -, signaling that data collection is complete.

Undertaking analysis of qualitative material includes art (Denzin & Lincoln, 2005) and imagination (Popay, 2003), involving a very time consuming learning process that only can be achieved by doing and by thinking about interpretation. It requires the ability to make links and a particular focus on issues of diversity and data saturation. Thus, excellence in qualitative research analysis depends on the experience and expertise of researchers.

The epidemiological imagination (Ashton, 1994), like the sociological imagination (Mills, 1959), is the capacity to shift from one perspective to another and requires the application of imaginative thought and new theoretical and practical knowledge to ask and answer unfamiliar and alternative research questions, taking into account the ways in which the wider social context (e.g. country, time period and social class), actors (e.g. norms, motives and values) and social actions shape outcomes, and how they interact and influence each other. As Popay argues in his paper *Qualitative research and the epidemiological imagination: A vital relationship*: "If epidemiology is to fully develop it imaginative potential then the intellectual frame that guides it and the methods it deploys must encompass both empirical observation and interpretation - measurement, meanings and context - and together these will provide both explanation and understanding" (Popay, 2003: 59).

Three main broader analytic strategies have been widely used to analyze and interpret qualitative data: an "editing approach", when researchers review, identify and interpret text segments like an editor; a "template approach", when investigators apply categories based on a code-book that results from prior research and theoretical perspectives; and an "immersion/crystallization approach", a less structured approach which involves several reflective cycles until interpretations intuitively crystallize (DiCicco-Bloom & Crabtree, 2006).

Content analysis is the most commonly used technique for qualitative data analysis. It involves the categorization and indexation of recurrent data or common major themes, allowing the identification of salient issues for particular groups or typical responses of all participants. Key issues and themes emerge as the researchers look in detail at transcripts, a task which may be developed through several processes:

- Systematic sorting of transcripts, line by line, to sift, chart, and sort material.
- Intensive scrutiny of notes and transcripts.

- Regular checking and re-checking of all the data, to evaluate the relevance of selected categories and their connection with data.
- Comparison of each segment in turn to appraise its relevance to categories and to map the range and variation of each category.
- Counting all references to certain issues or use of certain words.

When working in teams, data should be coding separately by two independent researchers and, as the analysis evolves, themes should be discussed between them. Sometimes a third expert solves potential disagreements. This process grounds the identification of theories and topics that should guide subsequent stages of data collection. Researchers start reading one transcript or the notes of one case, looking for one particular theme or question of the study or looking for stages in a sequence of events, and after a while subdivisions will emerge; for example:

"When people are talking about considering consent to brain surgery they may talk about feelings - hope, fear, disgust, dread. Each feeling can be marked with a different colour. Fear may begin to subdivide into what people fear, how afraid they say they are, and how despairing dread may gradually change towards anxious hope. After checking through one transcript several times, move on to the next. Does it fit the tentative subheadings-colours you have begun to use? Do you need to subdivide them further, or can you combine some? (…) The data begin to seem to form into groups as the analysis grows organically and the researcher can gain confidence that the analysis and theory generating are well grounded in the evidence" (Alderson, 2001: 24).

Thus, findings from qualitative research do not merely describe participants' narratives and experiences. They are based on a reflexive process, and researchers should be very knowledgeable about the subject under study.

3. Generalizability and validity

Lack of representativeness of qualitative studies is often criticized by traditional epidemiologists, although there are experiments in the natural sciences that are not based on random samples and large sample size, with findings contributing to a general theory of a certain phenomenon. In epidemiology generalizability or external validity refers to the extent to which findings from a study apply to a wider population or to different contexts. Qualitative studies rarely use random sampling, and the logic of generalizability is quite different from that of a sample survey. The qualitative findings are not supposed to be valid for population groups at large as they are descriptions, notions, or theories applicable within a specific setting but always within a wider context.

In qualitative research the generalizability of the findings is defined in relation to relevant literature, which enables researchers to show how far the research data and conclusions can be applied in other settings or to other groups. Thus, analytic generalization is associated with the generalization of a theory that explain the phenomenon being studied, or a theory that may have much wider applicability than the particular case studied.

Sampling procedures and determination of the sample size are relevant issues discussed in qualitative methodology, representing an active process of reflection. It involves thinking about the kind of relationship the study findings have to other populations and settings, and accurately extracting inferences that can be drawn from the data analysis. In this context, the concept of generalizability gives rise to the concept of transferability. Transferability refers to the degree to which the findings of qualitative research can be generalized or transferred to other contexts or settings, a responsibility of the researcher who is doing the generalization. The qualitative researcher can enhance transferability by doing a thorough job of describing the research context and its central assumptions. The person who wishes to "transfer" the findings to a different context is then responsible for making the judgment of how sensible the transfer is.

The scientific community has been discussing the value and legitimacy of a specific set of standards and guidelines for evaluating qualitative research. Popay (2003: 62) identified the following common "technical" quality assessment criteria:

- Appropriateness of the method to research question.
- Explicit link to theory.
- Clearly stated aims and objectives.
- Clear description of context, of sample and of fieldwork methods.
- Some validation of data analysis.
- Inclusion of sufficient data to support interpretation.

Many quantitative researchers see such criteria merely as a relabeling of the very successful quantitative criteria, a strategy aiming to accrue greater legitimacy for qualitative research. They suggest that a correct reading of the criteria for evaluating quantitative papers would show that these are also appropriate to appraise qualitative studies. According to this view, alternative criteria represent a different philosophical perspective that is subjectivist in nature, because scientific research presupposes some reality that is being observed and can be observed with more or less accuracy or validity, otherwise it is not scientific research.

Qualitative researchers commonly relate the well known principles of truth, respect, justice and avoiding harm with overlapping criteria for assessing research - validity, reliability and replicability, representativeness, and generalizability - taking into account bias as part of the methods and the findings. The following strategies have been used to guard against potentially adverse effects (Alderson, 2001: 10):

- Asking a balanced range of questions.
- Checking through all the data for how typical or exceptional each kind of response is.
- Examining the important unusual cases as to how and why they might be unusual, and the relevant examples that seem to challenge or disapprove a tentative general theory.
- Being aware of researchers' own prejudices and how they might affect the way the data are collected and interpreted.
- Selecting a broad sample of different types.

In sum, the following set of good practice guidelines will add credibility to the analysis and assure the validity of qualitative findings (Green & Thorogood, 2009; Popay et al., 1998):

- Transparency - The methods should be clearly stated and described in-depth to the audience, allowing other researchers to follow the same steps. An honest account of how the sample was chosen, how analysis was performed, and how the coding categories were developed should be provided.

- Maximizing validity - Validity means the truth of an interpretation, not in the sense of a positivist idea of a fixed truth, but a truth that is socially situated. Interpretations should be grounded both on theoretical approaches and empirical data, with relevant quotes to illustrate the typicality. The following strategies can contribute to maximize validity in qualitative studies: first, a simple count of answers can increase the audience's faith in validity, but it is not always appropriate; second, providing in-depth descriptions of the context with the purpose of facilitating the understanding of the interpretation, including, for example, the characteristics of the interviewers, the research setting and technical procedures.
- Maximizing reliability - Reliability relates to the repeatability of interpretation, that is, when the same methodological procedures are followed within a context with similar characteristics, the finding should be analogous. A strategy for improving reliability can include having more than one researcher coding and analyzing the data. At the same time, the line of thought behind codes and themes should be clearly recognized. However, qualitative research about personal experiences of health and illness are still harder to replicate, because people's knowledge and feelings may be complex, ambiguous and may depend on time, place and whom they are talking to. Thus, reliability also depends on giving a faithful report of peoples' changing accounts (Alderson, 2001: 9).
- Comparative - Qualitative researchers should compare all the narratives in order to find regularities in the data, and they should compare their findings with other findings attained in the same context or field or those that relate theoretically to the issue.
- Reflexivity - Taking into account that a qualitative researcher is part of the process of producing data and their meanings, reflexivity must guide his/her conducts. A reflexive awareness of the research process, the researcher's role, even the social setting or social context, would increase the rigor of analysis. Qualitative researchers should examine not only what people say and do, but also "why they might be saying these words and how the interview setting, the questions and themes, and the relationship between interviewee and interviewer might influence how each person reacts, as together they construct and re-construct their conversations" (Alderson, 2001: 14).

4. Mixed-methods research

The mixed-methods research approach, using qualitative and quantitative methods, has become unexceptional in recent years, and it has come to be seen by some writers as a distinctive research approach that warrants comparison with both quantitative and qualitative research (Creswell, 2008). However, the combination of quantitative and qualitative research in health studies remains scarce (Yamazaki et al., 2009). Indeed, bringing quantitative and qualitative research together in epidemiology is no easy task, because "too often the preoccupation of both sides (...) with the 'righteousness' of their cause - of their way of 'knowing' the world - deflects them from appreciating the value and power of research from the other tradition" (Popay, 2003: 59).

There are different types of mixed-methods research, depending on the following factors (see Bryman, 2006: 98):

- The quantitative and qualitative data may be collected simultaneously or sequentially.

- Priority may be given to quantitative or to qualitative data, depending on the study' design and objectives.
- The function of the integration may be, for example, triangulation, explanation or exploration.
- The mixed-methods research may occur at different stages in the research process, namely: question formulation; data collection; data analysis; or data interpretation.
- The number of research methods and hence sources of data.

Bryman (2006) devised a detailed scheme with the justifications that are found in both methodological writings and social science research articles for employing a mixed-method research approach, which arose from the following rationales: enhancement or building upon quantitative/qualitative findings; sampling; completeness; triangulation or greater validity; diversity of views; instrument development; different research questions; explanation; confirm and discover; context; offset; process; illustration; utility or improving the usefulness of findings; credibility; and unexpected results. The author concluded that the reasons given for using the mixed-methods research approach are not always aligned with their uses, thus calling for further theoretical and methodological thought on these rationales.

We are of the opinion that epidemiologists could add an important contribution to the discussion about the grounds on which mixed-methods research is conducted through the examination of concrete examples of research (e.g. Kessel et al., 2009; Krein et al. 2006). Fraga and colleagues, for example, combined quantitative and qualitative research when studying the case of alcohol use among adolescents, because the authors realized that both data were complementary and contributed to a better understanding of the problem (Fraga et al., 2011b). A cross-sectional study was carried out with 2036 adolescents where a structured questionnaire was administered; this made it possible to obtain the prevalence of alcohol use. Qualitative interviews with 30 of these adolescents were therefore conducted. The authors concluded that a high proportion of adolescents had experimented alcohol at 13 years of age, showing the importance of starting prevention at early life stages. While quantitative data showed that adolescents recognised that drinking alcohol is harmful, classifying alcohol as an addiction which is difficult to treat, qualitative interviews reveal some underlying misconceptions - adolescents were unable to identify serious consequences of alcohol use. In fact, they only reported minor temporary consequences of drinking alcohol, usually related to very high and acute consumption. Therefore, drinking behaviours of these adolescents are partly explained by social images that tended to devalue the major health consequences of alcohol use.

Qualitative research will be combined with a quantitative approach in an on-going research by Susana Silva and colleagues on the similarities and differences between the views and values of those in vitro fertilisation couples who agree to donate embryos for research and those who refuse to do so. A hospital-based survey has been performed after couples sign their informed consent sheet in order to indicate broad patterns of social, demographic, psychological, medical and treatment characteristics of in vitro fertilization couples. It will highlight the determinants of the acceptability of embryo research. All couples who are being asked to participate in the hospital-based survey will be contacted four months after receiving their pregnancy result, to request their participation in an in depth interview. The researchers will sample for maximum variation of views and experiences –heterogeneity sampling -, with the aim of recruiting sufficient participants to allow thematic saturation to be reached. The purpose of these in depth interviews is to address in vitro fertilization couples' negotiation of the personal and social dilemmas raised by the decision about the fates of their embryos, particularly the rights of prospective parents and children, notions of healthy embryos and child welfare, and expectations and concerns regarding the quality, safety, and efficacy of embryonic stem cell research. While this decision was made in advance, unanticipated consequences of combining quantitative and qualitative research may emerge when gathering the data due to surprising findings or unrealized potential in the data (Bryman, 2006).

5. Embodied experiences

The regulatory frameworks, legislation provisions and guidelines for ethical scientific procedures and guidance have been constructed worldwide over the last four decades (Montgomery & Oliver, 2009). In line with legal and professional ethical guidelines, qualitative researchers should state their engagement in informative and mutually respectful interactions and explain the benefits to those individuals participating in the study when submitting research proposals (Sandelowski & Barroso, 2003).

In fact, the process of establishing rapport, which involves a safe and comfortable environment, trust and a respect both for the participant and the information he/she shares, is essential to develop positive relationships during traditional ethnography, observation and qualitative interviews. As qualitative data is personal, context specific and likely to be identifiable, there can be three levels of informed consent: first, consent to take part in the research; second, consent the publication of the data; third, consent to secondary analysis (Alderson, 2001: 17-18).

DiCicco-Bloom and Crabtree (2006: 319) identified four main ethical issues related to the interview process:

- The risk of unanticipated harm should be reduced. Researchers must be prepared to provide psychological support, if it is needed.
- The interviewee's information must be protected through the maintenance of anonymity. However, qualitative researchers may be aware that "absolute confidentiality, that no-one would ever be written about in a way recognizable to their family, colleagues, doctor - or themselves - is rarely possible" (Alderson, 2001: 18).
- Ensuring adequate communication and effectively informing interviewees about the nature of the study and of the intent of the investigation. By asking for consent to participate several times in on-going interviews might reinforce participants' right to disengage from a research at any time.
- The risk of exploitation of the interviewees should be reduced, and their contributions to the success of the research process must be acknowledged.

Those ethical considerations tend to focus on the researcher-researched dyad (Aldred, 2008) and refer primarily to one side of the dialogue in developing guidelines for human subjects' protection - researched protection and risk management concerns (Connolly & Reid, 2007). At the same time, standard ethical practices that guide qualitative research represent work in progress, and "researchers need to consider the implications of their own research and use their experiences as a guide to enhance their own ethical standards" (DiCicco-Bloom & Crabtree, 2006: 319).

Conducting qualitative research is an embodied experience where researchers knowledgeable emotions and feelings. The discussion of methodological issues such as disclosure and reciprocity, listening to untold stories, reflexivity and management of emotions, as well as complex and shifting social and political relations with a focus on gender, power and organizations, is recent in qualitative health research (Aldred, 2008; Dickson-Swift et al., 2007, 2009). How to deal with these emotional costs and dilemmas associated with qualitative research experiences also needs to be discussed by epidemiologists.

One main issue concerns the gender of the participants in the study. In the context of studying infertility, for example, should the unit of analysis be woman, man or the couple? And should the interviewer be a woman or a man? In two studies conducted by Machado and Silva (2010), most of the men who participated were interviewed together with their wives (nineteen heterosexual couples, twenty-five women and one man) and the interviewers were females. While this interview context might have restricted the male participants' speeches and emotional repertoires, if we take into consideration that men tend to be socialized to silence their emotions and anxieties, in particular in the presence of women, it supports the understanding of the processes by which the social relationships and gender identities are deployed to construct meanings and to provide significance to personal experiences in the context of infertility.

Another subject is related with the presence of social inequalities in access and use of medical care in the field of in vitro fertilization treatments in Portugal, as well as the couples' narratives about cryopreservation of embryos (Silva & Machado, 2009b), which are usually accompanied by strong emotions. Silva still remembers an acute feeling of exhaustion at the end of an individual qualitative interview with a woman who was crying uncontrollably during the first five minutes of the interview. This female interviewee became so upset that Silva switched the tape recorder off and give the interviewee her hand. Like many others qualitative researchers, we think that it is very important to respond to the interviewees as human beings, touching them and offering support (Dickson-Swift et al., 2007: 336), grounded on mutual understanding and availability to look at and listen to them.

When feeling the weight of sharing human experiences characterized by social injustices, physical and psychological suffering and stigmatization, Silva felt the social responsibility to propose measures that can help to achieve social justice and equal citizenship (Sampson et al., 2008; Silva and Barros, 2011). While producing recommendations is not always seen by epidemiologists as scientific work, to understand the mediating factors accounting for the salience of statistical associations is essential, and these include the awareness and experience of inequities and emotional introversion as a response to life's difficulties (Behague & Goncalves, 2008).

Furthermore, while Silva studied other people´s fertility, her own was equally questionable. For most qualitative health researchers, it can be perceived as a context that ensures reciprocity in the research relationship (Liamputtong & Ezzy, 2005). However, Silva said to a female interviewee that "all went well" with the birth of her first child, although the ultrasound of the second trimester pregnancy exam revealed that her child's kidneys were dilated with what appeared to be multicystic dysplasia. The doctors detected bilateral hydronephrosis when the child was 3 days old and he underwent a surgical procedure at 10 days of age.

This particular research relationship caused some suffering, for two main reasons. First, she was asking to the interviewees to talk about their personal experiences, but she didn´t want to share her own experience. Second, some writers advocate researchers' self-disclosure as good research practice (Dickson-Swift et al., 2007: 332-334; Oakley, 1981). While Silva is now available to talk about this personal aspect of her life, when she conducted this qualitative interview, she intensely hated the stigmatized nature of how others projected meanings onto her unhealthy baby. Furthermore, she thought that her own research participant did not want to hear it.

In this particular decision-making process, Silva applied an embodied interpretation that touches both 'head' and 'heart' aspects of emotion work (Dickson-Swift et al., 2009), and formal methodological procedures and ethical guidelines seem of limited help to sustain or not sustain Silva's decision. We think that an embodied research approach in epidemiology should be promoted, including the analysis of the research relationships and researchers' emotions and feelings into reflections about research experiences, namely at the following levels: disclosure and reciprocity; reflexivity and management of emotions; rights and protection of both researchers and participants.

6. Conclusion

This chapter deals with how the underlying strategies and principles for data collection and textual interpretation are much the same as those of epidemiological research, with different procedures, because of the different type of data used and questions to be answered. Qualitative research is a science which depends upon conceptual analysis (Lambert & McKevitt, 2002) that aims to understand the basis of social action within wider heterogeneous social and material contexts. It is not just a limited set of specific methods always used in small scale studies and nor is it an easy option which contrasts with quantitative research (Popay, 2003).

There are multiple pathways of influence and causality that should underlie debate concerning the soundness of qualitative and quantitative methods. Qualitative methods contribute to the understanding of the complexities of human behavior which are sometimes dismissed by quantitative approaches. Thus, qualitative and quantitative methods are complementary tools that look for answers to different research questions in order to further epidemiological knowledge, aiming to describe, explain and understand the contexts we live in and to contribute to health improvement and to enhance social justice.

By highlighting the contributions that interpretative action can make in the wider body of published epidemiological research, epidemiology can reinforce the trustworthiness of qualitative research and its legitimacy, as well as the receptiveness of biomedical scientists towards social sciences. In doing so, epidemiology researchers produce evidence to improve the health of the population and reduce health inequalities.

7. Acknowledgments

This study was partly co-financed through FEDER funding from the Operational Programme Factors of Competitiveness - COMPETE and through national funding from the FCT - Foundation for Science and Technology (Portuguese Ministry of Education and Science) within the project "Health, governance and accountability in embryo research: couples' decisions about the fates of embryos" (FCOMP-01-0124-FEDER-014453). Sílvia Fraga holds a PhD fellowship from FCT - Foundation for Science and Technology (Portuguese Ministry of Education and Science) (SFRH/BD/44408/2008).

8. References

Agar, M. (2003). Toward a qualitative epidemiology. *Qualitative Health Research*, Vol. 13, No. 7, (September 2003), pp. 974-986, ISSN 1049-7323

Albert, M.; Laberge, S.; Hodges, B. D.; Regehr, G. & Lingard, L. (2008). Biomedical scientists' perception of the social sciences in health research. *Social Science & Medicine*, Vol. 66, No. 12, (June 2008), pp. 2520-2531, ISSN 0277-9536

Alderson, P. (2001). *On doing qualitative research linked to ethical healthcare*, The Wellcome Trust, Retrieved from <http://www.wellcome.ac.uk/stellent/groups/corporatesite/@msh_grants/documents/web_document/wtd003270.pdf>

Alderson, P.; Hawthorne, J. & Killen, M. (2006). Parents' experiences of sharing neonatal information and decisions: Consent, cost and risk. *Social Science & Medicine*, Vol. 62, No. 6, (March 2006), pp. 1319-1329, ISSN 0277-9536

Aldred, R. (2008). Ethical and political issues in contemporary research relationships. *Sociology-the Journal of the British Sociological Association*, Vol. 42, No. 5, (October 2008), pp. 887-903, ISSN 0038-0385

Ashton, J. (Ed.). (1994). *The epidemiological imagination*, Open University Press, ISBN 978-0-33519-100-0, Buckingham, United Kingdom

Baum, F. (1995). Researching Public-Health - Behind the qualitative quantitative methodological debate. *Social Science & Medicine*, Vol. 40, No. 4, (February 1995), pp. 459-468, ISSN 0277-9536

Béhague, D. P. & Goncalves, H. (2008). Exploring multiple trajectories of causality: collaboration between Anthropology and Epidemiology in the 1982 birth cohort, Pelotas, Southern Brazil. *Revista de Saúde Pública*, Vol. 42, No. Suppl. 2, (December 2008), ISSN 0034-8910

Black, N. (1994). Why we need qualitative research. *Journal of Epidemiology and Community Health*, Vol. 48, No. 5, (October 1994), pp. 425-426, ISSN 0143-005X

Bryman, A. (2006). Integrating quantitative and qualitative research: how is it done?. *Qualitative Research*, Vol. 6, No. 1, (February 2006), pp. 97-113, ISSN 1741- 3109

Campbell, M.; Fitzpatrick, R.; Haines, A.; Kinmonth, A. L.; Sandercock, P.; Spiegelhalter, D. & Tyrer, P. (2000). Framework for design and evaluation of complex interventions to improve health. *British Medical Journal*, Vol. 321, No. 7262, (September 2000), pp. 694-696, ISSN 0959-8138

Connolly, K. & Reid, A. (2007). Ethics review for qualitative inquiry: Adopting a values-based, facilitative approach. *Qualitative Inquiry*, Vol. 13, No. 7, (October 2007), pp. 1031-1047, ISSN 1552-7565

Creswell, J. (2008). *Research design: Qualitative, quantitative, and mixed methods approaches*, Sage Publication, ISBN 978-1-41296-557-6, Thousand Oaks, California, United States of America

Daly, J.; Willis, K.; Small, R.; Green, J.; Welch, N.; Kealy, M. & Hughes, E. (2007). A hierarchy of evidence for assessing qualitative health research. *Journal of Clinical Epidemiology*, Vol. 60, No. 1, (January 2007), pp. 43-49, ISSN 0895-4356

De Rouck, S. & Leys, M. (2009). Information needs of parents of children admitted to a neonatal intensive care unit: A review of the literature (1990-2008). *Patient Education and Counseling*, Vol. 76, No. 2, (August 2009), pp. 159-173, ISSN 0738-3991

Denzin, N. K. & Lincoln, Y. S. (2005). The art and practices of interpretation, evaluation, and representation, In: *Handbook of Qualitative Research*, N.K. Denzin & Y.S. Lincoln, (Eds), 909-914, Sage Publication, ISBN 978-0-76192-757-0, Thousand Oaks, California, United States of America

DiCicco-Bloom, B. & Crabtree, B. F. (2006). The qualitative research interview. *Medical Education*, Vol. 40, No. 4, (April 2006), pp. 314-321, ISSN 0308-0110

Dickson-Swift, V.; James, E. L.; Kippen, S. & Liamputtong, P. (2007). Doing sensitive research: What challenges do qualitative researchers face?. *Qualitative research*, Vol. 7, No. 3, (March 2007), pp. 327-353, ISSN 1741- 3109

Dickson-Swift, V.; James, E. L.; Kippen, S. & Liamputtong, P. (2009). Researching sensitive topics: Qualitative research as emotion work. *Qualitative research*, Vol. 9, No. 1, (January 2009), pp. 61-79, ISSN 1741- 3109

Economic and Social Research Council. (March 2010). *International Benchmarking Review of UK Sociology*, Economic and Social Research Council, British Sociological Association & Heads and Professors of Sociology Group, Retrieved from <http://www.esrc.ac.uk/_images/Int_benchmarking_sociology_tcm8-4556.pdf>

Ekman, A. & Litton, J. E. (2007). New times, new needs; e-epidemiology. *European Journal of Epidemiology*, Vol. 22, No. 5, (May 2007), pp. 285-292, ISSN 0393-2990

Fraga, S.; Ramos, E. & Barros, H. (2006). Smoking and its associated factors in Portuguese adolescent students. *Revista de Saúde Pública*, Vol. 40, No. 4, (August 2001), pp. 620-626, ISSN 0034-8910

Fraga, S.; Sousa, S.; Ramos, E.; Dias, I. & Barros, H. (2011a). Social representations of smoking behaviour in 13-year-old adolescents. *Revista Portuguesa de Pneumologia*, Vol. 17, No. 1, (January 2011), pp. 27-31, ISSN 0873-2159

Fraga, S.; Sousa, S.; Ramos, E.; Dias, S. & Barros, H. (2011b). Alcohol use among 13-year-old adolescents: Associated factors and perceptions. *Public Health*, Vol. 125, No. 7 (July 2011), pp. 448-456, ISSN 1476-5616

Green, J. & Britten, N. (1998). Qualitative research and evidence based medicine. *British Medical Journal*, Vol. 316, No. 7139, (April 1998), pp. 1230-1232, ISSN 0959-8138

Green, J. & Thorogood, N. (2009). *Qualitative methods for health research*, Sage Publications, ISBN 978-1-84787-074-2, London, United Kingdom

Greenhalgh, T. & Taylor, R. (1997). Papers that go beyond numbers (qualitative research). *British Medical Journal*, Vol. 315, No. 7110, (September 1997), pp. 740-743, ISSN 0959-8138

Jones, R. (2007). Strength of evidence in qualitative research. *Journal of Clinical Epidemiology*, Vol. 60, No. 4, (April 2007), pp. 321-323, ISSN 0895-4356

Kenny, D.A.; Kashy, D.A. & Cook, W.L. (2006). *Dyadic data analysis*, The Guilford Press, ISBN 978-1-57230-986-9, New York, USA

Kessel, A.; Green, J.; Pinder, R.; Wilkinson, R.; Grundy, C. & Lachowycz, K. (2009). Multidisciplinary research in public health: A case study of research on access to green space. *Public Health*, Vol. 123, No. 1, (January 2009), pp. 32-38, ISSN 0033-3506

Kesselheim, A. S.; Studdert, D. M. & Mello, M. M. (2010). Whistle-blowers' experiences in fraud litigation against pharmaceutical companies. *The New England Journal of Medicine*, Vol. 362, No. 19, (May 2010), pp. 1832-1839, ISSN 1533-4406

Krein, S. L.; Olmsted, R. N.; Hofer, T. P.; Kowalski, C.; Forman, J.; Banaszak-Holl, J. & Saint, S. (2006). Translating infection prevention evidence into practice using quantitative and qualitative research. *American Journal of Infection Control*, Vol. 34, No. 8, (October 2006), pp. 507-512, ISSN 0196-6553

Lambert, H. & McKevitt, C. (2002). Anthropology in health research: from qualitative methods to multidisciplinarity. *British Medical Journal*, Vol. 325, No. 7357, (July 2002), pp. 210-213, ISSN 0959-535X

Liamputtong, P. & Ezzy, D. (2005). *Qualitative research methods*, Oxford University Press, ISBN 978-0-19551-744-6, Oxford, United States of Amercia

Lloyd, M. (2000). Analysis on the move: Deconstructing troublesome health questions and troubling epidemiology. *Qualitative Health Research*, Vol. 10, No. 2, (March 2000), pp. 149-163, ISSN 1049-7323

Long, A. F. & Eskin, F. (1995). The new public health: Changing attitudes and practice. *Medical Principles and Practice*, Vol. 4, No. 3, (n.d.), pp. 171-178, ISSN 1011-7571

Machado, H. & Silva, S. (2009). Informed consent in forensic DNA databases: Volunteering, constructions of risk and identity categorization. *BioSocieties*, Vol. 4, No. 4, (December 2009), pp. 335-348, ISSN 1745-8552

Machado, H. & Silva, S. (2010). Gender and ethics in qualitative interviewing: research relationships in the context of a study of infertility in Portugal, In: *Feminism and women in leadership*, V. Nardi, (Ed.), 97-110, Nova Science Publishers, ISBN 978-1-61122-578-5, New York, United States of America

Machado, H.; Santos, F. & Silva, S. (2011). Prisoners' expectations of the national forensic DNA database: Surveillance and reconfiguration of individual rights. *Forensic Science International*, Vol. 210, No. 1-3, (July 2011), pp. 139-143, ISSN 0379-0738

Malterud, K. (2001). Qualitative research: standards, challenges, and guidelines. *Lancet*, Vol. 358, No. 9280, (August 2001), pp. 483-488, ISSN 0140-6736

Mays, N. & Pope, C. (1995). Qualitative research: Rigour and qualitative research. *British Medical Journal*, Vol. 311, No. 6997, (July 1995), pp. 109-112, ISSN 0959-8138

Mills, C.W. (1959). *The sociological imagination*, Oxford University Press, ISBN 978-0-19513-373-8, New York, United States of America

Montgomery, K. & Oliver, A. L. (2009). Shifts in guidelines for ethical scientific conduct: how public and private organizations create and change norms of research integrity. *Social Studies of Science*, Vol. 39, No. 1, (February 2009), pp. 137-155, ISSN 1460-3659

Muntaner, C. & Gómez, M.B. (2003). Qualitative and quantitative research in social epidemiology: is complementarity the only issue?. *Gaceta Sanitaria*, Vol. 17, No. Supl. 3, (n.d.), pp. 53-57, ISSN 0213-9111

Oakley, A. (1981). Interviewing women: a contradiction in terms?, In: *Doing feminist research*, H. Roberts, (Ed.), 30-61, Routledge & Kegan Paul, ISBN 0-415-02547-8, London, UK

Ploeg, I. V. D. (2001). *Prosthetic bodies: the construction of the fetus and the couple as patients in reproductive technologies*, Kluwer Academic Publishers, ISBN 1-4020-0116-9, Dordrecht, The Netherlands

Popay, J. (2003). Qualitative research and the epidemiological imagination: a vital relationship. *Gaceta Sanitaria*, Vol. 17, No. Suppl. 3, (n.d.), pp. 58-63, ISSN 0213-9111

Popay, J.; Rogers, A. & Williams, G. (1998). Rationale and standards for the systematic review of qualitative literature in health services research. *Qualitative health research*, Vol. 8, No. 3, (May 1998), pp. 341-351, ISSN 1049-7323

Reisinger, H. S. (2004). Counting apples as oranges: Epidemiology and ethnography in adolescent substance abuse treatment. *Qualitative Health Research*, Vol. 14, No. 2, (February 2004), pp. 241-258, ISSN 1049-7323

Renfrew, M. J.; Dyson, L.; McCormick, F.; Misso, K.; Stenhouse, E.; King, S. E. & Williams, A. F. (2010). Breastfeeding promotion for infants in neonatal units: a systematic review. *Child Care Health and Development*, Vol. 36, No. 2, (March 2010), pp. 165-178, ISSN 0305-1862

Sampson, H.; Bloor, M. & Fincham, B. (2008). A price worth paying?: Considering the 'cost' of reflexive research methods and the influence of feminist ways of 'doing'. *Sociology-the Journal of the British Sociological Association*, Vol. 42, No. 5, (October 2008), pp. 919-933, ISSN 0038-0385

Sandelowski, M. & Barroso, J. (2003). Writing the proposal for a qualitative research methodology Project. *Qualitative health research*, Vol. 13, No. 6, (July 2003), pp. 781-820, ISSN 1049-7323

Shuval, K.; Harker, K.; Roudsari, B.; Groce, N.E.; Mills, B.; Siddiqi, Z. & Shachak, A. (2011). Is qualitative research second class science? A quantitative longitudinal examination of qualitative research in medical journals. *PLoS ONE*, Vol. 6, No. 2, (February 2011), pp. e16937, eISSN-1932-6203

Silva, S. & Barros, H. (2011). Users' perspectives on accessibility to IVF treatments in Portugal: a qualitative study. *Revista de Saúde Pública* (in press), ISSN 0034-8910

Silva, S. & Machado, H. (2009a). Trust, morality and altruism in the donation of biological material - the case of Portugal. *New genetics and society*, Vol. 28, No. 2, (n.d.), pp. 103-118, ISSN 1469-9915

Silva, S. & Machado, H. (2009b). A compreensão jurídica, médica e "leiga" do embrião em Portugal: um alinhamento com a biologia?. *Interface - Comunicação, Saúde, Educação*, Vol. 13, No. 30, (July/September 2009), pp. 31-43, ISSN 1414-3283

Silva, S. & Machado, H. (2010). Uncertainty, risks and ethics in unsuccessful in vitro fertilization treatment cycles. *Health, Risk & Society*, Vol. 12, No. 6 (n.d.), pp. 531-545, ISSN 1469-8331

Silva, S. & Machado, H. (2011a). The construction of meaning by experts and would-be parents in assisted reproductive technology. Sociology of Health & Illness, Vol. 33, No. 6, (September 2011), pp. 853-868, ISSN 1467-9566

Silva, S. & Machado, H. (2011b). Heterosexual couples' uses and meanings of ovarian stimulation: Relatedness, embodiment and emotions. *Health (London)*, Vol. 15, No. 6, (November 2011), pp. 626-638, ISSN 1461-7196

Vermeulen, E. (2004). Dealing with doubt: Making decisions in a neonatal ward in The Netherlands. *Social Science & Medicine*, Vol. 59, No. 10, (November 2004), pp. 2071-2085, ISSN 0277-9536

Williamson, D. L.; Choi, J.; Charchuk, M.; Rempel, G. R.; Pitre, N.; Breitkreuz, R. & Kushner, K. E. (2011). Interpreter-facilitated cross-language interviews: a research note. *Qualitative research*, Vol. 11, No. 4, (August 2011), pp. 381-394, ISBN 1468-7941

Yamazaki, H.; Slingsby, B. T.; Takahashi, M.; Hayashi, Y.; Sugimori, H. & Nakayama, T. (2009). Characteristics of qualitative studies in influential journals of general medicine: a critical review. *Bioscience Trends*, Vol. 3, No. 6, (December 2009), pp. 202-209, ISSN 1881-7823

5

Between Epidemiology and Basic Genetic Research – Systems Epidemiology

Eiliv Lund
University of Tromsø
Norway

1. Introduction

Systems epidemiology can be considered as an attempt to implement functional genomic analyses into the common prospective design. Functional genomics cover research on genes, genomes and the products of genes such as gene transcripts (mRNA and microRNA) and proteins. Methods include gathering, integrating, and analyzing complex data from high throughput technologies such as genomics, epigenomics, transcriptomics, proteomics, and metabolomics (often collectively named "the 'omics"). A main goal is to build models to better understand the complex interactions taking place within cells, tissues or whole organisms, using mathematical, statistical and computational approaches. Some of these high throughput techniques can be run in available material, some need new biological sampling. The expansion of the information available through these methods has created a challenge for the analyses both in terms of laboratory analyses, statistical analyses and functional interpretations. At the same time it will mirror the current dichotomy in research between epidemiology and basic research. The goal of this chapter is to point to the alternative research direction of functional genomics created by the new technological opportunities. The time should have come for including functional measures in both blood and tissues in prospective observations studies of humans. With this as a background the design and current analytical approaches of the Norwegian Women and Cancer postgenome cohort will be discussed in relation to carcinogenesis. The chapter will deal more with study design and related aspects than with statistics or biology.

2. Background

Modern technology has over the last decade given epidemiologists the opportunity for expanding their field of science from the studies of associations between exposures and disease till gene-environment analyses of single nucleotide polymorphisms, SNPs, as part of molecular epidemiology (1). The genome wide association studies, GWAS, created both the need for huge collaborative efforts, high throughput technologies and novel statistical approaches due to the large number of comparisons done. One example of the collaborative efforts could be the Consortium of cohorts (2), and the adjustment of p-values to keep an adequate false discovery rate is an example of novel statistical methods for the GWAS analyses (3). As part of the gene-environment exploration the scientific approach has changed from single gene analyses based on biological knowledge of the function till inductive or hypothesis generating approaches by looking at all genes simultaneously (1). This is also named the agnostic approach (4). So far the GWAS studies in cancer have discovered around 200 SNPs that most have a relative risk less than two. The post-GWAS strategy is under discussion, and the direction recommended is towards studies of functional aspects of these SNPs (4).

This development should be held against the common view behind the agnostic GWAS strategy which strongly points to the lack of exact biological information for making exact single genes or pathways approaches fruitful. In fact, the lack of *in vivo* derived information on most genes and pathways as part of carcinogenesis could hamper the search for mechanisms of carcinogenesis.

Another approach to expand the field of traditional epidemiology is systems epidemiology (5). This scientific discipline is the equivalent of systems biology, but performed in an epidemiological scale. In systems biology, high throughput 'omics' technologies are combined with computational analyses to investigate the metabolism of cells, tissues or organisms during health and disease. The aim of systems epidemiology is to study molecular mechanisms of disease in epidemiological studies. Systems epidemiology implicate better collections of biological material for functional studies and a carcinogenic model more relevant for epidemiology - an exposure driven functional model (6).

3. Status of functional genomics in epidemiology

The extent to which systems epidemiology is a realistic approach depends on the underlying assumption that blood and tissues communicate through gene expression and that the communication from cells undergoing a disease process through the blood might be trace signals from distorted metabolic pathways. This approach depends on adequately collected and stored biological material suitable for high throughput technologies used for studies of functional changes during the development of chronic diseases. Transcriptomics consists of two major classes of gene expression functions. mRNA is a copy or a messenger of the gene code information stored as DNA for the production of proteins in the cell. It is rapidly degraded by the Rnase. microRNAs are not coding for proteins, but regulates the expression of mRNAs. It is more resistance to degradation and can be used as biomarkers (7). New studies of the transport and delivery of microRNA are rapidly growing, strongly supporting the view that blood is an important channel for communication between cells. Thus, the basic assumption of systems epidemiology gains momentum.

The extent to which mRNA and microRNA are transported in the blood stream as information carriers can only be verified in humans through a prospective study design. There exist many studies with repeated blood samples with DNA from plasma/serum, but few with biological material suitable for gene expression analyses of mRNA simultaneously of peripheral blood and tumour tissue. One serious objection is the time frame for the function of gene expression which could differ, so the snapshot through one blood sample could give a confusing picture. But, those important cell regulations that are disturbed in the disease process should be expected to have some constancy over time since most exert the effects as a consequence of substantial exposures over a prolonged time. The success of this approach could depend on repeated measurements in order to be able to study changes in gene functions over a lifetime.

There is growing evidence that gene expression in peripheral blood reflects different lifestyle factors. Several cross-sectional studies of gene expression have been published highlighting numerous and interconnected pathways or gene sets affected in blood by defined lifestyle factors or exposure variables e.g. smoking (8), hormones (9) or organic pollutants (10). Important objections are the level of technical noise (11). Although blood gene expression profiling promises molecular-level insight into disease mechanisms, there remains a lack of baseline data describing the nature and extent of variability in blood gene expression in the general population. Characterizations of this variation and the underlying factors that most influence gene expression amongst healthy individuals play an important role in the feasibility, design and analysis of future blood-based studies. The number of studies with lifestyle exposures related to microRNA is absent and only a few studies exist for epigenetics "e.g". DNA methylation (12). In addition, a few case-control studies (13) have been published. So far these cross-sectional studies have not been transformed into prospective studies. At the same time a large number of studies have been publish based on clinical cohorts relating gene expression patterns in tumour tissue to survival and prognosis. Several studies have shown the usefulness of more functional classification of breast cancer (14). This might be important for etiological research as a means to improve the classification of breast cancer tumours.

4. An example of a biological model and the relationship to epidemiology: The two-stage model of carcinogenesis

In cancer epidemiology, the estimations of the carcinogenic multistage model is more than fifty years old (15). The situation today is not different from the early papers, namely that there is a lack of observational data of the stages of carcinogenesis. Due to this lack of observed data the parameters in the mathematical model can not be solved uniquely (16). At the same time the importance of fixing one parameter in the mathematical model has been stressed, this could be the duration or changes related to the last stage. There exist at least five models (15), some of them clearly more explored than others like the two-stage clonal growth model (17), figure 1.

The biological model considers that the carcinogenic process starts with a mutation which is a change in one of the DNA sequences of a gene. The cell with this mutation then will undergo a rapid growth named the clonal phase. A second mutation will be necessary in order to have a transformed cancer cell that will grow as a tumour through the promotional, last stage. Dependent on the exposure which drives the carcinogenic process a stop or withdrawal of exposure could bring the promotional stage into arrest or the cancer cells could die through a process named apoptosis.

5. The functional genomics of prospective studies – The globolomic design

The structure of a globolomic study design could be as shown in figure 2. On the left different sources of exposure information are given, from questionnaires, blood samples, tissue samples and pathological paraffin blocks. The differences between the traditional cohort study and the globolomic one is given at the right side of the figure 2. The richness of biological material multiplies the possible analytical strategies, at the same time the complexity is far beyond current epidemiological methodology.

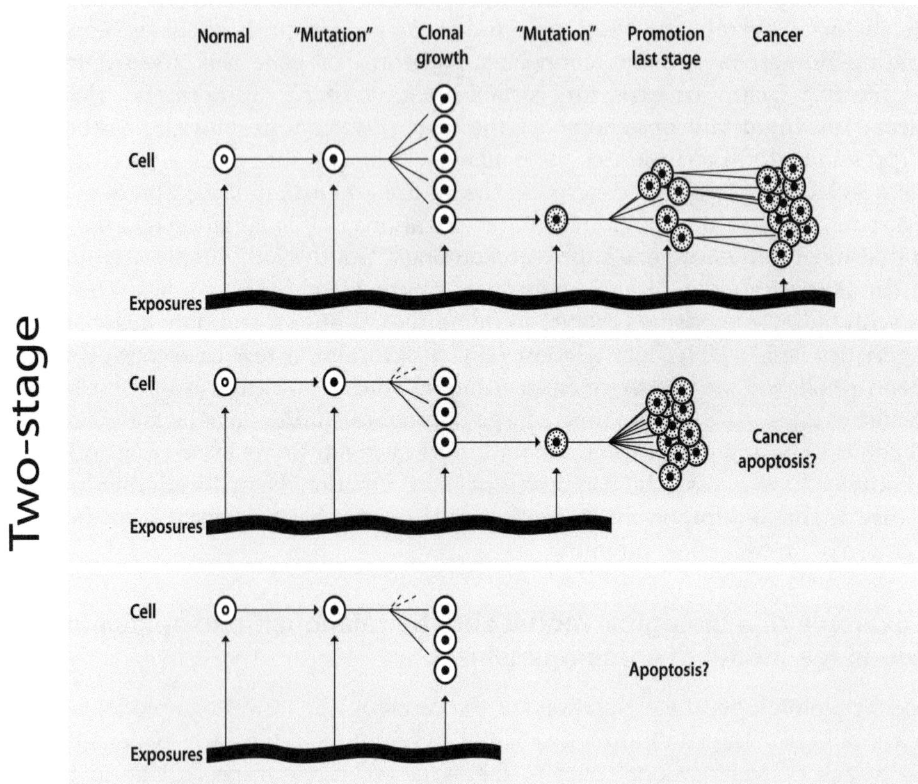

Fig. 1. Schematic description of the relationship between the clonal two-stage model and different scenarios of exposures.

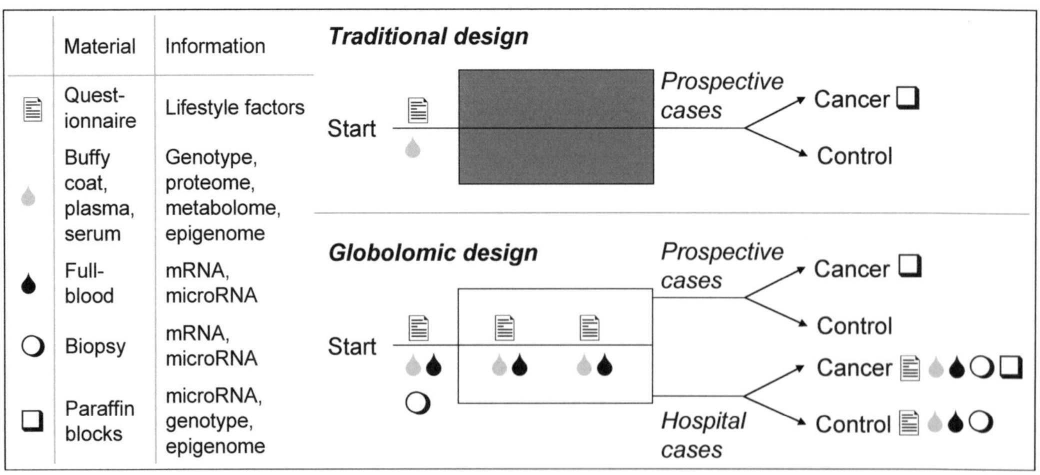

Fig. 2. The globolomic prospective study design.

As an example of the need for new and extended collection of both biological material and questionnaire information is given the structure of the Norwegian Women and Cancer cohort in Box 1, for more detailed information see (18).

1. Women sampled at random from the Norwegian population register, 172 000 women were enrolled.
2. Mailed letter of invitation and a questionnaire.
3. The postgenome biobank. Women born 1943-57 were eligible since they were invited or would be invited to participate in the Norwegian national mammographic screening program covering women 50-69 years, altogether 148 000.
4. Women were asked if they were willing to donate a blood sample to the study and at the same time give consent to update information on place of living. Approximately 95% of those returning the eight pages questionnaire answered yes to both questions.
5. Blood sampling. A package containing equipment for blood sampling and a two-paged questionnaire were mailed by groups of 500 random women. Participants brought the blood collection kit to their physicians office for blood sampling; one standard citrate tube and one collection tube containing a buffer for preservation of mRNA and microRNA. The blood samples give us access to mRNA and microRNA for gene expression, DNA from "buffy coat" for SNPs analyses, plasma for studies of metabolomics and proteomics.
6. The *passive follow-up* was completed through linkage to the national cancer registry in Norway based on the unique birth number and to registers of death and emigration. The information on cancer can then be used as end-points.
7. Collection of tumour biopsies through an *active follow-up* of all 148 000 women born 1943-57 at the time of diagnosis in collaboration with 10 of the major hospitals throughout Norway covered around 40% of the study sample. When a woman presented at the hospital with a lump in her breast, or one was diagnosed at the mammographic screening unit, all women were asked if they had participated in the NOWAC study. If they answered yes they were asked to give informed consent for a second biopsy for research use. At the same time they gave a blood sample and filled in a one page questionnaire.
8. For each of these women five random controls were drawn from the NOWAC postgenome cohort matched by age and date of the original blood donation. From these blood samples the same information can be extracted as from those blood samples collected originally. From the biopsy one can obtain microRNA, mRNA and tumour DNA.
9. For all cases of breast cancer the paraffin blocks stored in the pathological bio-banks are searched for to obtain microRNA and DNA.
10. Collection of breast tissue biopsies from healthy women participating in the NOWAC study and living in the north of Norway.

Box 1. Design, approaches and content of the Norwegian Women and Cancer postgenome study.

6. Challenges of systems epidemiology

The following will discuss several challenges raised by the introduction of functional genomics in prospective studies as part of systems epidemiology. The total amount of information is challenging the ordinary epidemiological analytical systems. From the DNA one can extract information for 500 000 SNPs, the same from tumour DNA, for each of the blood samples there will be a unique set of 25 000 gene expressions of mRNA and around 1 000 microRNAs. The methylation chips for epigenetic analyses cover around 500 000 variants. The number of measurements of metabolomics could be tens till hundreds. The proteomic screening analyses is just underway. Lastly, the questionnaire information could cover around 1 000 variables. In addition, there are scanned pictures from the microarrays and many files with technical information. Altogether, the storing and use of such large data sets will be dependent on computer science and cluster computers.

6.1 The nature of gene expression as exposure variable

In a prospective study gene expression could be classified as exposure. In a traditional design one would then use a Cox proportional model to estimate the relative hazard. This has typically been the procedure with the GWAS studies of SNPs. A SNP is a lifelong lasting characteristic that does not change over time or during follow-up. As such, SNPs could look as an ideal exposure variable being reliable and constant over the follow-up time. The analyses of gene expression in a follow-up study will be complicated by the possibilities of different population distributions throughout the follow-up period of the differences between cases and controls for each of the single of the 25 000 genes. Suppose we expect the gene expression in the controls to be similar over time. The hypothesis for a mutagen could be that the gene expression in the cases changes during follow-up as a consequence of events related to the disease process. We would then search for a change in the distribution of the differences in gene expression between cases and controls. These differences could have many potential distributions. The proportional hazard function would not be adequate.

The novel design gives us several challenges:

Challenge one: Biologically, the gene expression measured as the difference between the cases and the controls could either be the consequence of the exposure i.e. smoking changes the expression of a large number of genes, or the ongoing carcinogenic process due to the same exposures. This raises some methodological and statistical problems; how to estimate the changes in gene expression due to the carcinogenic process independently of the changes due to the carcinogen not necessarily linked to the carcinogenic process. If a mutation took place then the exponential increase in cancer cells could give a similar increase in expression of the affected genes. The differences in gene expression would then be an exponential function over time. Just putting both the gene expression variables and the exposure variables into the same model could give an unmeasured *over adjustment* of some of these variables. This can be handled by stratification which on the other hand would decrease the statistical power. Again, the analyses should be run agnostic before the information from basic research on gene function should be used.

Challenge two: As mentioned the traditional GWAS studies have been based mainly on the Cox proportional hazard model or using logistic regression analyses. The use of proportional hazard has the assumptions of proportionality and multiplicative risk estimation. There is no basic or epidemiological evidence of proportional hazard over time for the gene expression. In contrast, several other time-dependant models could be used.

The null hypothesis of no differences over time between the gene expression of cases and controls would in a linear model be closely parallel lines, eventually with the same beta-coeffisient.

One plausible model could be an increasing level of gene expression in cases compared to the controls as an effect of the mutations giving a clonal growth. This would give an exponential curve in an additive model or a straight line in a logarithmic model. There are many potential models that should be explored, but at the moment no strong preferences for the models exists from observational studies.

Challenge three: In traditional epidemiology including the gene-environment analyses of GWAS the search has been for the highest relative risks or the lowest p-values. This simple assumption does not hold for functional analyses. There is no evidence that important functional changes due to the disease process should be more clearly expressed than other ongoing cellular functions or effects of lifestyle. The search would be for genes that exerts a given time dependant pattern. The first analyses in systems epidemiology would be to sort the time-dependant functions of the 25 000 genes keeping in mind the consequences of the multiple testing. To sort out the highest p-values could remove very important information.

Challenge four: The time-dependant analysis of the gene expression could need new statistical tests and adaption of new functions for the follow-up studies. A major task both of design, laboratory work and statistical methods would be to improve the sensitivity of the analyses.

Challenge five: There is an obvious concern about the complexity of the total data structure of the functional information possible to obtain for a small number of cases and controls. This is a work that is ongoing in systems biology and several methods should be possible to adapt in order to improve the biological explanations of findings in the epidemiological studies.

7. Discussion

The design of a prospective study including trancriptomic options has only recently been implemented in the globolomic design of NOWAC. In the discussion of *pro et cons* for building new cohort studies the option for gene expression analyses are mostly neglected (19, 20, 21), but has been proposed by some (22).

The notion of gene-expression as exposures confronts the epidemiologists with approximately 25 000 possibly time-dependant exposure variables. This adds to the well known uniqueness of each woman's lifestyle. Consider data from the NOWAC study taking the mode of six well known factors that either increase or decrease the risk of breast cancer. Based on information from 172 000 women combining the mode value for age at menarche, parity, age at first full term pregnancy, age at menopause, age at first use of hormonal replacement therapy and age at first use of oral contraceptive left no one to share the same lifetime exposure pattern. Even with so few variables the risk profiles of the women are highly different. It is under such conditions that the time dependant changes exert effects through the functioning of the genes. In order to focus on the overall importance of the exposures we would sum up over a person's lifetime the continuously changing lifestyle with both risk and preventive factors. The diversity of exposures gives a diversity of functional changes and an individual may at the same time have several potential carcinogenic processes ongoing even within the same tissue "e.g" the effect of smoking and radiation exposure on lung tissue.

It is well known that different exposures have different effect on the diseases. In cancer the carcinogenic process is different for exposures like radiation, chemicals, bacteria, and virus. In addition, several chemicals act as hormone imitators. There is no strong reason to believe in exact the same model of carcinogenesis for all exposures. Radiation hits the DNA in a different manner from use of hormones in postmenopausal women. Heterogeneity of exposures drives heterogeneity of functional changes and in the end the expression profiles.

7.1 Trans-etiological research

So far etiological or causal research has been done almost independently in basic cell biology and epidemiology except for the gene-environment analysis. One could call this a dichotomy, see Box 2.

	Epidemiology	basic genetic research
Common approaches		
Gene-enviroment analyses	exposure and gene interactions	
Bioinformatics	gene functions	
Dualism		
Model of carcinogenesis	multistage	mutational
Driving forces	exposures	mutations
Exposures	yes	mostly none
Methods	observational	experimental
Mechanistic/functional	no	yes, main focus
Scientific approach	whole genome scan	
Time relationship	prospective	cross-sectional end-point related
Causality	criteria for statistical association time order	experimental verification mRNA, oncogenes etc
Time relationship		

Box 2. Examples of common approaches and the dualism between epidemiology and basic cancer research.

In almost every aspect of scientific work these two disciplines have different views, methods and models. The expansion of functional genomics into epidemiology could improve the communications far beyond the current. While methodologies and designs of studies differ greatly, this could be considered as a natural consequence of the research fields. But behind this is the deeper conflict in science between those used to put up deductive hypothesis and test them in experiments versus the agnostic approach to the observational studies in epidemiology. The history of genomic analysis, SNPs, going from single gene studies over annotated genes till pathways analyses and ending up in GWAS clearly demonstrates the very different approaches scientifically in basic genetic research and epidemiology - from deductive designs of experiments till observational studies searching for associations. In order to improve collaboration between basic genetic research and epidemiology mutual understanding of methodological approaches in each discipline would be important.

8. Concluding remarks

A unique opportunity to expand design and interpretations of statistical associations in epidemiological studies has been given due to new technologies. At the same time this opportunity will depend on a closer collaboration between basic researchers in different biological disciplines and epidemiologist, giving us a possibility of a new trans-etiological research.

9. References

[1] Spitz MR, Bondy ML. The evolving discipline of molecular epidemiology of cancer. Carcinogenesis 2010; 31; 127-34

[2] Haiman CA, Dossus L, Setiawan VW, Stram DO, Dunning AM, Thomas G, Thun MJ, Albanes D, Altshuler D, Ardanaz E, Boeing H, Buring J, Burtt N, Calle EE, Chanock S, Clavel-Chapelon F, Colditz GA, Cox DG, Feigelson HS, Hankinson SE, Hayes RB, Henderson BE, Hirschhorn JN, Hoover R, Hunter DJ, Kaaks R, Kolonel LN, Le Marchand L, Lenner P, Lund E, Panico S, Peeters PH, Pike MC, Riboli E, Tjonneland A, Travis R, Trichopoulos D, Wacholder S, Ziegler RG. Genetic variation at the CYP19A1 locus predicting circulating oestrogen levels but not breast cancer risk in postmenopausal women. Cancer Res 2007; 67: 1-5.

[3] Reiner A, Yekutieli D, Benjamini Y. Identifying differentially expressed genes using false discovery rate controlling procedures. Bioinformatics 2003; 19: 368-75.

[4] Freedman ML et al. principles for the post-GWAS functional characterization of cancer risk loci. Nature Genetics 2011; 43; 513-18.

[5] Lund E, Dumeaux V: Towards a more functional concept of causality in cancer research. Int J Mol Epi Genet 2010; 1:124-133.

[6] Lund E. An exposure driven functional model of carcinogenesis. Med Hypoteses 2011 May 5. [Epub ahead of print]

[7] Cortez MA et al. MicroRNAs in body fluids - the mix of hormones and biomarkers. Nat Rev Clin Onc 2011; 8; 467-77.

[8] Lampe JW, Stepaniants SB, Mao M, Radich JP, Dai H, Linsley PS, Friend SH, Potter JD. Signature of environmental exposures using peripheral leukocyte gene expression: tobacco smoke. Cancer Epidemiol Biomarkers Prev 2004; 13: 445-53.

[9] Waaseth M, Olsen KS, Rylander C, Lund E, Dumeaux V. Sex hormones and gene expression signatures in peripheral blood from postmenopausal women - the NOWAC postgenome study.BMC Med Genomics. 2011 Mar 31;4:29

[10] Terasaka S, Aita Y, Inoue A, Hayashi S, Nishigaki M, Aoyagi K, Sasaki H, Wada-Kiyama Y, Sakuma Y, Akaba S, Tanaka J, Sone H, Yonemoto J, Tanji M, Kiyama R. Using a customized DNA microarray for expression profiling of the estrogen-responsive genes to evaluate estrogen activity among natural estrogens and industrial chemicals. Environ Health Perspect 2004; 112: 773-81.

[11] Dumeaux V, Olsen SK, Paulssen RH, Børresen-Dale AL, Lund E. Deciphering blood gene expression variation – The postgenome NOWAC study. PLoS Genetics 2009 (in press)

[12] Vaissière T, Cuenin C, Paliwal A, Vineis P, Hoek G, Krzyzanowski M, Airoldi L, Dunning A, Garte S, Hainaut P, Malaveille C, Overvad K, Clavel-Chapelon F, Linseisen J, Boeing H, Trichopoulou A, Trichopoulos D, Kaladidi A, Palli D, Krogh V, Tumino R, Panico S, Bueno-De-Mesquita HB, Peeters PH, Kumle M, Gonzalez CA, Martinez C, Dorronsoro M, Barricarte A, Navarro C, Quiros JR, Berglund G, Janzon L, Jarvholm B, Day NE, Key TJ, Saracci R, Kaaks R, Riboli E, Hainaut P, Herceg Z. Quantitative analysis of DNA methylation after whole bisulfitome amplification of a minute amount of DNA from body fluids. Epigenetics. 2009 May 16;4(4):221-30. Epub 2009 May 24.

[13] Sharma P, Sahni NS, Tibshirani R, Skaane P, Urdal P, Berghagen H, Jensen M, Kristiansen L, Moen C, Sharma P, Zaka A, Arnes J, Sauer T, Akslen LA, Schlichting E, Børresen-Dale AL, Lönneborg A Early detection of breast cancer based on gene-expression patterns in peripheral blood cells. Breast Cancer Res 2005; 7: R634-44.

[14] Sørli T. Molecular portraits of breast cancer: tumour subtypes as distinct disease entities. Eur J Cancer 2004; 40: 2667-75

[15] Vineis P, Schatzkin A, Potter JD. Model of carcinogenesis: an overview. Carcinogenesis 2010; 31; 1703-9

[16] Cox LA, Huber WA. Symmetry, identifiability, and prediction uncertainties in multistage clonal expansion (MSCE) models of carcinogenesis. Risk Analysis 2007; 27; 1441-53.

[17] Moolgavkar SH, Day NE, Stevens RG. Two-stage model for carcinogenesis: epidemiology of breast cancer in females. JNCI 1980; 65: 559-569.

[18] Lund, E; Dumeaux, V; Braaten T; Hjartåker, Engeset D; Skeie, G; Kumle, M. Cohort profile: The Norwegian women and cancer study - NOWAC - Kvinner og kreft. International Journal of Epidemiology 2008; 37; 36-41

[19] Collins FS, Manolio TA. Necessary but not sufficient. Nature 2007; 445: 259.

[20] Willett WC, Blot WJ, Colditz GA, Folsom AR, Henderson BE, Stampfer MJ. Merging and emerging cohorts: not worth the wait. Nature 2007: 445; 257-258.

[21] Colditz GA, Sellers TA, Trapido E. Epidemiology – identifying the causes and preventability of cancer? Nature Rev 2006; 75-83.

[22] Potter JD. Epidemiology informing clinical practice; from bills of mortality to population laboratories. Nat Clin Pract Oncol 2005; 2: 625-34.

6

Molecular Epidemiology of Parasitic Diseases: The Chagas Disease Model

Juan David Ramírez and Felipe Guhl
Centro de Investigaciones en Microbiología y Parasitología Tropical (CIMPAT), Universidad de los Andes, Bogotá, Colombia

1. Introduction

Parasitic diseases represent one of the most important issues in public health. More than one billion people worldwide are infected by parasites causing different disease scenarios. Parasitic diseases are closely related to geographic, social and economic factors driving the prevalence and incidence of these pathologies (WHO, 2010). These represent a broad group of eukaryotic organisms that may cause severe diseases in animal and human populations. Parasites are the causative agents of pathologies such as Malaria. In 2008, there were 247 million cases of Malaria and nearly one million deaths from the disease, mostly among children living in Africa. In Africa, a child dies of Malaria every 45 seconds; the disease accounts for 20% of all childhood deaths. Leishmaniasis threatens approximately 350 million men, women and children in 88 countries around the world. As many as 12 million people are believed to be currently infected by this disease, with approximately 1–2 million estimated new cases occurring every year. Additionally, an estimated of 10 million people are infected worldwide by Chagas disease (American trypanosomiasis), mostly in Latin America, where Chagas disease is endemic. More than 25 million people are at risk of acquiring this disease. It is estimated that in 2008, Chagas disease killed more than 10,000 people. Schistosomiasis is a chronic, parasitic disease caused by blood flukes (trematode worms) of the genus *Schistosoma*. More than 207 million people are infected with these organisms worldwide, with an estimated 700 million people at risk in 74 endemic countries. Lymphatic filariasis affects more than 1.3 million people in 81 countries. Approximately 65% of those infected live in Southeast Asia, 30% in Africa and the remainder in other tropical areas. Lymphatic filariasis afflicts over 25 million men with genital disease and over 15 million people with lymphoedema. Because the prevalence and intensity of infection are linked to poverty, elimination can contribute to achieving the United Nations Millennium Development Goals. Human African Trypanosomiasis (HAT) affects mostly poor populations living in remote rural areas of Africa. If untreated, it is usually fatal. Travellers also risk becoming infected if they venture through regions where the insect vector (tse tse flies) is common. Generally, the disease is not found in urban areas, although some cases have been reported in suburban areas of Kinshasa, the capital of the Democratic Republic of Congo, and Luanda, the capital city of Angola. In 2004, the number of new reported cases fell to 17,616, which the WHO considered to be due to increased control, estimating the cumulative rate to be between 50,000 and 70,000 cases (WHO, 2010). These trends show the importance of developing strategies to mitigate the prevalence of these parasitic diseases, and molecular epidemiology arises as a potential tool to understand disease dynamics.

Molecular epidemiology is considered a powerful tool for understanding the genetic variation and evolution of pathogens. The use of the technologies based on molecular biology techniques has allowed the scientific community to reveal disease determinants and the genetic structure of parasites that provoke diseases and cause millions of deaths each year. In recent years, new studies have been conducted with the purpose of elucidating the genetic structure of the etiological agents of these pathologies with the aim of designing strategies that could help to mitigate the associated diseases in human and animal populations. Molecular epidemiology and population genetics have shown to be powerful strategies to understand the genetic structure of parasites, with special emphasis on understanding disease and transmission dynamics. The objective of this chapter is to illustrate for the reader the paramount importance of molecular epidemiology in parasitic diseases, showing some clear examples of parasite disease and transmission dynamics. The focus will be on how molecular epidemiology can be a helpful tool to mitigate disease transmission, prevalence and incidence and can be used as a reliable tool for disease surveillance as well as the need to create synergy between molecular epidemiology and public health programmes to reduce the prevalence of parasitic diseases.

2. Importance and relevance of molecular epidemiology

Molecular epidemiology may be defined as a tool focused on the contribution of potential genetic factors identified by molecular techniques to the aetiology, distribution and prevention of disease across populations (Kilbourne, 1973). It is a field of study that has recently emerged from the integration of molecular biology, epidemiology, biochemistry and public health systems (Figure 1). This approach has been useful in attempting to determine the pathogenesis of certain diseases as well as the genetic variation and genetic structure of pathogens.

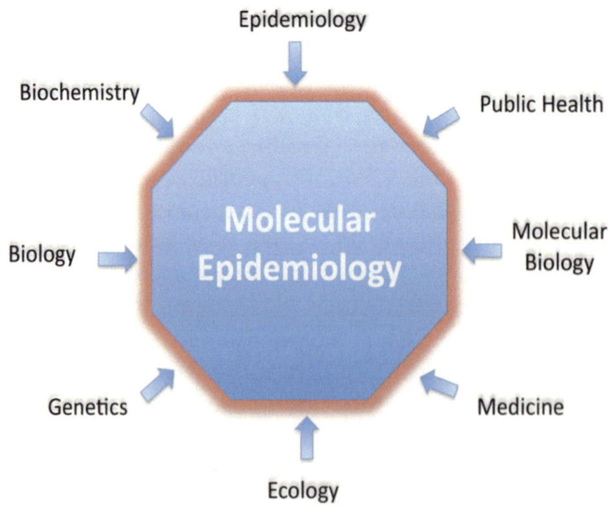

Fig. 1. Molecular epidemiology is considered an interdisciplinary science that is a composite of different sciences.

Molecular epidemiology has recently gained paramount importance in the fields of human genetics and in molecular virology. One clear example of this is the use of molecular epidemiology to track viruses that generate severe acute respiratory syndrome (SARS). This allowed researchers to develop strategies with the purpose of tracking the transmissibility and dispersal of this virus, observing that the positive selection pressure associated with human hosts resulted in the emergence of lineages of the virus that became readily transmissible between humans, causing the epidemic outbreak of 2002-2003 (Zhao, 2007). The use of molecular markers also permitted the establishment of prevention and control strategies to mitigate the transmission of these genotypes, thus avoiding increased disease prevalence. Thus, this example shows how traceable pathogens can be and clearly demonstrates the great utility of molecular biology on the basis of molecular epidemiology in obtaining a deeper understanding regarding parasitic diseases.

Molecular epidemiology has been established as a promising science for studying the contribution of potential genetic markers and environmental risk factors of parasitic diseases representing a close synergy between molecular biology and epidemiology. Some of the main objectives of molecular epidemiology focused on the study of parasitic diseases are as follows:

- To enhance our understanding of the pathogenesis of parasitic diseases: Some authors have used the *Toxoplasma gondii* model to describe relationships between nucleoside triphosphate hydrolase (NTPase) isoforms and *Toxoplasma* strain virulence in human toxoplasmosis, reporting that different isoforms are involved in clinical forms of this parasitic disease (Johnson et al., 2003).
- To define genetic susceptibility with genetic markers: The use of human pedigrees to observe patterns of susceptibility to visceral leishmaniasis in Brazil has allowed researchers to develop action plans to mitigate this tropical disease in endemic areas (Jamieson et al., 2007).
- To allow evaluation of subclinical or early disease markers: Prognostic markers are one of the milestone deliverables in molecular epidemiology. In the case of *T. gondii*, a quantitative real-time PCR assay for amniotic fluid has been developed to provide a prognostic marker of foetal infection in pregnant women (Romand et al., 2004)
- To provide new standards for descriptive epidemiology: Some of the problems involved in descriptive epidemiology show how difficult it is to track some kinds of diseases. In particular, the parasites that cause gastrointestinal syndromes fall into this category, such as *Entamoeba histolytica, Taenia solium, Ascaris lumbricoides, Giardia intestinalis, Enterobius vermicularis* and others. Microscopic identification becomes tedious and, in some case confusing due to similar morphologies among some parasites. Molecular detection based on PCR assays has provided the field of descriptive epidemiology with a more reliable way to analyse data in population descriptive studies (Singh et al., 2009; Pecson et al., 2006).
- To improve precision in analytical epidemiology: While descriptive epidemiology provides the what, who, when and where; analytical epidemiology attempts to provide the why and how. Few examples are listed related to the detection of emergent genotypes in disease surveillance. A good example is that of HAT, which is caused by two sympatric subspecies (*Trypanosoma brucei rhodesiense* and *T. b. gambiense*); each subspecies is involved in disease severity causing a large number of annual deaths in Africa (Morrison et al., 2011).

As has been shown thus far, molecular epidemiology as applied to the study of parasites is considered an important and relevant tool to investigate these organisms. The important point to focus is on the correct use of the information obtained. Molecular methods are currently available and becoming cheaper every day, and the emergence of new accurate and feasible molecular methods shows promising results for the molecular epidemiology field; however, in molecular epidemiology, the clinical question must be always highlighted to obtain the most reliable results. Thus, the income data become the critical point in the study of parasitic diseases and the basis for obtaining a good outcome that can be translated to meet the main aims of molecular epidemiology studies (Figure 2). This chapter will discuss the molecular methods available to develop molecular epidemiology studies focused on parasites, with some clear examples of how useful and necessary molecular epidemiology is for understanding disease outcomes, transmission dynamics and the current genetic structure of parasitic diseases.

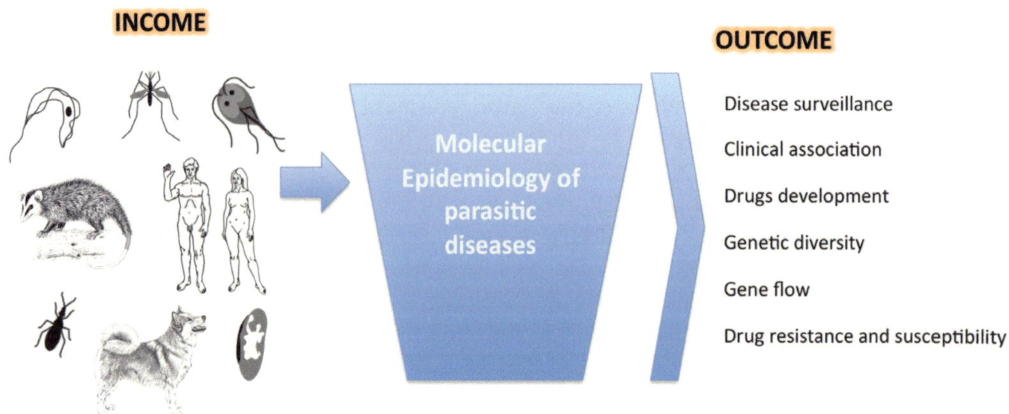

Fig. 2. Flow of information based on the accurate and reliable use of molecular epidemiology focused on the study of parasitic diseases.

3. Molecular biology tools applied in the analysis of parasitic diseases

Molecular biology has made important contributions in the last ten years with respect to understanding the genetics of parasites causing human illness. A broad description of the markers used in molecular epidemiology and their features is presented in Table 1. The first techniques used to track pathogens and disease dispersal were based on biochemical markers, with Multilocus Enzyme Electrophoresis (MLEE) being broadly used to study parasites such as *T. cruzi*, *Leishmania* spp, *E. histolytica* and *T. brucei* (Miles et al., 1977; Pinto et al., 2005; Mathews et al., 1983; Nijokou et al., 2004). This technique is based on differences between loci; according to the obtained banding pattern, it is possible to distinguish among lineages. In the case of *Leishmania,* this technique was used to differentiate species of the genus involved in visceral and cutaneous leishmaniasis (Bañuls et al., 2000; Bañuls et al., 2002; Zhang et al., 2006). A drawback of this technique is the need to culture large quantities of parasites, which are quite difficult to obtain in most parasitic diseases. Subsequently, molecular biology techniques based on the use of DNA were developed, among which RAPDs (Random Amplified Polymorphic DNA), AFLPs (Amplified Fragment Length Polymorphism), PFGE (Pulse Field Gel Electrophoresis) and RFLPs (Restriction Fragment Length Polymorphism) were the most used techniques within the scientific community. In this sense, analysis of ribosomal markers using RAPDs was of paramount importance in attempting to develop assays to distinguish among morphologically similar amoebas. *E. histolytica* and *E. dispar*, which represent pathogenic and non-pathogenic amoeba species, respectively, have been suggested by many authors to have evolved identically up to the point when a mutation generated a cryptic speciation pattern (Clark et al., 2006). The use of RAPD techniques has also been an important aid in understanding genetic variation within *E. histolytica* isolated from different hosts (Gomes et al., 2000; Prakash et al., 2000). AFLPs and RFLPs are the most recent techniques to be employed to track pathogen dispersal and elucidate their genetic diversity. Fingerprinting based on AFLPs has been useful in differentiating subspecies of *T. brucei*, which is the aetiological agent of sleeping sickness, a pathology that affects more than 8 million people in Africa. These techniques have shown great reproducibility in distinguishing *T. b. rhodesiense* and *T. b. gambiense*, two sympatric species that generate different symptomatologies, demonstrating how molecular epidemiology can assist in understanding disease outcomes in certain pathologies, thus aiding in developing proper treatment and management measures (Agbo et al., 2002; Masiga et al., 2006). RFLPs have been applied to parasites such as *T. gondii* and *Trichinella spiralis*, which are two species for which pigs play an important role in transmission dynamics. *T. gondiii* is considered to display a clonal population, but its isolates have been divided into three types that are geographically clustered and, in some cases, are involved in disease outcomes (Wang et al., 1995; Su et al., 2002; Fuentes et al., 2001). These molecular markers have been shown to be important in discriminating species as well as evaluating genetic variability among isolates from the same species. The great advantage of these molecular markers is that they can be used to show the pattern of variation across the whole genome of a pathogen, rather than just a specific region, as will be shown later.

Feature	**MLEE[1]**	**RAPD[2] and AFLP[3]**	**RFLP[4] and PFGE[5]**	**Microarrays**	**MLMT[6]**	**MLST[7]**	**qPCR[8]**	**Genome Sequencing**
Culturing	Yes	No	No	No	No	No	No	No
Analysis of distinct loci	Yes	No	No	Yes	Yes	Yes	Yes	No
Cost	Low	Low	Low	High	Medium	Medium	Medium	High
Labor	High	Low	Low	High	Low	Low	Low	Medium
Informative	Low	Low	Low	High	High	High	High	High
Portability	Low	Medium	Medium	Low	High	High	Medium	Low

[1] Multilocus Enzyme Electrophoresis, [2] Random Amplified Polymorphic DNA, [3] Amplified Fragment Length Polymorphisms, [4] Restriction Fragment Length Polymorphisms, [5] Pulse Field Gel Electrophoresis, [6] Multilocus Microsatellite Typing, [7] Multilocus Sequence Typing, [8] Quantitative Real Time PCR

Table 1. Molecular markers used in molecular epidemiology studies.

The development of Polymerase Chain Reaction (PCR) was of great importance and represents an incredible advance in molecular biology. Since 1990, PCR has been broadly used to study parasites. Modifications of PCR, such as PCR-RFLP, Nested PCR, RT-PCR, AP-PCR (Allele Polymorphic Polymerase Chain Reaction), SHELA-PCR (Solution Hybridization Enzyme-Linked Assay Polymerase Chain Reaction) and qPCR (Quantitative Real Time Polymerase Chain Reaction), have been applied to study parasites. In these tests, the only thing that a researcher requires is a few aliquots of DNA, which simplifies the analysis. The use of PCR-RFLP is widely reported in discriminating *Leishmania* species. In these studies, the use of Heat Shock proteins with different molecular weights allows discrimination based on PCR amplification of genes that are subsequently digested with restriction endonucleases. According to the band patterns obtained in such analyses, it has been possible to distinguish between the subgenera *Viannia* and *Leishmania* as well as species from the different subgenera in some cases (Volpini et al., 2004; Montalvo et al., 2006). Discrimination among *Leishmania* species or their complexes is necessary in conducting studies on treatment resistance and clinical manifestations associated with leishmaniasis, in which some species cause cutaneous forms, and others cause visceral forms. One of the most important advances in the modification of PCR assays has been the development of quantitative Real-Time PCR (qPCR). This assay involves the quantification of DNA copies in each PCR cycle. The first applications of this technique have been for diagnostic purposes in cases where it has been possible to estimate parasitic loads in infected patients. In the case of *L. infantum*, the species involved in visceral leishmaniasis manifestations, assays have been developed to estimate parasitic loads in biopsies of infected patients and, thus, to estimate the efficacy of treatment using qPCR (Mary et al., 2004; Bretagne et al., 2001; Ranasinghe et al., 2008). Additionally, qPCR using SYBR green and Hybridisation probe chemistry has allowed the development of melting temperature (Tm) analysis according to a dissociation curve. This permits screening for genotypes or species according to the specific temperature of an amplicon and enables observation of single nucleotide polymorphisms, all in the same reaction. Thus, a qPCR Real Time protocol has been proposed to identify *Leishmania* species focused on spliced leader genes and minicircle kDNA regions; according to distinct temperatures, investigators were able to discriminate *Leishmania* species (Wortmann et al., 2005). This approach has also been applied to other parasites, such as *Giardia,* for which qPCR assays were developed to detect *G. lamblia* and to discriminate its genotypes in stool specimens (Guy et al., 2004). Additionally, it has been used to study schistosomiasis, an helminthic disease that affects populations in Africa, Asia and America, with qPCR assays being developed to discriminate species in water where the infective form (cercariae) lives and is transmitted to humans (Lier et al., 2006). qPCR has been shown to be a reliable, feasible, fast and accurate method in molecular epidemiology to discriminate species as well as to determine genotypes within species. This suggests the need to pursue studies involving this method, though in some cases, validation studies are required, and further research is needed. A problem involved in working on parasites is sensitivity because in some parasite diseases, the parasitic loads are quite low and even undetectable in some cases, such that concentration methods must be applied or it may be necessary to analyse the whole sample.

Other molecular markers include microarrays and Southern blot and northern blot techniques. The drawback of microarrays is that they are time consuming, expensive, and in some cases, they do not provide the desired information. In the last decade, the rise of sequencing procedures has been an important addition to molecular epidemiology investigations. The ability to obtain DNA sequences has allowed researchers to unravel the genetic structure of parasites and to go further in the analyses that can be applied. Thus, molecular phylogenetics and population genetics have provided molecular epidemiology with certain, reliable tools for understanding the genetic structure of parasites. Molecular phylogenetics is the science focused on understanding the evolutionary relationships among groups of organisms based on molecular sequences, and these techniques have been broadly applied to parasites. Hence, molecular phylogenetics has allowed the reconstruction of phylogenetic trees based on maximum parsimony and/or maximum composite likelihood methods with the aim of understanding the evolutionary history of parasites and, in some cases, developing analysis involving loci. Based on the use of DNA sequences and phylogenetic reconstructions, new methods such as MLST (Multilocus Sequence Typing) have arisen. MLST has been broadly used in bacteria and yeast but has only recently been applied to parasites; the drawback of MLST in addressing protozoan parasites associated with working with clonal diploids instead of clonal haploids, such as bacteria. The genetic structure of clonal diploid pathogenic organisms is important in terms of elucidating the drivers of disease prevalence, installation and outcomes as well as the virulence factors and geographical distribution related to the disease. In recent years, the population structure of microorganisms such as *Plasmodium*, *Giardia*, *Entamoeba*, Trypanosomes (*T. brucei*, *T. congolense* and *T. cruzi*), *Candida*, *Leishmania* and *Toxoplasma* has gained paramount relevance due to the discussion of clonal propagation versus sexual recombination (De Meeus et al., 2006; Benett et al., 2010; Grigg and Suzuki, 2003; Morrison et al., 2009; Rougeron et al., 2010; Mzilahowa et al., 2007). There are three hypotheses that describe the genetic structure observed in clonal diploid organisms. In 1987, Harvey and Keymer suggested a panmictic population structure in which sexual recombination is frequent. In 1991, Tibayrenc et al. proposed the clonal theory of parasitic protozoa, suggesting that these organisms display a clonal propagation mode associated with infrequent sexual recombination events. Finally, in 1993, Maynard-Smith et al. proposed an epidemic population structure with a background level of frequent sexual recombination and with occasional clonal expansion of particular genotypes. These hypotheses have been tested using a large number of parasitic protozoa; however, the debate still continues.

The use of new methods for typing and elucidating the genetic variability of parasites like MLST has gained importance because it can be considered to be an improvement of MLEE. MLST makes use of different loci involved in parasite metabolism. Thus, MLST strategies have been developed in *Leishmania* for species identification using five metabolic enzymes that are able to discriminate species and genotypes within complexes (Zemanova et al., 2007). An MLST approach has also recently been described for discriminating among subtypes of *Blastocystis*, which is a protozoan parasite involved in bowel inflammation and acute diarrhoea in immunodeficient patients (Stensvold and Clark, 2011). MLST analyses are not only used to discriminate genotypes of species but also to detect recombination or likely genetic exchanges among parasite populations (diploid clonals). In the case of sexual parasites such as helminthes, these approaches are employed to discriminate among species or to detect genotypes. Another important development in molecular epidemiology has been the use of microsatellite markers in developing MLMT (Multilocus Microsatellite Typing) strategies. Microsatellite markers are defined as tandem repetitions of 1-6 base pair segments of DNA; they are neutral and co-dominant and are useful in developing population genetics analyses. The variability of microsatellites is due to their higher rate of mutation compared to other neutral regions of DNA. The use of microsatellite markers is widely reported for purposes ranging from species identification to detection of recombination based on population genetics statistics. In *P. vivax,* polymorphic microsatellite markers have been amplified and analysed to unravel the genetic structure of this parasite and to understand its co-evolution with other *Plasmodium* species (Gomes et al., 2003; Imgwon et al., 2006). Population genetics tools present a limitation when working with clonal diploids related to the assumption of Hardy-Weinberg equilibrium and other statistics, such as *Fis* and *Fst*.

In recent years, DNA sequencing has become an important tool in understanding microorganisms, particularly those involved in human pathologies. Sequencing procedures have been improved, and pyrosequencing has become an important method to obtain more feasible and accurate DNA sequences. Pyrosequencing is a method of DNA sequencing based on the "sequencing by synthesis" principle. It differs from Sanger sequencing in that it relies on the detection of pyrophosphate release upon nucleotide incorporation, rather than chain termination with dideoxynucleotides. Genome sequencing methods developed in bacteria have also been applied to sequence whole genomes in parasites. The first parasite genome sequenced was that of *P. falciparum* (Gardner et al., 2002), followed by the genomes of other parasites, such as *Leishmania, T. brucei, T. cruzi* and *T. gondii* (Ivens et al., 2005; Elsayed et al., 2005; Bontell et al., 2009). New initiatives have been developed to sequence larger genomes, such as those from helminthes including *Ascaris, Taenia, Schistosoma* and *Echinococcus*. These approaches have allowed scientists to develop projects aimed at annotating parasite genomes for the purpose of detecting possible pharmaceutical markers to develop drugs against these microorganisms. Genome sequencing is becoming cheaper due to the advances made by Illumina, which will allow the scientific community to begin sequencing genomes instead of single genes. The possibility of obtaining this type of metadata permits the application of tools in bioinformatics, metabolomics, immunomics, vaccinomics, proteomics and other field with the purpose of transitioning into the OMICS era. The OMICS era is considered to be associated with the most advanced techniques for understanding the molecular epidemiology of parasitic diseases. These tools will be of paramount importance in developing new drugs against parasites as well as evaluating surveillance disease markers or prognostic disease markers to understand the relatedness between disease outcomes and parasite genetic variability, which is one of the main objectives in molecular epidemiology.

4. Comparative molecular epidemiology: The Chagas disease model

Chagas disease, which is caused by the parasite *T. cruzi*, is a complex zoonosis that is widely distributed throughout the American continent. The infection can be acquired through triatomine faeces, blood transfusion, oral and congenital transmission and laboratory accidents. Chagas disease represents an important public health problem, with estimates by the Pan American Health Organization in 2005 of at least 7.7 million people being infected with *T. cruzi* and another 110 million being at risk (WHO, 2007). Additionally, immigration of infected people from endemic countries is now making Chagas disease a relevant health issue in other regions, including Europe and the United States (Rassi et al., 2009). Chagas disease is comprised of two stages, with the acute phase occurring approximately one week after the initial infection and approximately 30-40% of infected patients developing the chronic phase of the disease, in which cardiomyopathy is the most frequent and severe clinical manifestation (Rassi et al., 2009). Chagas has lately gained more importance due to recent reports of imported cases in Europe, the United States and Canada (Schmunis and Yadon, 2010).

Obtaining a full understanding of the aetiology and epidemiology of Chagas disease across its distribution has proved elusive and complex and remains the subject of intense investigation to the present day. The difficulty in completely defining the epidemiology of Chagas disease is attributable to several factors. First, Chagas disease is a zoonosis, and a variety of widely distributed mammals serve as reservoirs for *T. cruzi*. Moreover, all mammals are susceptible to *T. cruzi* infection. An additional factor that contributes to the complexity of Chagas disease as a zoonosis is the variety of vectors involved, as they are not simply represented by a range of related species or genera, as is the case for all other known insect vector-associated diseases. Triatomine bugs are a subfamily of insects, and across this relatively broad taxonomic range, there are members from all groups that can harbour *T. cruzi*. However, most transmission is attributable to three main genera: *Rhodnius, Panstrongylus*, and *Triatoma*, but this diversity still represents two different tribes of the subfamily (Rhodniini and Triatomini). Furthermore, the insects vary in more than their ancestry, being associated with a diverse range of vertebrate hosts and ecological associations. The third factor that complicates the epidemiology of Chagas disease and accounts for variation in the clinical manifestation of the disease is the subspecific diversity of *T. cruzi* itself. Much work has been conducted over the past 40 years to elucidate the variation of *T. cruzi* across its geographical distribution and associations with hosts and vector species.

The *T. cruzi* parasite comprises a heterogeneous population that displays clonal propagation due to its different cycles of transmission and the possibility of recombination exchanges, which can be found in nature and have previously been reported *in vitro* (Gaunt et al., 2003, Sturm et al., 2003; Westenberger et al., 2002). *T. cruzi* is genetically diverse and is classified into a series of strains or subtypes. This genetic diversity was initially discovered using a panel of isoenzyme markers to investigate differences between parasites involved in domestic and sylvatic cycles in Bahia state in Brazil (Miles et al., 1977). This study represented a breakthrough, revealing that in Bahia, there were substantial genetic differences between the parasites involved in sympatric sylvatic and domestic transmission cycles. These variants were designated zymodemes I and II (ZI and ZII). Soon thereafter, it was revealed that the widespread strain associated with the sylvatic cycle in Brazil (ZI) was the predominant cause of human disease in Venezuela (Miles et al., 1981). These groundbreaking findings paved the way for investigating the aetiology of Chagas disease, allowing host-vector-parasite associations and comparative geographical distributions to be explored, as reviewed by Miles et al. (2009). Subsequently, four additional zymodemes were described from Brazil, Paraguay, and Bolivia. In the following two decades, various authors proceeded to characterise strains of *T. cruzi*, applying other molecular methods as they became available. As a result, further diversity was discovered within the original zymodemes. However, the designations of subtypes in the literature began to become confusing. Recently, a new nomenclature for *T. cruzi* has been adopted that includes six Discrete Taxonomic Units (DTUs) designated *T. cruzi* I (TcI), *T. cruzi* II (TcII), *T. cruzi* III

(TcIII), *T. cruzi* IV (TcIV), *T. cruzi* V (TcV) and *T. cruzi* VI (TcVI) based on different molecular markers and biological features (Zingales et al., 2009). These DTUs are broadly distributed in the American continent in diverse ecotopes (Figure 3). Discrimination of the six DTUs has become an important issue in the molecular epidemiology of *T. cruzi*. There are many reports showing algorithms for the molecular characterisation of these DTUs by performing RAPD, PCR-RFLP, qPCR, MLST, MLMT and DNA sequencing analyses, but to date, there is no consensus protocol for strain typing (Lewis et al., 2009; Rozas et al., 2007; Ramírez et al., 2010; Duffy et al., 2009; Yeo et al., 2011; Llewelly et al., 2009). One of the most recent and reliable algorithms for *T. cruzi* typing was reported by Ramírez et al., 2010 and has been applied on biological samples (Figure 4).

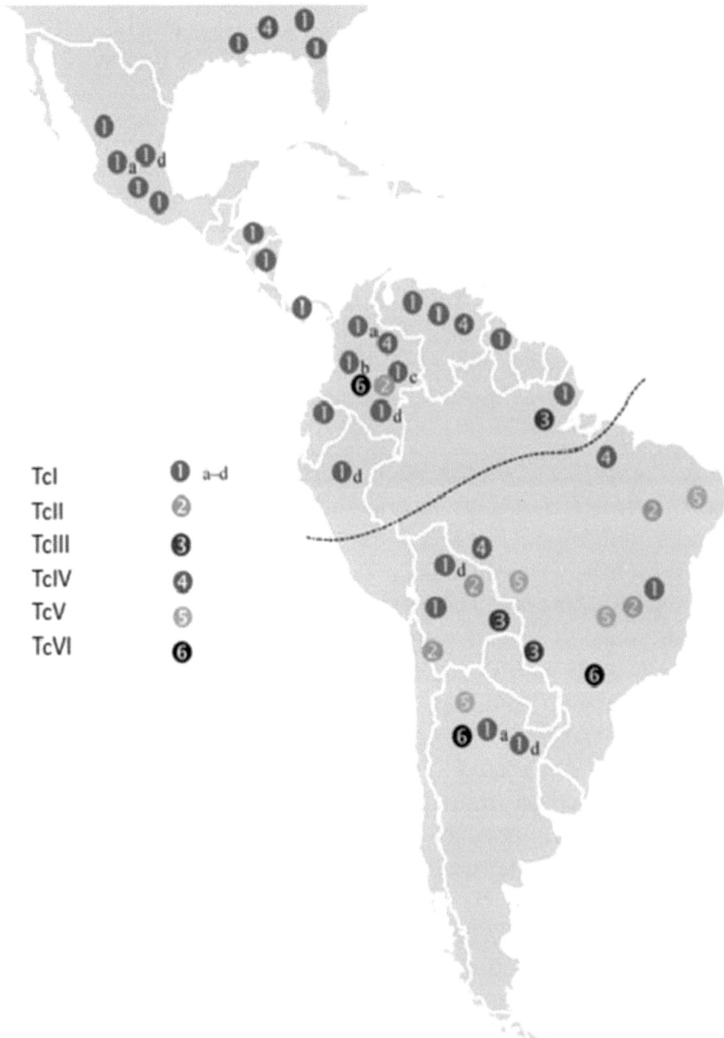

Fig. 3. Geographical distribution of *T. cruzi* DTUs in the American continent based on Patterson and Guhl, 2010.

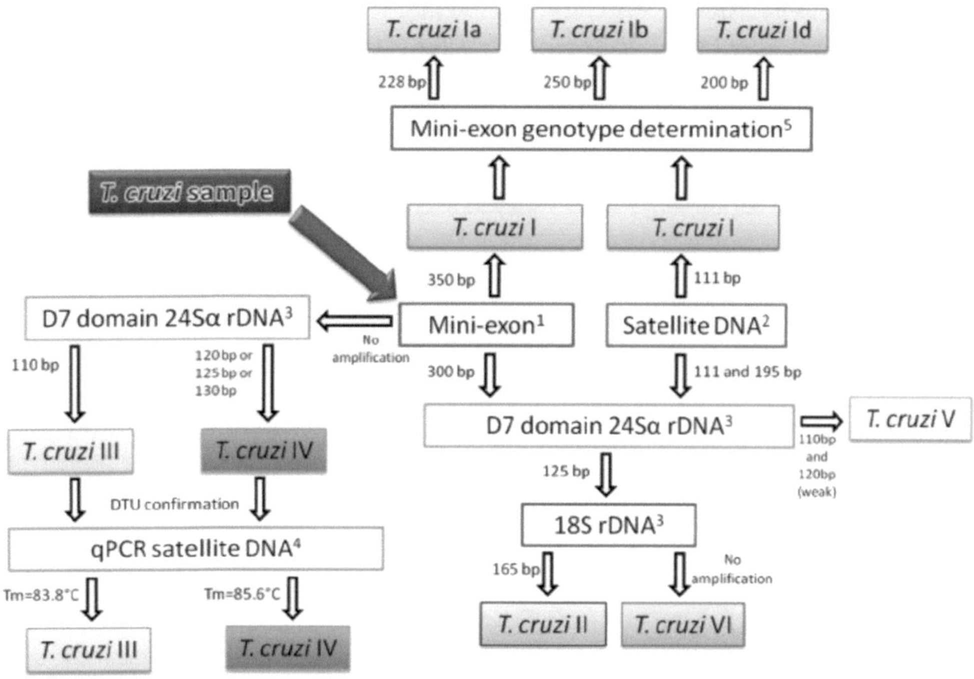

Fig. 4. Algorithm for typing *T. cruzi* DTU´s based on five molecular markers and also used to genotype biological samples (Ramírez et al., 2010).

In a sense, the findings of Miles et al. (1977) were the tip of the iceberg in unravelling the genetic structure of *T. cruzi*, but at the same time, they hit the nail on the head. The observed predominance of TcI in the human populations in Venezuela and Colombia and TcII, TcV, and TcVI mostly infecting human hosts in Brazil was to prove representative (i.e., it has since been demonstrated that TcI predominates in countries north of the Amazon and TcII-TcVI in Southern Cone countries, but this distribution is not absolute). This is particularly illuminating given that there are distinct clinical differences between patients presenting with Chagas disease in these two geographical regions. Strains appear to differ in terms of both their pathogenicity and response to treatment. TcI and TcII-VI are all associated with cardiac lesions in human infections, but it appears that only TcII, TcV, and TcIV are also associated with digestive tract lesions (Prata, 2001), despite the recent report of digestive tract lesions in Colombia caused by TcI (Mantilla et al., 2010). TcI is generally considered to be less pathogenic with lower parasitemia (Burgos et al., 2007) and more chronic cases being asymptomatic compared to Chagas caused by TcII, TcV, and TcVI in Argentina, Brazil, Chile, Paraguay, and Uruguay. TcI is almost the only form found in human infections north of the Amazon region. Moreover, there is an observed general partitioning of former TcII subtypes between sylvatic and domestic transmission cycles; the human disease is associated with TcII, while TcV is rarely associated with sylvatic hosts (Yeo et al., 2005), and TcIII and TcIV are predominantly sylvatic.

TcI has remained a constant grouping in the nomenclature since it was first described. However, recent studies based on mini-exon gene (SL-IR) sequences have shown polymorphism on this region, with four genotypes being reported within TcI. These genotypes have also been reported in various regions of South America, where five TcI genotypes have been detected (Figure 5) (Cura et al., 2010; Herrera et al., 2007; Guhl and Ramírez, 2011). Different molecular markers, including a 48 set of microsatellite loci, have also shown the great diversity in TcI (Guhl and Ramírez, 2011; Llewellyn et al., 2009; Spotorno et al., 2008; Ramírez et al., 2011). Primers designed based on TcI sequences confirmed the existence of three genotypes (Ia, Ib and Id) and a new genotype found in the Southern cone countries designated TcIe (Cura et al., 2010; Falla et al., 2009).

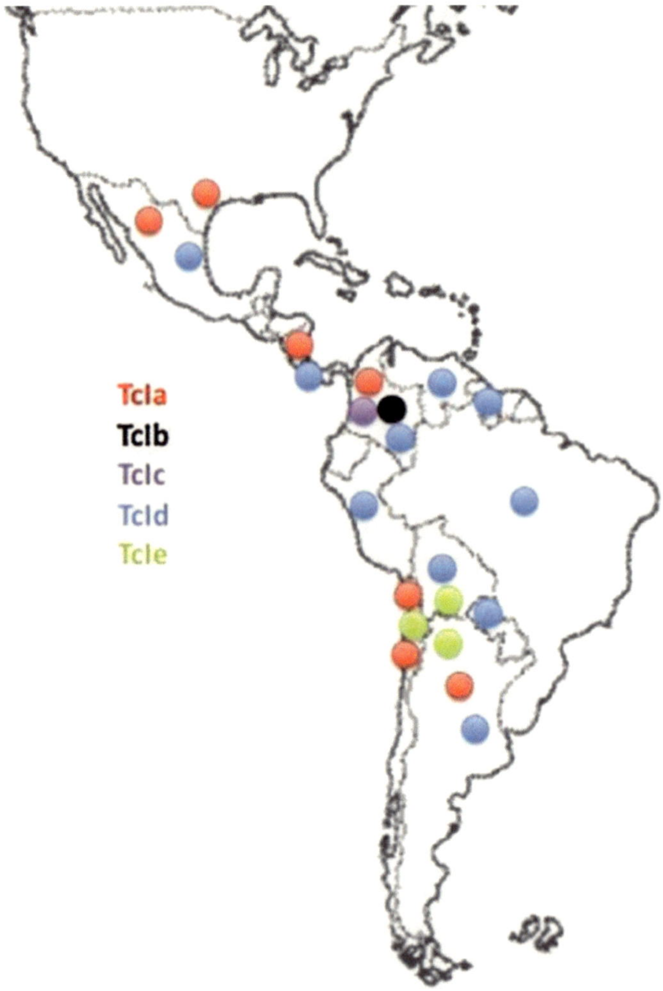

Fig. 5. Geographical distribution of *T. cruzi* I genotypes based on SL-IR region (Guhl and Ramírez, 2011)

Genetic variability has been clearly demonstrated in *T. cruzi*, with reports of homogeneous (TcII) and heterogeneous groups considered to be hybrids due to recombination events (TcIII-TcVI) (Gaunt et al., 2003, Sturm et al., 2003; Westenberger et al., 2002). It has been shown that TcIII and TcIV are likely to be a product of recombination of TcI and TcII and

TcIV-TcVI to be a product of recombination of TcII and TcIII/TcIV (Brisse et al., 2003), although this last statement is still controversial. The recent advances in sequencing procedures have allowed three complete *T. cruzi* genomes to be obtained. The first strain fully sequenced was CL Brener (TcVI), which showed a large number of repetitive elements along the core genome (Elsayed et al., 2005). Likewise, the recent sequencing of the Esmeraldo (TcII) and Sylvio X10 (TcI) genomes has shown the relationship between repetitive elements and mucin-like proteins, which are closely associated with parasite cell invasion and survival, showing this area of inquiry to be quite promising with respect to obtaining more information about the genetic structure of *T. cruzi* DTUs (Franzen et al., 2011; Andersson, 2011).

The molecular epidemiology and distribution of *T. cruzi* genotypes may have important implications with respect to characteristics of the disease. However, few correlations have related *T. cruzi* genetic variability and disease outcome, though it has been shown that TcI is more closely related to patients with cardiomyopathy in Colombia and Venezuela, while TcII-TcVI are more associated with patients with digestive syndrome (megaesophagus/megacolon) (Mantilla et al., 2011; Rassi et al., 2009). The distribution of *T. cruzi* genotypes and reservoirs is implicated in the genetic epidemiology of the disease. In the southern part of the American continent, infection of *Canis familiaris* has been found to be related to TcIV, V and VI, whereas infections in the north are associated with genotypes Ia and Ib (Falla et al., 2009; Herrera et al., 2009). Furthermore, a significant number of *D. marsupialis* are infected with the TcId genotype, which suggests an association with the sylvatic transmission cycle. Similar studies in primates have demonstrated that TcI predominantly infects arboreal reservoirs (Cura et al., 2010; Falla et al., 2009). There are several hypotheses regarding the distribution of different genetic groups of *T. cruzi*, suggesting that reservoirs belonging to arboreal ecotopes are preferentially infected with TcI and that terrestrial ecotopes are infected with TcII-TcVI (Yeo et al., 2005). This hypothesis is controversial in light of recent reports demonstrating that the arboreal ecotope reservoirs *Monodelphis brevicaudata, Philander frenata and Didelphis aurita* are infected with TcIII, TcIV and TcII, respectively (Marcili et al., 2009; Llewellyn et al., 2009b).

However, the associations are not absolute, and in the case of TcI, there is no apparent clustering of particular TcI genotypes with *Didelphis* in comparison to isolates from other arboreal mammals (Llewellyn et al., 2009b). Additionally, with respect to phylogeographical analyses of TcIII, the results indicate that isolates cluster according to geography rather than host association (Marcili et al., 2009; Llewellyn et al., 2009b). This could also be supported by the recent analysis developed in mammals naturally infected with TcI using microsatellite markers revealing the role of mammalian reservoirs in diversifying selection on *T. cruzi* (Llewellyn et al., 2011). Two interesting studies on host responses to different strains have confirmed, by comparative artificial infection, that in the southern USA, two species of opossum (*Monodelphis domestica* and *Didelphis virginiana*) seem to be resistant to TcIV (Roellig et al., 2009; Roellig et al., 2010). This highlights a mechanism for the association of a vertebrate host with one strain over others. The strong association between TcI and *Rhodnius* species can be explained by a similar mechanism: comparative studies on artificial infection of *R. prolixus* with various strains revealed a tendency for this species to be resistant to infection by TcII (Mello et al., 1995). In triatomines, susceptibility or resistance to trypanosome infections seems to be modulated by intestinal symbionts that are vital for development. *T. cruzi* is considered to be subpathogenic for triatomines, whereas *Trypanosoma rangeli* is a species that commonly infects *Rhodnius* species and causes pathogenicity based on reduction of the number of symbionts (Vallejo et al., 2009). Studies using different species of triatomines, such as *R. pallescens, T. dimidiata, R. colombiensis* and *P. geniculatus*, have shown the affinity of TcI for infecting these species in comparison with TcII (Mejia-Jaramillo et al., 2009). At least half of all species of triatomine bugs have been found to be naturally infected with *T. cruzi* (Lent and Wygodzinsky, 1979; Schofield, 1994). Unfortunately, the vast majority of these records do not include specific strain associations. This is clearly an area of potential research. In the context of dispersal triggered by starvation, there is evidence that starvation decreases *T. cruzi* infection in triatomines (Kollien and Schaub, 1998), and in some species, starvation may clear the infection altogether (Phillips et al., 1967; Vargas et al., 1985). This factor could help to explain paradigms such as that observed in Venezuela, where sylvatic and domestic bugs seem to be in panmixia, but TcI shows discrete general clustering of sylvatic and domestic cycles (Fitzpatrick et al., 2009; Llewellyn et al., 2009b). Triatomine bugs directly determine the aetiology of the strains of *T. cruzi* involved in human transmission cycles. This is clear because despite TcI and *Didelphis* being widespread, it is the northern distribution of *Rhodnius* that corresponds with its occurrence in human cycles. Overall, the aspects of epidemiological relevance are that associations between terrestrial ecology, *T. infestans*, terrestrial mammals, and *T. cruzi* strains TcII/TcIV have led to the prominence of TcII, TcV, and TcIV in human infections in the southern cone countries of South America. In the northern cone countries of South America, human American Trypanosomiasis infections seem to stem from TcI associated with arboreal *Rhodnius* and arboreal mammals.

The definition of *T. cruzi* nomenclature must be related to the biological, clinical and pathological characteristics associated with specific populations of *T. cruzi* (Campbell et al., 2004; Zafra et al., 2009). To our knowledge, few correlations reported have been demonstrated to date regarding differences of the host humoral response to specific *T. cruzi* genotypes; however, these findings were flawed because of the low reliability of the diagnostic tests used, leading to a high proportion of false negatives due to variability in the *T. cruzi* strain used for the diagnosis. The implication of TcI in severe forms of myocarditis in cardiac samples from chronic chagasic patients in Argentina and the lack of any specific clinical manifestation related to *T. cruzi* DTUs in Bolivian chagasic patients indicate the pleomorphism of *T. cruzi* (Ramírez et al., 2009; Moncayo and Ortiz, 2006; Burgos et al., 2010; del Puerto et al., 2010). There have been studies reporting detection of *T. cruzi* in blood samples. Direct detection of *T. cruzi* DTUs in the blood of chronic Chagasic patients was carried out by amplification of the 24Sα rDNA divergent domain and the use of mitochondrial house-keeping genes (Zafra et al., 2009). In this study, molecular characterisation of *T. cruzi* DTUs showed that most of the patients were infected with TcI, while some patients were found to be infected with TcII (9.9%). Recently, a new approach to *T. cruzi* DTU detection in chronic Chagasic patients was developed indicating that TcI is the predominant DTU, though TcII was also detected, and it was reported that the genetic characteristics of TcII parasites found in Colombia were similar to those of TcII found in Bolivia and Chile (González et al., 2010). Regarding the genetic variability of the parasite, prognostic markers based on mitochondrial genes where the presence of specific mutations can trigger complications of the chronic phase of the disease in asymptomatic patients have also been demonstrated (dos Santos et al., 2009; Carranza et al., 2009). Despite the observed genetic variability, it is important to consider the presence of *T. cruzi* clones that can be found in different tissues. Several studies have demonstrated a specific histiotropism of *T. cruzi* in mice showing differences in the pathological, immunological and clinical features that the parasite can elicit in the host (Andrade et al., 2002; Ramírez et al., 2010; Manoel-Caetano et al., 2008). Moreover, some authors have shown that the *T. cruzi* population in a patient's bloodstream could be dissimilar to the parasite population that causes tissue damage (Vago et al., 2000). Differences were found in *T. cruzi* populations in the bloodstreams of patients with chronic Chagasic cardiomyopathy and those of Chagasic patients without cardiomyopathy (Venegas et al., 2009). Microsatellite analyses have also shown multiclonality in heart samples and in the bloodstreams of infected patients, demonstrating that specific populations of *T. cruzi* can probably determine disease outcome (Burgos et al., 2007; Valadares et al., 2008).

Molecular epidemiological studies on *T. cruzi* have attempted to establish the effects of different DTUs in the clinical progression of Chagas disease. Several studies have shown the effect of genetic variability on the host immune response (dos Santos et al., 2009; Melquiades-Rodriguez et al., 2010; Ramírez et al., 2009). It was previously known that cardiopathies in southern cone countries were caused by TcII, TcV and TcVI, but it has recently been demonstrated that TcI can play an important role specifically in severe cardiopathies related to Chagas disease. Studies of cardiac biopsies from Argentinean patients revealed that patients with severe myocarditis were infected with TcI, whereas those with moderate or absent myocarditis were infected with TcII, TcV or TcVI (Burgos et al., 2010). At the same time that the TcI genotype was found in severe myocarditis patients, it was demonstrated that in patients with chronic chagasic cardiopathy, the TcIa genotype was most commonly found in the bloodstream, whereas TcId was most commonly found in cardiac biopsies. These results are consistent with reports from patients in Colombia, where the least and most prevalent TcI genotypes in adult patients with chronic chagasic cardiopathy were TcId and TcIa, respectively (Ramírez et al., 2010). This suggests a possible type of histotropism associated with TcI genotypes as well as the epidemiological importance of this DTU in southern countries, where cardiopathies were previously thought to be caused primarily by TcII, TcV and TcVI. A model of clonal histiotropism has been previously reported showing how a composite of clones is related to disease outcome. Recently reported results from Colombia support this premise, with cardiac biopsies being observed to be infected with TcId, while TcIa is found circulating in the bloodstream (Zafra et al., 2011; Ramírez et al., 2010). This suggests the need to pursue studies to correlate the association between *T. cruzi* genotypes and clinical manifestations of Chagas disease. New studies are also necessary to determine the specific *T. cruzi* populations generating tissue damage in infected patients.

Most of the research performed in Chagas disease is related to understanding the molecular epidemiology of this endemic pathology. Many questions are continually emerging every day in this field based on epidemiological circuits with the aim of better estimating the transmission dynamics of *T. cruzi* in endemic areas. The involvement of *T. cruzi* genetic variability in clinical manifestations is of paramount importance and could resolve the question regarding the high pleomorphism displayed by this clinical entity. New initiatives must be created with interdisciplinary groups with the purpose of unravelling the molecular comparative epidemiology of Chagas disease and attempting to mitigate this pathology in endemic countries.

5. Concluding remarks

In this chapter, many examples regarding the usefulness of molecular epidemiology in parasitic diseases were addressed. These examples illustrated different applications of molecular methods to understand the pathogens that cause human parasitic diseases. It is important to consider the need for synergy between descriptive, analytical and molecular epidemiological methods to develop robust and unbiased data. As a relevant example, we presented the case of *T. cruzi* and described how molecular methods have been useful in defining hypotheses about the parasite's geographical distribution, host associations and the implications of different genotypes for clinical manifestations related to the heart. Despite the studies reported in the literature on molecular epidemiology in parasites, public health systems do not consider the importance of integration between these two areas. We propose the integration of molecular epidemiology and public health systems to mitigate and reduce the prevalence of tropical diseases caused mainly by parasites, and this combination could become a potential tool for disease prevention and control as well as for the development of appropriate programmes for disease surveillance in endemic countries.

6. References

Agbo E, E., C., Majiwa PAO, Claassen HJ, Te Pas MF (2002) Molecular variation of *Trypanosoma brucei* subspecies as revealed by AFLP fingerprinting. Parasitology 124:349-358.

Andersson B. (2011). The *Trypanosoma cruzi* genome; conserved core genes and extremely variable surface molecule families. Research in Microbiology 162:619-625

Andrade LO, Machado CRS, Chiari E, Pena SDJ, Macedo AM (2002) *Trypanosoma cruzi*: role of host genetic background in the differential tissue distribution of parasite clonal populations. Experimental Parasitology 100:269-275

Bañuls A-L, Dujardin J-C, Guerrini F, De Doncker S, Jacquet D, Arevalo J, Noel S, Le Ray D, Tibayrenc M (2000) Is *Leishmania (Viannia) peruviana* a Distinct Species? A MLEE/RAPD Evolutionary Genetics Answer. Journal of Eukaryotic Microbiology 47:197-207.

Bañuls AL, Hide M, Tibayrenc M (2002) Evolutionary genetics and molecular diagnosis of *Leishmania* species. Transactions of the Royal Society of Tropical Medicine and Hygiene 96:S9-S13.

Bennett RJ (2010) Coming of Age—Sexual Reproduction in *Candida* Species. PLoS Pathog 6:e1001155

Bertram NS (1967) Laboratory studies of *Trypanosoma cruzi* infections in: *Rhodnius prolixus*--larvae and adults in: *Triatoma infestans, T. protracta* and *T. maculata*--adults. J Med Entomol 4:167-170.

Bontell I, Hall N, Ashelford K, Dubey J, Boyle J, Lindh J, Smith J (2009) Whole genome sequencing of a natural recombinant *Toxoplasma gondii* strain reveals chromosome sorting and local allelic variants. Genome Biology 10:R53.

Bretagne S, Durand R, Olivi M, Garin J-F, Sulahian A, Rivollet D, Vidaud M, Deniau M (2001) Real-Time PCR as a New Tool for Quantifying *Leishmania infantum* in Liver in Infected Mice. Clin Diagn Lab Immunol 8:828-831.

Brisse S, Henriksson J, Barnabé C, Douzery EJP, Berkvens D, Serrano M, De Carvalho MRC, Buck GA, Dujardin J-C, Tibayrenc M (2003) Evidence for genetic exchange and hybridization in *Trypanosoma cruzi* based on nucleotide sequences and molecular karyotype. Infection, Genetics and Evolution 2:173-183.

Burgos JM, Altcheh J, Bisio M, Duffy T, Valadares HMS, Seidenstein ME, Piccinali R, Freitas JM, Levin MJ, Macchi L, Macedo AM, Freilij H, Schijman AG (2007) Direct molecular profiling of minicircle signatures and lineages of *Trypanosoma cruzi* bloodstream populations causing congenital Chagas disease. International Journal for Parasitology 37:1319-1327.

Burgos JM, Diez M, Vigliano C, Bisio M, Risso M, Duffy Ts, Cura C, Brusses B, Favaloro L, Leguizamon MaS, Lucero RH, Laguens R, Levin MJ, Favaloro R, Schijman AG Molecular Identification of *Trypanosoma cruzi* Discrete Typing Units in End-Stage Chronic Chagas Heart Disease and Reactivation after Heart Transplantation. Clinical Infectious Diseases 51:485-495.

Campbell DA WS, Sturm NR. (2004) The determinants of Chagas disease: connecting parasite and host genetics. Curr Mol Med 4:549-562.

Carranza JC, Valadares HMS, D'Ávila DA, Baptista RP, Moreno M, Galvão LMC, Chiari E, Sturm NR, Gontijo ED, Macedo AM, Zingales B (2009) Trypanosoma cruzi maxicircle heterogeneity in Chagas disease patients from Brazil. International Journal for Parasitology 39:963-973

Clark CG, Ali IKM, Zaki M, Loftus BJ, Hall N (2006) Unique organisation of tRNA genes in *Entamoeba histolytica*. Molecular and Biochemical Parasitology 146:24-29.

Cura CI, Mejía-Jaramillo AM, Duffy T, Burgos JM, Rodriguero M, Cardinal MV, Kjos S, Gurgel-Gonçalves R, Blanchet D, De Pablos LM, Tomasini N, da Silva A, Russomando G, Cuba CAC, Aznar C, Abate T, Levin MJ, Osuna A, Gürtler RE, Diosque P, Solari A, Triana-Chávez O, Schijman AG *Trypanosoma cruzi* I genotypes in different geographical regions and transmission cycles based on a microsatellite motif of the intergenic spacer of spliced-leader genes. International Journal for Parasitology 40:1599-1607.

da Silva Manoel-Caetano F, Carareto CMA, Borim AA, Miyazaki K, Silva AE (2008) kDNA gene signatures of *Trypanosoma cruzi* in blood and oesophageal mucosa from chronic chagasic patients. Transactions of the Royal Society of Tropical Medicine and Hygiene 102:1102-1107.

del Puerto R, Nishizawa JE, Kikuchi M, Iihoshi N, Roca Y, Avilas C, Gianella A, Lora J, Gutierrez Velarde FU, Renjel LA, Miura S, Higo H, Komiya N, Maemura K, Hirayama K Lineage Analysis of Circulating *Trypanosoma cruzi* Parasites and Their Association with Clinical Forms of Chagas Disease in Bolivia. PLoS Negl Trop Dis 4:e687.

Duffy T, Bisio M, Altcheh J, Burgos JM, Diez M, Levin MJ, Favaloro RR, Freilij H, Schijman AG (2009) Accurate Real-Time PCR Strategy for Monitoring Bloodstream Parasitic Loads in Chagas Disease Patients. PLoS Negl Trop Dis 3:e419.

El-Sayed NM, Myler PJ, Bartholomeu DC, Nilsson D, Aggarwal G, Tran A-N, Ghedin E, Worthey EA, Delcher AL, Blandin Gl, Westenberger SJ, Caler E, Cerqueira GC, Branche C, Haas B, Anupama A, Arner E, Ã...slund L, Attipoe P, Bontempi E, Bringaud Fdr, Burton P, Cadag E, Campbell DA, Carrington M, Crabtree J, Darban H, da Silveira JF, de Jong P, Edwards K, Englund PT, Fazelina G, Feldblyum T, Ferella M, Frasch AC, Gull K, Horn D, Hou L, Huang Y, Kindlund E, Klingbeil M, Kluge S, Koo H, Lacerda D, Levin MJ, Lorenzi H, Louie T, Machado CR, McCulloch R, McKenna A, Mizuno Y, Mottram JC, Nelson S, Ochaya S, Osoegawa K, Pai G, Parsons M, Pentony M, Pettersson U, Pop M, Ramirez JL, Rinta J, Robertson L, Salzberg SL, Sanchez DO, Seyler A, Sharma R, Shetty J, Simpson AJ, Sisk E, Tammi MT, Tarleton R, Teixeira S, Van Aken S, Vogt C, Ward PN, Wickstead B, Wortman J, White O, Fraser CM, Stuart KD, Andersson Br (2005) The Genome Sequence of Trypanosoma cruzi, Etiologic Agent of Chagas Disease. Science 309:409-415.

Falla A, Herrera C, Fajardo A, Montilla M, Vallejo GA, Guhl F (2009) Haplotype identification within *Trypanosoma cruzi* I in Colombian isolates from several reservoirs, vectors and humans. Acta Tropica 110:15-21.

Fitzpatrick S, Feliciangeli MD, Sanchez-Martin MJ, Monteiro FA, Miles MA (2008) Molecular Genetics Reveal That Silvatic *Rhodnius prolixus* Do Colonise Rural Houses. PLoS Negl Trop Dis 2:e210.

Franzen O, Ochaya S, Sherwood E, Lewis MD, Llewellyn MS, Miles MA, Andersson Br Shotgun Sequencing Analysis of *Trypanosoma cruzi* I Sylvio X10/1 and Comparison with *T. cruzi* VI CL Brener. PLoS Negl Trop Dis 5:e984.

Fuentes I, Rubio JM, Ramirez C, Alvar J (2001) Genotypic Characterization of *Toxoplasma gondii* Strains Associated with Human Toxoplasmosis in Spain: Direct Analysis from Clinical Samples. J Clin Microbiol 39:1566-1570.

Gardner MJ, Hall N, Fung E, White O, Berriman M, Hyman RW, Carlton JM, Pain A, Nelson KE, Bowman S, Paulsen IT, James K, Eisen JA, Rutherford K, Salzberg SL, Craig A, Kyes S, Chan M-S, Nene V, Shallom SJ, Suh B, Peterson J, Angiuoli S, Pertea M, Allen J, Selengut J, Haft D, Mather MW, Vaidya AB, Martin DMA, Fairlamb AH, Fraunholz MJ, Roos DS, Ralph SA, McFadden GI, Cummings LM, Subramanian GM, Mungall C, Venter JC, Carucci DJ, Hoffman SL, Newbold C, Davis RW, Fraser CM, Barrell B (2002) Genome sequence of the human malaria parasite *Plasmodium falciparum*. Nature 419:498-511.

Gaunt MW, Yeo M, Frame IA, Stothard JR, Carrasco HJ, Taylor MC, Mena SS, Veazey P, Miles GAJ, Acosta N, de Arias AR, Miles MA (2003) Mechanism of genetic exchange in American trypanosomes. Nature 421:936-939.

Gomes MA, Melo MN, Macedo AM, Furst C, Silva EF (2000) RAPD in the analysis of isolates of *Entamoeba histolytica*. Acta Tropica 75:71-77 .

Gomez JC, McNamara DT, Bockarie MJ, Baird JK, Carlton JM, Zimmerman PA (2003) Identification of a polymorphic *Plasmodium vivax* microsatellite marker. The American Journal of Tropical Medicine and Hygiene 69:377-379.

González CI, Ortiz S, Solari A Colombian *Trypanosoma cruzi* major genotypes circulating in patients: Minicircle homologies by cross-hybridization analysis. International Journal for Parasitology 40:1685-1692.

Grigg ME, Suzuki Y (2003) Sexual recombination and clonal evolution of virulence in *Toxoplasma*. Microbes and Infection 5:685-690 .

Guhl F, Ramírez JD (2011) *Trypanosoma cruzi* I diversity: Towards the need of genetic subdivision? Acta Tropica 119:1-4.

Guy RA, Payment P, Krull UJ, Horgen PA (2003) Real-Time PCR for Quantification of *Giardia* and *Cryptosporidium* in Environmental Water Samples and Sewage. Appl Environ Microbiol 69:5178-5185 .

Harvey PH, Keymer AE (1987) Sex among the parasites. Nature 330:317-318.

Herrera C, Bargues MD, Fajardo A, Montilla M, Triana O, Vallejo GA, Guhl F (2007) Identifying four *Trypanosoma cruzi* I isolate haplotypes from different geographic regions in Colombia. Infection, Genetics and Evolution 7:535-539.

Herrera C, Guhl F, Falla A, Fajardo A, Montilla M, Adolfo Vallejo G, Bargues MD (2009) Genetic Variability and Phylogenetic Relationships within *Trypanosoma cruzi* I Isolated in Colombia Based on Miniexon Gene Sequences. Journal of Parasitology Research 2009 DOI 10.1155/2009/897364.

Imwong M, Sudimack D, Pukrittayakamee S, Osorio L, Carlton JM, Day NPJ, White NJ, Anderson TJC (2006) Microsatellite Variation, Repeat Array Length, and Population History of *Plasmodium vivax*. Molecular Biology and Evolution 23:1016-1018.

Ivens AC, Peacock CS, Worthey EA, Murphy L, Aggarwal G, Berriman M, Sisk E, Rajandream M-A, Adlem E, Aert R, Anupama A, Apostolou Z, Attipoe P, Bason N, Bauser C, Beck A, Beverley SM, Bianchettin G, Borzym K, Bothe G, Bruschi CV, Collins M, Cadag E, Ciarloni L, Clayton C, Coulson RMR, Cronin A, Cruz AK, Davies RM, De Gaudenzi J, Dobson DE, Duesterhoeft A, Fazelina G, Fosker N, Frasch AC, Fraser A, Fuchs M, Gabel C, Goble A, Goffeau A, Harris D, Hertz-Fowler C, Hilbert H, Horn D, Huang Y, Klages S, Knights A, Kube M, Larke N, Litvin L, Lord A, Louie T, Marra M, Masuy D, Matthews K, Michaeli S, Mottram JC, Muller-Auer S, Munden H, Nelson S, Norbertczak H, Oliver K, O'Neil S, Pentony M, Pohl TM, Price C, Purnelle Bnd, Quail MA, Rabbinowitsch E, Reinhardt R, Rieger M, Rinta J, Robben J, Robertson L, Ruiz JC, Rutter S, Saunders D, SchÃ¤fer M, Schein J, Schwartz DC, Seeger K, Seyler A, Sharp S, Shin H, Sivam D, Squares R, Squares S, Tosato V, Vogt C, Volckaert G, Wambutt R, Warren T, Wedler H, Woodward J, Zhou S, Zimmermann W, Smith DF, Blackwell JM, Stuart KD, Barrell B, Myler PJ (2005) The Genome of the Kinetoplastid Parasite, Leishmania major. Science 309:436-442 .

Jamieson SE, Miller EN, Peacock CS, Fakiola M, Wilson ME, Bales-Holst A, Shaw MA, Silveira F, Shaw JJ, Jeronimo SM, Blackwell JM (2006) Genome-wide scan for visceral leishmaniasis susceptibility genes in Brazil. Genes Immun 8:84-90.

Johnson M, Broady K, Angelici MC, Johnson A (2003) The relationship between nucleoside triphosphate hydrolase (NTPase) isoform and *Toxoplasma* strain virulence in rat and human toxoplasmosis. Microbes and Infection 5:797-806.

Kilbourne ED (1973) The Molecular Epidemiology of Influenza. Journal of Infectious Diseases 127:478-487.

Kollien AH and Schaub AGA (1998) Development of *Trypanosoma cruzi* after starvation and feeding of the vector - a review. Tokai J Exp Clin Med 23:335-340.

Lehane MJ (1994) TRIATOMINAE: BIOLOGY and CONTROL. By C. J. Schofield. Medical and Veterinary Entomology 8:218-218 DOI 10.1111/j.1365-2915.1994.tb00501.x.

Lent and Wygodzinsky (1979) Revision of the Triatominae, Hemiptera Reduviidae and their significance as vectors of Chagas' disease. Bull Am Mus Nat Hist 163:123-520.

Lewis MD, Ma J, Yeo M, Carrasco HnJ, Llewellyn MS, Miles MA (2009) Genotyping of *Trypanosoma cruzi*: Systematic Selection of Assays Allowing Rapid and Accurate Discrimination of All Known Lineages. The American Journal of Tropical Medicine and Hygiene 81:1041-1049.

Lier T, Simonsen GS, Wang T, Lu D, Haukland HH, Vennervald BJ, Hegstad J, Johansen MV (2009) Real-Time Polymerase Chain Reaction for Detection of Low-Intensity Schistosoma japonicum Infections in China. The American Journal of Tropical Medicine and Hygiene 81:428-432

Llewellyn MS, Lewis MD, Acosta N, Yeo M, Carrasco HJ, Segovia M, Vargas J, Torrico F, Miles MA, Gaunt MW (2009b) *Trypanosoma cruzi* IIc: Phylogenetic and Phylogeographic Insights from Sequence and Microsatellite Analysis and Potential Impact on Emergent Chagas Disease. PLoS Negl Trop Dis 3:e510.

Llewellyn MS, Miles MA, Carrasco HJ, Lewis MD, Yeo M, Vargas J, Torrico F, Diosque P, Valente V, Valente SA, Gaunt MW (2009) Genome-Scale Multilocus Microsatellite Typing of *Trypanosoma cruzi* Discrete Typing Unit I Reveals Phylogeographic Structure and Specific Genotypes Linked to Human Infection. PLoS Pathog 5:e1000410.

Llewellyn MS, Rivett-Carnac JB, Fitzpatrick S, Lewis MD, Yeo M, Gaunt MW, Miles MA Extraordinary *Trypanosoma cruzi* diversity within single mammalian reservoir hosts implies a mechanism of diversifying selection. International Journal for Parasitology 41:609-614.

Mantilla JC, Zafra GA, Macedo AM, González CI (2010) Mixed infection of *Trypanosoma cruzi* I and II in a Colombian cardiomyopathic patient. Human Pathology 41:610-613.

Marcili A, Lima L, Valente VC, Valente SA, Batista JS, Junqueira ACV, Souza AI, da Rosa JA, Campaner M, Lewis MD, Llewellyn MS, Miles MA, Teixeira MMG (2009) Comparative phylogeography of *Trypanosoma cruzi* TCIIc: New hosts, association with terrestrial ecotopes, and spatial clustering. Infection, Genetics and Evolution 9:1265-1274.

Mary C, Faraut F, Lascombe L, Dumon H (2004) Quantification of *Leishmania infantum* DNA by a Real-Time PCR Assay with High Sensitivity. J Clin Microbiol 42:5249-5255.

Masiga DK, Ndung'u K, Tweedie A, Tait A, Turner CMR (2006) *Trypanosoma evansi*: Genetic variability detected using amplified restriction fragment length polymorphism (AFLP) and random amplified polymorphic DNA (RAPD) analysis of Kenyan isolates. Experimental Parasitology 114:147-153.

Mathews HM, Moss DM, Healy GR, Visvesvara GS (1983) Polyacrylamide gel electrophoresis of isoenzymes from *Entamoeba* species. J Clin Microbiol 17:1009-1012.

Mejía-Jaramillo AM, Peña VH, Triana-Chávez O (2009) *Trypanosoma cruzi*: Biological characterization of lineages I and II supports the predominance of lineage I in Colombia. Experimental Parasitology 121:83-91.

Mello CB, Garcia ES, Ratcliffe NA, Azambuja P (1995) *Trypanosoma cruzi* and *Trypanosoma rangeli*: Interplay with Hemolymph Components of Rhodnius prolixus. Journal of Invertebrate Pathology 65:261-268.

Miles MA, Llewellyn MS, Lewis MD, Yeo M, Baleela R, Fitzpatrick S, Gaunt MW, Mauricio IL (2009) The molecular epidemiology and phylogeography of *Trypanosoma cruzi* and parallel research on Leishmania: looking back and to the future. Parasitology 136:1509-1528.

Miles MA, Povoa MM, De Souza AA, Lainson R, Shaw JJ, Ketteridge DS (1981) Chagas's disease in the Amazon Basin: II. The distribution of *Trypanosoma cruzi* zymodemes 1 and 3 in Pará State, north Brazil. Transactions of the Royal Society of Tropical Medicine and Hygiene 75:667-674.

Miles MA, Toye PJ, Oswald SC, Godfrey DG (1977) The identification by isoenzyme patterns of two distinct strain-groups of *Trypanosoma cruzi*, circulating independently in a rural area of Brazil. Transactions of the Royal Society of Tropical Medicine and Hygiene 71:217-225.

Moncayo A, Ortiz Yanine MI (2006) An update on Chagas disease (human American trypanosomiasis). Annals of Tropical Medicine and Parasitology 100:663-677.

Montalvo AM, Fraga J, Aylema Romero J, Monzote L, Montano I, Dujardin JC (2006) PCR-RFLP/Hsp70 para identificar y tipificar *Leishmania* de la región neotropical. Revista Cubana de Medicina Tropical 58:0-0.

Morrison LJ (2011) Parasite-driven pathogenesis in *Trypanosoma brucei* infections. Parasite Immunology 33:448-455.

Morrison LJ, Tait A, McLellan S, Sweeney L, Turner CMR, MacLeod A (2009) A Major Genetic Locus in *Trypanosoma brucei* Is a Determinant of Host Pathology. PLoS Negl Trop Dis 3:e557.

Mzilahowa T, McCall PJ, Hastings IM (2007) "Sexual" Population Structure and Genetics of the Malaria Agent *P. falciparum*. PLoS ONE 2:e613.

Njiokou F, Nkinin SW, Grébaut P, Penchenier L, Barnabé C, Tibayrenc M, Herder S (2004) An isoenzyme survey of Trypanosoma brucei s.l. from the Central African subregion: population structure, taxonomic and epidemiological considerations. Parasitology 128:645-653.

Patterson JS, Guhl F (2010) Geographical Distribution of Chagas DiseaseAmerican Trypanosomiasis. Elsevier, London, pp. 83-114.

Pecson BM, Barrios JA, Johnson DR, Nelson KL (2006) A Real-Time PCR Method for Quantifying Viable *Ascaris* Eggs Using the First Internally Transcribed Spacer Region of Ribosomal DNA. Appl Environ Microbiol 72:7864-7872 .

Pinto M, Rosa JD, Fernandes Z, Graminha M, Mine J, Allegretti S, Delort S, Riedel C, Paes E, Cupolillo E (2005) Isolation and isoenzyme characterization of *Leishmania (Viannia) braziliensis* from a case of human cutaneous leishmaniasis in northeast centre of the state of São Paulo. Memórias do Instituto Oswaldo Cruz 100:733-734.

Prakash A, Chakraborti A, Mahajan RC, Ganguly NK (2000) *Entamoeba histolytica*: Rapid Detection of Indian Isolates by Cysteine Proteinase Gene-Specific Polymerase Chain Reaction. Experimental Parasitology 95:285-287.

Prata A (2001) Clinical and epidemiological aspects of Chagas disease. The Lancet Infectious Diseases 1:92-100.

Quan J-H, Kim TY, Choi I-U, Lee Y-H (2008) Genotyping of a Korean isolate of *Toxoplasma gondii* by multilocus PCR-RFLP and microsatellite analysis. Korean J Parasitol 46:105-108.

Ramírez JD, Duque MC, Guhl F (2011) Phylogenetic reconstruction based on Cytochrome b (Cytb) gene sequences reveals distinct genotypes within Colombian Trypanosoma cruzi I populations. Acta Tropica 119:61-65.

Ramírez JD, Guhl F, Rendón LM, Rosas F, Marin-Neto JA, Morillo CA (2010) Chagas Cardiomyopathy Manifestations and *Trypanosoma cruzi* Genotypes Circulating in Chronic Chagasic Patients. PLoS Negl Trop Dis 4:e899.

Ramírez JD, Guhl F, Umezawa ES, Morillo CA, Rosas F, Marin-Neto JA, Restrepo S (2009) Evaluation of Adult Chronic Chagas' Heart Disease Diagnosis by Molecular and Serological Methods. J Clin Microbiol 47:3945-3951.

Ranasinghe S, Rogers ME, Hamilton JGC, Bates PA, Maingon RDC (2008) A real-time PCR assay to estimate *Leishmania chagasi* load in its natural sand fly vector *Lutzomyia longipalpis*. Transactions of the Royal Society of Tropical Medicine and Hygiene 102:875-882.

Rassi A, Marin-Neto JA Chagas disease. The Lancet 375:1388-1402.

Rodrigues CM, Valadares HMS, Francisco AF, Arantes JM, Campos CFa, Teixeira-Carvalho Aa, Martins-Filho OA, Araujo MrSS, Arantes RME, Chiari E, Franco GrR, Machado CR, Pena SrDJ, Faria AMC, Macedo AM (2010) Coinfection with Different *Trypanosoma cruzi* Strains Interferes with the Host Immune Response to Infection. PLoS Negl Trop Dis 4:e846.

Roellig DM, Ellis AE, Yabsley MJ (2009) Genetically different isolates of *Trypanosoma cruzi* elicit different infection dynamics in raccoons (*Procyon lotor*) and *Virginia* opossums (*Didelphis virginiana*). International Journal for Parasitology 39:1603-1610.

Roellig DM, McMillan K, Ellis AE, Vandeberg JL, Champagne DE, Yabsley MJ (2010) Experimental infection of two South American reservoirs with four distinct strains of Trypanosoma cruzi. Parasitology 137:959-966 .

Romand S, Chosson M, Franck J, Wallon M, Kieffer F, Kaiser K, Dumon H, Peyron F, Thulliez P, Picot S (2004) Usefulness of quantitative polymerase chain reaction in amniotic fluid as early prognostic marker of fetal infection with *Toxoplasma gondii*. American Journal of Obstetrics and Gynecology 190:797-802 DOI 10.1016/j.ajog.2003.09.039.

Rougeron V, De Meeûs T, Hide M, Waleckx E, Bermudez H, Arevalo J, Llanos-Cuentas A, Dujardin J-C, De Doncker S, Le Ray D, Ayala FJ, Bañuls A-L (2009) Extreme inbreeding in *Leishmania braziliensis*. Proceedings of the National Academy of Sciences 106:10224-10229.

Rozas M, De Doncker S, Adaui V, Coronado X, Barnabé C, Tibyarenc M, Solari A, Dujardin J-C (2007) Multilocus Polymerase Chain Reaction Restriction Fragmentâ€"Length Polymorphism Genotyping of *Trypanosoma cruzi* (Chagas Disease): Taxonomic and Clinical Applications. Journal of Infectious Diseases 195:1381-1388.

Santos DM, Talvani A, da Mata Guedes PM, Machado-Coelho GLL, de Lana M, Bahia MT (2009) *Trypanosoma cruzi*: Genetic diversity influences the profile of immunoglobulins during experimental infection. Experimental Parasitology 121:8-14.

Schmunis GA, Yadon ZE Chagas disease: A Latin American health problem becoming a world health problem. Acta Tropica 115:14-21.

Singh U, Ehrenkaufer GM (2009) Recent insights into *Entamoeba* development: Identification of transcriptional networks associated with stage conversion. International Journal for Parasitology 39:41-47 .

Smith JM, Smith NH, O'Rourke M, Spratt BG (1993) How clonal are bacteria? Proceedings of the National Academy of Sciences 90:4384-4388.

Spotorno O AE, Córdova L, Solari I A (2008) Differentiation of *Trypanosoma cruzi* I subgroups through characterization of cytochrome b gene sequences. Infection, Genetics and Evolution 8:898-900.

Stensvold C, Clarck G (2011) Multilocus sequence typing of *Blastocystis* sp. subtype 3. 21st European Congress of Clinical Microbiology and Infectious Diseases (ECCMID), 27th International Congress of Chemotherapy (ICC).

Sturm NR, Vargas NS, Westenberger SJ, Zingales B, Campbell DA (2003) Evidence for multiple hybrid groups in *Trypanosoma cruzi*. International Journal for Parasitology 33:269-279.

Su C, Zhang X, Dubey JP (2006) Genotyping of *Toxoplasma gondii* by multilocus PCR-RFLP markers: A high resolution and simple method for identification of parasites. International Journal for Parasitology 36:841-848 .

Tibayrenc M, Ayala FJ (1991) Towards a population genetics of microorganisms: The clonal theory of parasitic protozoa. Parasitology Today 7:228-232.

Vago AR, Andrade LO, Leite AA, d'Ávila Reis D, Macedo AM, Adad SJ, Tostes Jr S, Moreira MCV, Filho GB, Pena SDJ (2000) Genetic Characterization of *Trypanosoma cruzi* Directly from Tissues of Patients with Chronic Chagas Disease: Differential Distribution of Genetic Types into Diverse Organs. The American Journal of Pathology 156:1805-1809.

Valadares HMS, Pimenta JR, de Freitas JM, Duffy T, Bartholomeu DC, de Paula Oliveira R, Chiari E, Moreira MdCV, Filho GB, Schijman AG, Franco GR, Machado CR, Pena SDJ, Macedo AM (2008) Genetic profiling of *Trypanosoma cruzi* directly in infected tissues using nested PCR of polymorphic microsatellites. International Journal for Parasitology 38:839-850.

Vallejo GA, Guhl F, Schaub GA Triatominae-*Trypanosoma cruzi/T. rangeli*: Vector-parasite interactions. Acta Tropica 110:137-147.

Vargas LG, Zeledon R (1985) Effect of fasting on *Trypanosoma cruzi* infection in *Triatoma dimidiata* (Hemiptera: Reduviidae). Journal of Medical Entomology 22:683-683.

Venegas J, Coñoepan W, Pichuantes S, Miranda S, Apt W, Arribada A, Zulantay I, Coronado X, Rodriguez J, Reyes E, Solari A, Sanchez G (2009) Differential distribution of Trypanosoma cruzi clones in human chronic chagasic cardiopathic and non-cardiopathic individuals. Acta Tropica 109:187-193.

Volpini ÂC, Passos VMA, Oliveira GC, Romanha AJ (2004) PCR-RFLP to identify *Leishmania (Viannia) braziliensis* and *L. (Leishmania) amazonensis* causing American cutaneous leishmaniasis. Acta Tropica 90:31-37.

Westenberger SJ, Barnabé C, Campbell DA, Sturm NR (2005) Two Hybridization Events Define the Population Structure of *Trypanosoma cruzi*. Genetics 171:527-543.

WHO (2007) Report of scientific group in Chagas disease. Buenos Aires, Argentina, April 17-20, 2005. Special Programme for Research and Training in Tropical Diseases (TDR).

WHO (2010) Millennium Development Goals: progress towards the health-related Millennium Development Goals .

Wortmann G, Hochberg LP, Arana BA, Rizzo NR, Arana F, Ryan JR (2007) Diagnosis of cutaneous Leishmaniasis in Guatemala using a Real-Time Polymerase Chain Reaction assay and the smartcycler. The American Journal of Tropical Medicine and Hygiene 76:906-908.

Yeo M, Acosta N, Llewellyn M, Sánchez H, Adamson S, Miles GAJ, López E, González N, Patterson JS, Gaunt MW, Arias ARd, Miles MA (2005) Origins of Chagas disease: Didelphis species are natural hosts of *Trypanosoma cruzi* I and armadillos hosts of *Trypanosoma cruzi* II, including hybrids. International Journal for Parasitology 35:225-233.

Yeo M, Mauricio IL, Messenger LA, Lewis MD, Llewellyn MS, Acosta N, Bhattacharyya T, Diosque P, Carrasco HJ, Miles MA Multilocus Sequence Typing (MLST) for Lineage Assignment and High Resolution Diversity Studies in *Trypanosoma cruzi*. PLoS Negl Trop Dis 5:e1049.

Zafra G, Mantilla J, Valadares H, Macedo A, GonzÃ¡lez C (2008) Evidence of *Trypanosoma cruzi* II infection in Colombian chagasic patients. Parasitology Research 103:731-734.

Zafra G, Mantilla JC, Jácome J, Macedo AM, González CI (2011) Direct analysis of genetic variability in *Trypanosoma cruzi* populations from tissues of Colombian chagasic patients. Human Pathology 42:1159-1168.

Zemanová E, Jirku M, Mauricio IL, Horák A, Miles MA, Lukes J (2007) The *Leishmania donovani* complex: Genotypes of five metabolic enzymes (ICD, ME, MPI, G6PDH, and FH), new targets for multilocus sequence typing. International Journal for Parasitology 37:149-160.

Zhang W-W, Miranda-Verastegui C, Arevalo J, Ndao M, Ward B, Cuentas AL, Matlashewski G (2006) Development of a Genetic Assay to Distinguish between *Leishmania viannia* Species on the Basis of Isoenzyme Differences. Clinical Infectious Diseases 42:801-809.

Zhao G-p (2007) SARS molecular epidemiology: a Chinese fairy tale of controlling an emerging zoonotic disease in the genomics era. Philosophical Transactions of the Royal Society B: Biological Sciences 362:1063-1081.

Zingales B, Andrade S, Briones M, Campbell D, Chiari E, Fernandes O, Guhl F, Lages-Silva E, Macedo A, Machado C, Miles M, Romanha A, Sturm N, Tibayrenc M, Schijman A (2009) A new consensus for *Trypanosoma cruzi* intraspecific nomenclature: second revision meeting recommends TcI to TcVI. MemÃ³rias do Instituto Oswaldo Cruz 104:1051-1054.

7

Viral Evolutionary Ecology: Conceptual Basis of a New Scientific Approach for Understanding Viral Emergence

J. Usme-Ciro[1,2*], R. Hoyos-López[1,2,3*] and J.C. Gallego-Gómez[1,2†]
[1]*Viral Vector Core and Gene Therapy (Neurosciences Group of Antioquia), Faculty of Medicine, University of Antioquia, Medellin,*
[2]*Translational and Molecular Medicine Group, Faculty of Medicine, University of Antioquia, Medellin,*
[3]*Molecular Systematics Group, National University of Colombia, Medellin, Colombia*

1. Introduction

Kilbourne first applied the term of Molecular Epidemiology in 1973 in a paper on influenza [1], since then the term has been extensively used for other diseases caused by viruses [2-4], bacteria [5-7], parasites [8-10] and even non-infectious diseases [11, 12]. Molecular epidemiology was subsequently accompanied by a more integrative definition of eco-epidemiology [13, 14] with little impact in scientific literature.

Although molecular epidemiology and eco-epidemiology are important in the understanding of disease and disease emergence [15, 16], we postulate here that the medical science community needs to consider a new conceptual approach to epidemiological studies of emerging infectious diseases (e.g. viral diseases). Emerging viral diseases are mainly caused by RNA viruses whose transmission cycles involve the ecological interaction with several actors and the evolutionary responses through time.

The new approach called Viral Evolutionary Ecology (VEE) [17, 18] combined with epidemiology will help us to better explain many emerging viral diseases by encompassing the complex interface between such factors as genetic structure, evolutionary biology and ecology of pathogens [19], and environmental aspects such as biodiversity, society, and human impact on natural ecosystems, all of them closely interplaying in ways often as yet unknown [20, 21]. This complimentary approach has been previously considered under the field of Evolutionary Epidemiology [22-24], however, the impact in the study of viral emergence needs to be highlighted.

Under the VEE framework where the real actors are the viruses instead of human beings, we can recognize our main role in disturbing the environment and offering conditions for new

---

*These authors contributed equally
†Corresponding Author

viruses to emerge. Viruses do not live for causing disease to humans, animals, plants or other organisms, they are simply naturally selected to increase their viral fitness, a process in which ecology and evolutionary biology play the main role, so viral emergence and disease are mere consequences of this dynamic.

In this sense, public health problems (e.g. several viral diseases) are the unexpected consequence of new ecological niches promoted by human actions on natural systems. In Luria's words "…each virus disease is potentially a different form of virus life…" [25]. Over the last 10 to 15 thousand years, humankind has been changing the planet, triggering the "Butterfly Effect" with dramatic alterations [26], producing new ecological landscapes called emerging or novel ecosystems [27], and the subsequent emergence of viral diseases.

Today, emerging viral diseases caused by respiratory, encephalitic and haemorrhagic viruses, and others like AIDS, have a severe impact on public health and economy not only in developing countries but also worldwide [28]. It is necessary to integrate current knowledge on VEE, with epidemiological and surveillance programmes to assess new public health policies.

2. The study of risk factors and eco-epidemiology

Epidemiology is a field focused on estimation of distribution and frequency of risk factors, prediction of the public health impact, and finally, offering control and prevention strategies for reducing the effects of disease in human populations [29]. In a restricted sense, the emphasis of this scientific discipline is directed to the study of factors, in a closer contact among the infectious agent with humans, such as social, cultural, biological, environmental, etc.

The causes underlying the rise of disease are at macro (socio-cultural) and micro (cellular and molecular) levels, but they are indeed acting over the individuals, populations and communities [30, 31]. There are several lines of evidence on the relationship between natural ecosystems intervention and re/emergence of diseases produced by bacteria, parasites and viruses [32-37]. Specifically, for understanding viral emergence it is important to understand the sylvatic cycle of viruses, the transition to human populations, the relationship between vectors, pathogens and reservoirs in wildlife ecosystems, the change in the distribution of vectors and reservoirs after natural habitat fragmentation, and how these conditions are generating potential new roles and ecological niches for species.

Wild ecosystems historically disturbed by agricultural and industrial activities with changes in biotic and abiotic factors (water bodies distribution, soil profiles, plant coverage, breeding microclimate, vertebrate and invertebrate populations, etc.) [38], constitute new selective pressures for pathogens and therefore new opportunities for adaptation [39]. It allows vectors/reservoirs to exploit the new resources, favouring viral contact with potentially new host populations (humans). In fact, evidence of distribution and abundance of mosquitoes in intervened areas demonstrates the high frequency of endophilic species and parasites transmission [34, 40-42].

For instance, blood-sucking mosquitoes may constitute the connectors between real and potential transmission cycles as they allow arboviruses (Arthropod-borne Viruses) to circulate in different geographical regions [43], involving human and wild reservoir species (mainly Rodentia and Didelphimorphia) [44-46].

On the other hand, Eco-epidemiology has been defined in two ways: first, as a paradigm that can integrate multiple levels of causes to reconsider the risk factors for disease in a human population [14, 30]; second, as the study of ecological effects perceived as having adverse effects on populations, ecosystems and the services provided by nature [13, 47, 48]. Despite the breadth of the eco-epidemiological approach, interactions of the virus-vector-host triad, their complex cycles, incidence and prevalence of diseases in geographic areas, ecological dynamics and historical (evolutionary) factors must be considered using a more integrative approach that helps us to predict the pathogen distribution and potential emergence of disease.

When a virus is introduced into a new host population, or quickly expands its range with a corresponding increase in cases of the disease, it is considered an Emerging Virus [36, 49]. There are three ways for a virus to emerge: *De novo* evolution of a new virus; the introduction of an existing virus from another species; and spread of a virus from a smaller population in which the virus may have previously emerged or have been introduced [50]. In any case, emerging viruses are descents from those lineages that circulate naturally.

The study of emerging viruses is often invoked by Molecular Epidemiology, using phylogenetic methods to infer the origin, emergence, spread and disease dynamics [16, 39, 51]. Evolutionary and ecological dynamics of emerging viruses are so linked that viral diversity is correlated with the epidemic dynamics [52].

Although Epidemiology considers the risk factors and Eco-Epidemiology introduces ecological factors under causal thought, it is still necessary to include the evolutionary variable, which is the goal of the VEE approach.

3. Viral evolutionary ecology

Viruses are not considered living beings but biological entities that evolve [53], and depending on the population size, their evolution can be determined in a higher or lower proportion by genetic drift or natural selection, respectively. Considering a natural transmission cycle of a virus between hosts, maybe involving an invertebrate vector, it is expected that adaptive evolution allows an efficient replication of the virus in such an environment [54]. If the ecosystem is stable and the transmission cycle has been established for a long time, it is expected that the rate of infection and mortality does not critically affect the host population [55]. The genetic background of current viruses evolved in such conditions possibly reflects the interaction of their ancestors with the whole environment, being better explained by an evolutionary ecology approach.

Ecology studies contemporary interactions, while Evolutionary Biology is concerned with historical issues. In this sense, Evolutionary Ecology is focused on the integration of these two disciplines to understand the most complicated issues, for example the causes of abundance and distribution of organisms, in relationship with abiotic and biotic dynamical variables [56-58].

VEE studies the impact of the evolutionary response of viruses to the hosts, and other interacting environmental factors, which are shaping their observed diversity and distribution patterns [18]. Although the role of evolutionary processes in driving viruses to new or more severe outcomes of diseases is known, the study of ecological and historical scenario, in which pathogen–host interaction evolves, is not always so well considered. VEE is becoming necessary for understanding and explaining the different patterns of disease in the human population, like acute-to-chronic [59], asymptomatic-to-lethal infections [55, 60] and the emergence of new viruses in humans [61, 62].

Under VEE, the virulence of pathogens is conceived as a process, in which a specific genotype or lineage is selected, which is translated into differential fitness and expansion of the disease [63]. The potential change in virulence resulting from selective pressures imposed by changes in host ecology has motivated the introduction of a new dimension within the objectives of epidemiology, incorporating ideas from the evolutionary ecology of parasites [64].

Viruses necessarily use the cellular machinery for their life cycles, however, the cell is only one component of the whole environment a virus has to face. Depending on the virus, a specific life history commonly involves replication in a specific cell type and tissue, the survivorship of viral particles in the external environment and specific transmission mode (e.g. aerosols, arthropod vectors, etc.) [65]. These features are some of the components of the Hutchinsonian niche of a virus allowing adaptation through time [66]. If every feature above is taken into account, virus-derived problems to humans could be easily understood, not like a virus-derived but a human-derived virus-driven problem (disease and/or disease emergence).

Several processes, such as transmission, host-shift, co-evolutionary arms race, resource tracking, competitive interactions and life histories, highlight the importance of ecology to explain past and current variation and distribution of viruses. Variables, such as host species, host density, competition with other viruses, genetic trade-offs on adaptation and physicochemical conditions, determine transmission and the final success of a virus in a specific host [67].

At present, the geno/phenotype of viruses is being challenged to overcome new changes, such as new host availability and loss of the original ecosystem. Thinking about the high diversity and adaptive potential of viruses, mainly because of their high mutation rates, large population sizes, short generation times and population dynamics [68-70], we expect from novel host and/or vector availability the adaptive evolution of new genetic variants in viral populations capable of exploiting the new environments and emerging in new transmission cycles involving new actors like humans, domestic and even wild animals.

Let us consider the AIDS epidemic whose responsible viruses are HIV-1 and -2. It was estimated that SIVs (Simian Immunodeficiency Viruses) had been circulating in African monkeys for at least 32,000 years [71] and HIV probably originated from them in the 1930s, with the most common recent ancestor (MRCA) estimated by mean of molecular clock analysis and coalescence theory, and the jump of species barrier probably due to the confluence of several factors [72].

Several hypotheses have been postulated to explain the emergence of HIV epidemic in humans. The first one related to hunters killing monkeys, natural reservoirs of SIV in a non-pathological relationship. The increase of dead monkeys in the forest and several events in Africa such as civil wars, human displacements, sexual violence, poverty and prostitution, could have produced an increase in size of SIV populations, contact between monkeys, their products and humans, altogether leading to the jump of SIV to human beings and originating the pandemic virus of the Twentieth Century [73].

On the other hand, not all SIV strains in Africa are closely related to posterior epidemic HIV strains. It was recently found that several GUD (Genital Ulcers Diseases, like syphilis, chancroid and lymphogranuloma venereum), prostitution and possibly lack of circumcision in African human populations, could have favoured the jump of species barrier or host-shift of SIV from monkeys to humans [74].

It could be more comprehensible using an illustration that represents the multidimensional space (hyper-volume) of environmental factors, that affect the performance of a species, as postulated by Evelyn Hutchinson [75]. In Figure 1, these n-dimensions are converted into only three coordinates for clarity. Performance of a viral species or genotype can be represented by a mountain (adaptive peaks in Simpsons' conception [76]), in which every peak corresponds to the maximum viral fitness of every viral species, or the maximum number of viruses produced by that specific genotype or species. Taking into account that fitness is a relative measure, viral fitness could change through evolutionary time as environmental conditions also change. Viral species in this model move over the surface of the adaptive landscape. If adequate environmental factors converge, the species could have real existence.

In our example, there are two mountains representing two viral species (Species A and Species B), existing in two different lapses of evolutionary time and infecting two different hosts (Sigma and Phi), respectively. Species A is the ancestor and could have originated Species B by successful adaptation after colonization of a new host. The probability of Species A exploiting the new host species (Phi) could be null (zero) or maximal (one). When environmental conditions dramatically change, as mentioned above with SIV, the probability of the Species A jumping to the host species Phi and the opportunity for adaptation to this new host are very high. The resulting virus (Species B) playing a new role in the ecosystem (new ecological niche) can be considered an emerging virus.

The trajectory of the virus jumping from one species to another could be represented using a curved arrow, in which fitness decrease is associated with poor adaptation to the new host at the initial contact [77]. After this process the adaptation allows a gradual fitness increase up to the highest peak, in which the phylogenetic nearness of the donor and the recipient host species is extremely important [78].

Figure 1 has the limitation of assuming that Species A disappears once the adaptation to the new host occurs. This is not always true as this ancestral virus could continue infecting the original host (Sigma) and co-exist with the descent virus (Species B) in evolutionary time. The same has occurred with emergent HIV and contemporary SIV strains, closely related to the ancestor of HIV.

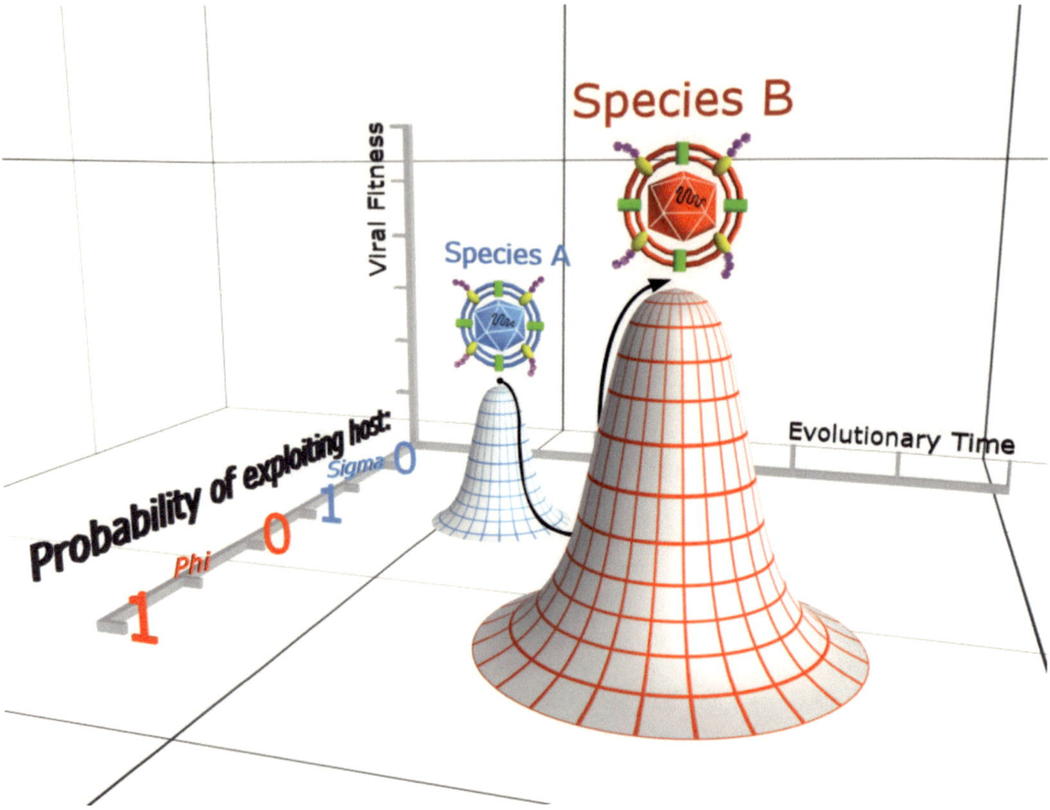

Fig. 1. Ecological niche, adaptive landscape and the jump of species barrier: adaptive landscape representing the fitness of two viral species (A and B) in their specific hosts (Sigma and Phi, respectively). Species A is the ancestor of B, generated after colonization of a new host species (Phi). The probability of Species A exploiting host Phi could be null (zero) or maximal (one) and depends on n-dimensions of the environment. Viral emergence occurs when species B originates from adaptation of the species B to the new host, with a new ecological niche.

4. The new multidisciplinary and integrated approach: Viral emergence using the VEE framework

Over the last 50 years of virological research, many fine details in the cellular and molecular biology of viral infection, immunology, viral morphogenesis and other topics have been elucidated. In spite of these tremendous advances, the interface between intra-host and inter-host dynamics has not been so well addressed. The causes and process of emergence of viral diseases have to be necessarily studied at the genetic and ecological levels in which several factors related with the ecology and evolutionary biology of pathogens, hosts and the pathogen-host relationship are undeniable.

In natural ecosystems, many viruses have natural transmission cycles, involving vectors and wild reservoirs, however, transformation of the landscape leads to changes in their abundance and distribution [79, 80]. With these changes, some viral species could exploit the ecological resources, adapting to new hosts (e.g. humans), making possible the emergence of viruses [78, 81].

Viruses exist in a high variety of ecosystems, in which numerous elements are implied in their trafficking and disease dynamics [80]. An important group of viruses implied in emergent and re-emergent diseases belong to the families *Togaviridae* (genus *Alphavirus*), *Flaviviridae* (genus *Flavivirus*) and *Bunyaviridae* (genera *Orthobunyavirus* and *Phlebovirus*) [32, 35-37]. These viruses are transmitted by haematophagous arthropods, mainly mosquitoes (Diptera: *Culicidae*). The family *Culicidae* of insect vectors is often associated with sylvatic areas, historically modified by human activities like artificial landscapes (agriculture, livestock, mining, house building and urbanization) [32, 35-37].

Viral diseases are the evolutionary consequence of our historical landscape alteration. Considering the very ancient origin of SIV (several thousands of years), the recent emergence of HIV (1930s) and the Acquired Immune Deficiency Syndrome (AIDS) as a new pathological entity, viral disease emergence can be considered as an evolutionary event, precipitated by changes in landscape ecology, due to human activity after the rise of agriculture (10 to 15 thousand years ago) [82]. If the ecological niche for species A (in Figure 1) is represented by the corresponding mountain, then new variables will be shaping the ecological niche for species B.

SIV has been infecting monkeys in Africa over thousands of years and HIV has recently arisen by SIV jumping and adapting from monkeys to humans. In this sense, the HIV epidemic could have been due to successful colonization and virus adaptation to the new host, and several other factors mediating transmission in the last host, all of them allowing the generation of a new ecological niche.

It is important to establish the phylogenetic relationship between virus isolates from different geographical regions (phylogeography), emphasizing the fact that ecological factors could explain the presence of a virus in the ecosystem and the necessary interactions for potential emergence (niche). Landscape ecology studies how landscape structure affects the abundance and distribution of organisms [83-85]. Combining landscape ecology with VEE will be a powerful tool for understanding the epidemiology of viral diseases that have devastating effects on the human population.

For epidemiology, it is important to identify any emergent pathogen for establishment of public health policies. It is worrisome that viral diversity in wild tropical areas is almost unknown. It is necessary to establish new and fast tools for taxonomic identification of both viruses and their arthropod vectors [86]. The study of ecologic variables mediating the transmission cycle (viral trafficking) will be useful in finding patterns and predictive factors for the emergence of new viruses.

VEE studies the responsible elements for maintaining viral circulation in wild ecosystems, as well as the patterns generated from ecosystem perturbation, which determine the convergence of conditions (ecological and evolutionary) in the new or emergent ecosystem favouring the co-existence of viruses, reservoirs and vectors [79, 87], and mediating viral disease emergence.

5. Conclusion

Emerging viral diseases are seriously affecting human populations and our current epidemiological tools are insufficient to explain the emerging process. Viruses are not living organisms, but they have genomes and their evolution is governed by the same factors driving evolution in all other living beings. The emergence can be well understood as a biological process by applying concepts of evolutionary biology such as adaptation. If we also consider the environmental changes enabling new selective pressures (novel ecosystems), we can expect the appearance of new virus-host interactions (ecological niches). Therefore, epidemiological and evolutionary ecology studies must be integrated to obtain a better explanation of viral emergence and establishment of measures for the prediction and control of these devastating diseases.

6. Acknowledgments

This work was funded by COLCIENCIAS (Colombia) grants: 11150418079, 111540820511, 111549326198 and 111545921525. Special acknowledgement to Dr. Christon J. Hurst at Xavier University, Cincinnati, Ohio (USA), for his continuous encouragement and support, including partial review of a preliminary version of this manuscript. JUC received a Doctoral Fellowship from COLCIENCIAS. The Neuroscience Group was granted by the Programa de Sostenibilidad 2009-2010 of the Universidad de Antioquia.

7. References

[1] Kilbourne ED. The molecular epidemiology of influenza. The Journal of infectious diseases. 1973 Apr;127(4):478-87.
[2] Holmes EC, Zhang LQ, Robertson P, Cleland A, Harvey E, Simmonds P, et al. The molecular epidemiology of human immunodeficiency virus type 1 in Edinburgh. The Journal of infectious diseases. 1995 Jan;171(1):45-53.
[3] Rota JS, Heath JL, Rota PA, King GE, Celma ML, Carabana J, et al. Molecular epidemiology of measles virus: identification of pathways of transmission and implications for measles elimination. The Journal of infectious diseases. 1996 Jan;173(1):32-7.
[4] Saiz JC, Sobrino F, Dopazo J. Molecular epidemiology of foot-and-mouth disease virus type O. The Journal of general virology. 1993 Oct;74 (Pt 10):2281-5.
[5] Handsfield HH, Totten PA, Fennel CL, Falkow S, Holmes KK. Molecular epidemiology of Haemophilus ducreyi infections. Annals of internal medicine. 1981 Sep;95(3):315-8.
[6] Goarant C, Reynaud Y, Ansquer D, de Decker S, Saulnier D, le Roux F. Molecular epidemiology of Vibrio nigripulchritudo, a pathogen of cultured penaeid shrimp (Litopenaeus stylirostris) in New Caledonia. Systematic and applied microbiology. 2006 Nov;29(7):570-80.
[7] Kazwala RR, Kusiluka LJ, Sinclair K, Sharp JM, Daborn CJ. The molecular epidemiology of Mycobacterium bovis infections in Tanzania. Veterinary microbiology. 2006 Feb 25;112(2-4):201-10.
[8] Banuls AL, Hide M, Tibayrenc M. Molecular epidemiology and evolutionary genetics of Leischmania parasites. International journal for parasitology. 1999 Aug;29(8):1137-47.

[9] Ghosh S, Frisardi M, Ramirez-Avila L, Descoteaux S, Sturm-Ramirez K, Newton-Sanchez OA, et al. Molecular epidemiology of Entamoeba spp.: evidence of a bottleneck (Demographic sweep) and transcontinental spread of diploid parasites. Journal of clinical microbiology. 2000 Oct;38(10):3815-21.
[10] Thompson RC, Colwell DD, Shury T, Appelbee AJ, Read C, Njiru Z, et al. The molecular epidemiology of Cryptosporidium and Giardia infections in coyotes from Alberta, Canada, and observations on some cohabiting parasites. Veterinary parasitology. 2009 Feb 5;159(2):167-70.
[11] Hyman BT, Tanzi R. Molecular epidemiology of Alzheimer's disease. The New England journal of medicine. 1995 Nov 9;333(19):1283-4.
[12] Lower GM, Jr., Nilsson T, Nelson CE, Wolf H, Gamsky TE, Bryan GT. N-acetyltransferase phenotype and risk in urinary bladder cancer: approaches in molecular epidemiology. Preliminary results in Sweden and Denmark. Environmental health perspectives. 1979 Apr;29:71-9.
[13] Bro-Rasmussen F, Lokke H. Ecoepidemiology--a casuistic discipline describing ecological disturbances and damages in relation to their specific causes: exemplified by chlorinated phenols and chlorophenoxy acids. Regul Toxicol Pharmacol. 1984 Dec;4(4):391-9.
[14] Susser M, Susser E. Choosing a future for epidemiology: II. From black box to Chinese boxes and eco-epidemiology. American journal of public health. 1996 May;86(5):674-7.
[15] Kilpatrick AM, Daszak P, Goodman SJ, Rogg H, Kramer LD, Cedeno V, et al. Predicting pathogen introduction: West Nile virus spread to Galaipagos. Conserv Biol. 2006 Aug;20(4):1224-31.
[16] Vasconcelos HB, Nunes MR, Casseb LM, Carvalho VL, Pinto da Silva EV, Silva M, et al. Molecular epidemiology of Oropouche virus, Brazil. Emerging infectious diseases. 2011 May;17(5):800-6.
[17] Dennehy JJ. Bacteriophages as model organisms for virus emergence research. Trends in microbiology. 2009 Oct;17(10):450-7.
[18] DeFillipis VR, Villareal LP. An Introduction to the Evolutionary Ecology of Viruses. In: Hurst C, ed. *Viral Ecology*. New York: Academic Press 2000.
[19] Schrag SJ, Wiener P. Emerging infectious disease: what are the relative roles of ecology and evolution? Trends in ecology & evolution. 1995 Aug;10(8):319-24.
[20] McMichael AJ. Environmental and social influences on emerging infectious diseases: past, present and future. Philosophical transactions of the Royal Society of London. 2004 Jul 29;359(1447):1049-58.
[21] Ostfeld RS, Keesing F. Biodiversity and disease risk: the case of Lyme Disease. Conservation Biology. 2000;14(3):722-8.
[22] Ewald PW. Cultural vectors, virulence and the emergence of evolutionary epidemiology. In: Harvey PH, Partridge L, eds. *Oxford Surveys in Evolutionary Biology*: Oxford University Press 1988.
[23] Restif O. Evolutionary epidemiology 20 years on: challenges and prospects. Infect Genet Evol. 2009 Jan;9(1):108-23.
[24] Mideo N, Alizon S, Day T. Linking within- and between-host dynamics in the evolutionary epidemiology of infectious diseases. Trends in ecology & evolution. 2008 Sep;23(9):511-7.

[25] Luria SE. General Virology. New York: Wiley 1953.
[26] Reiners WA, Driese KL. Transport of energy, information, and material through the Biosphere. Ann Rev Environm Res. 2003;28:107-35.
[27] Hobbs RJ, Higgs E, Harris JA. Novel ecosystems: implications for conservation and restoration. Trends in ecology & evolution. 2009 Nov;24(11):599-605.
[28] Palumbi SR. Humans as the world's greatest evolutionary force. Science (New York, NY. 2001 Sep 7;293(5536):1786-90.
[29] Carr S, Unwin N, Pless-Mulolli T. An Introduction to Public Health and Epidemiology. Open University Press. New York: McGraw-Hill 2007.
[30] March D, Susser E. The eco- in eco-epidemiology. Int J Epidemiol. 2006 Dec;35(6):1379-83.
[31] Susser E. Eco-epidemiology: thinking outside the black box. Epidemiology. 2004 Sep;15(5):519-20; author reply 27-8.
[32] Carver S, Bestall A, Jardine A, Ostfeld RS. Influence of hosts on the ecology of arboviral transmission: potential mechanisms influencing dengue, murray valley encephalitis, and ross river virus in Australia. Vector Borne Zoonotic Dis. 2009 Feb;9(1):51-64.
[33] Cassis G. Biodiversity loss: a human health issue. Med J Aust. 1998 Dec 7-21;169(11-12):568-9.
[34] Keesing F, Belden LK, Daszak P, Dobson A, Harvell CD, Holt RD, et al. Impacts of biodiversity on the emergence and transmission of infectious diseases. Nature. 2010 Dec 2;468(7324):647-52.
[35] Morens DM, Folkers GK, Fauci AS. Emerging infections: a perpetual challenge. Lancet Infect Dis. 2008 Nov;8(11):710-9.
[36] Morse SS. Factors in the emergence of infectious diseases. Emerging infectious diseases. 1995 Jan-Mar;1(1):7-15.
[37] Subbarao SK, Kumar KV, Nanda N, Nagpal BN, Dev V, Sharma VP. Cytotaxonomic evidence for the presence of Anopheles nivipes in India. J Am Mosq Control Assoc. 2000 Jun;16(2):71-4.
[38] Robertson AI. The gaps between ecosystem ecology and industrial agriculture. Ecosystems. 2000;3:413-8.
[39] Holmes EC. The Evolution and Emergence of RNA Viruses. New York: Oxford University Press 2009.
[40] Connell JH. Diversity in tropical rain forests and coral reefs. Science (New York, NY. 1978 Mar 24;199(4335):1302-10.
[41] Koren HS, Crawford-Brown D. A framework for the integration of ecosystem and human health in public policy: two case studies with infectious agents. Environ Res. 2004 May;95(1):92-105.
[42] Montes J. [Culicidae fauna of Serra da Cantareira, Sao Paulo, Brazil]. Rev Saude Publica. 2005 Aug;39(4):578-84.
[43] Forattini OP. Culicidologia médica: identificação, biologia, epidemiologia. São Paulo: Editora da Universidade de São Paulo 2002.
[44] Balter M. Virus from 1959 sample marks early years of HIV. Science (New York, NY. 1998 Feb 6;279(5352):801.
[45] de Thoisy B, Dussart P, Kazanji M. Wild terrestrial rainforest mammals as potential reservoirs for flaviviruses (yellow fever, dengue 2 and St Louis encephalitis viruses) in French Guiana. Trans R Soc Trop Med Hyg. 2004 Jul;98(7):409-12.

[46] de Thoisy B, Lacoste V, Germain A, Munoz-Jordan J, Colon C, Mauffrey JF, et al. Dengue infection in neotropical forest mammals. Vector Borne Zoonotic Dis. 2009 Apr;9(2):157-70.
[47] Cormier S, Norton SB, Suter GW. The U.S. Environmental Protection Agency's Stressor Identification Guidance: A process for determining the probable causes of biological impairments. Human and Ecological Risk Assessment. 2003;9:1431-44.
[48] Fox GA. Practical causal inference for ecoepidemiologists. J Toxicol Environ Health. 1991 Aug;33(4):359-73.
[49] Morse SS. Emerging viruses: defining the rules for viral traffic. Perspect Biol Med. 1991 Spring;34(3):387-409.
[50] Morse S. Emerging Viruses. New York: Oxford University Press 1993.
[51] Sall AA, Zanotto PM, Vialat P, Sene OK, Bouloy M. Molecular epidemiology and emergence of Rift Valley fever. Memorias do Instituto Oswaldo Cruz. 1998 Sep-Oct;93(5):609-14.
[52] Pybus OG, Rambaut A. Evolutionary analysis of the dynamics of viral infectious disease. Nat Rev Genet. 2009 Aug;10(8):540-50.
[53] van Regenmortel MH, Mahy BW. Emerging issues in virus taxonomy. Emerging infectious diseases. 2004 Jan;10(1):8-13.
[54] Greene IP, Wang E, Deardorff ER, Milleron R, Domingo E, Weaver SC. Effect of alternating passage on adaptation of sindbis virus to vertebrate and invertebrate cells. J Virol. 2005 Nov;79(22):14253-60.
[55] Pfennig KS. Evolution of pathogen virulence: the role of variation in host phenotype. Proc Biol Sci. 2001 Apr 7;268(1468):755-60.
[56] Fox CW, Roof DA, Fairbairn D. Evolutionary Ecology: Concepts and Case Studies Oxford University Press 2001.
[57] Krebs CJ. Ecology: The Experimental Analysis of Distribution and Abundance. 6 ed. San Francisco: Benjamin Cummings 2009.
[58] Pianka ER. Evolutionary Ecology. California: Benjamin Cummins 1999.
[59] Grenfell BT, Pybus OG, Gog JR, Wood JL, Daly JM, Mumford JA, et al. Unifying the epidemiological and evolutionary dynamics of pathogens. Science (New York, NY. 2004 Jan 16;303(5656):327-32.
[60] Ebert D. Experimental evolution of parasites. Science (New York, NY. 1998 Nov 20;282(5393):1432-5.
[61] Antia R, Regoes RR, Koella JC, Bergstrom CT. The role of evolution in the emergence of infectious diseases. Nature. 2003 Dec 11;426(6967):658-61.
[62] Pepin KM, Lass S, Pulliam JR, Read AF, Lloyd-Smith JO. Identifying genetic markers of adaptation for surveillance of viral host jumps. Nature reviews. 2010 Nov;8(11):802-13.
[63] Hurst CJ. Viral Ecology. London: Academic Press 2000.
[64] Galvani AP. Epidemiology meets evolutionary ecology. Trends in Ecology and Evolution. 2003;18:132-9.
[65] De Paepe M, Taddei F. Viruses' life history: towards a mechanistic basis of a trade-off between survival and reproduction among phages. PLoS Biol. 2006 Jul;4(7):e193.
[66] Holt RD. Bringing the Hutchinsonian niche into the 21st century: ecological and evolutionary perspectives. Proc Natl Acad Sci U S A. 2009 Nov 17;106 Suppl 2:19659-65.
[67] Holmes EC. The phylogeography of human viruses. Mol Ecol. 2004 Apr;13(4):745-56.

[68] Moya A, Holmes EC, Gonzalez-Candelas F. The population genetics and evolutionary epidemiology of RNA viruses. Nature reviews. 2004 Apr;2(4):279-88.
[69] Sanjuan R, Nebot MR, Chirico N, Mansky LM, Belshaw R. Viral mutation rates. J Virol. 2010 Oct;84(19):9733-48.
[70] Domingo E. Virus Evolution. In: Knipe DM, Howley PM, eds. *Fields Virology*. Philadelphia: Wolkers Kluwer/Lippincott Williams and Wilkins 2007.
[71] Worobey M, Telfer P, Souquiere S, Hunter M, Coleman CA, Metzger MJ, et al. Island biogeography reveals the deep history of SIV. Science (New York, NY. 2010 Sep 17;329(5998):1487.
[72] Lemey P, Pybus OG, Wang B, Saksena NK, Salemi M, Vandamme AM. Tracing the origin and history of the HIV-2 epidemic. Proc Natl Acad Sci U S A. 2003 May 27;100(11):6588-92.
[73] Ujvari SC. The History of the Dissemination of Microorganisms. Estudos Avançados. 2008;22(64):171-82.
[74] de Sousa JD, Muller V, Lemey P, Vandamme AM. High GUD incidence in the early 20 century created a particularly permissive time window for the origin and initial spread of epidemic HIV strains. PloS one. 2010;5(4):e9936.
[75] Hutchinson E. Concluding Remarks. Cold Spring Harbor Symposia on Quantitative Biology. 1957;22(2):415-27.
[76] Simpsons GG. Tempo and mode in evolution. New York: Columbia University Press 1944.
[77] Dennehy JJ, Friedenberg NA, Holt RD, Turner PE. Viral ecology and the maintenance of novel host use. Am Nat. 2006 Mar;167(3):429-39.
[78] Hurst CJ. Defining the Ecology of Viruses. In: Hurst CJ, ed. *Studies in Viral Ecology*. Hoboken, New Jersey: John Wiley & Sons, Inc. 2011.
[79] Yanoviak SP, Paredes JE, Lounibos LP, Weaver SC. Deforestation alters phytotelm habitat availability and mosquito production in the Peruvian Amazon. Ecol Appl. 2006 Oct;16(5):1854-64.
[80] Weaver SC, Reisen WK. Present and future arboviral threats. Antiviral Res. 2010 Feb;85(2):328-45.
[81] Cleaveland S, Haydon DT, Taylor L. Overviews of pathogen emergence: which pathogens emerge, when and why? Current topics in microbiology and immunology. 2007;315:85-111.
[82] Barrett R, Kuzawa CW, McDade T, Armelagos GJ. Emerging and re-emerging infectious diseases: the third epidemiologic transition. Annual Review of Anthropology. 1998;27:247-71.
[83] Turner MG. Landscape ecology: the effect of pattern on process. Annual Review of Ecology and Systematics. 1989;20:171–97.
[84] Wiens JA, Moss MR. Issues and Perspectives in Landscape Ecology. Cambridge: Cambridge University Press 2005.
[85] Ostfeld RS, Glass GE, Keesing F. Spatial epidemiology: an emerging (or re-emerging) discipline. Trends in ecology & evolution. 2005 Jun;20(6):328-36.
[86] Childs JE. Pre-spillover prevention of emerging zoonotic diseases: what are the targets and what are the tools? Current topics in microbiology and immunology. 2007;315:389-443.
[87] Vasilakis N, Cardosa J, Hanley KA, Holmes EC, Weaver SC. Fever from the forest: prospects for the continued emergence of sylvatic dengue virus and its impact on public health. Nature reviews. 2011 Jul;9(7):532-41.

8

Overview of Pharmacoepidemiological Databases in the Assessment of Medicines Under Real-Life Conditions

Carla Torre[1] and Ana Paula Martins[2]
[1]*Centre for Health Evaluation & Research (CEFAR), National Association of Pharmacies (ANF),*
[2]*Institute for Research in Medicines and Pharmaceutical Sciences (iMed.UL), Faculty of Pharmacy, University of Lisbon, Portugal*

1. Introduction

Pharmacoepidemiology studies the use and effects, both beneficial and adverse, of medicines in large numbers of people. It applies the methods of Epidemiology to the area of Clinical Pharmacology (Strom, 2005a). This field seeks to further the knowledge and science underlying post marketing drug surveillance (studies conducted after a medicine has been released into the market).

The *raison d'être* of these studies is to bridge the gap between the information generated by clinical pre-marketing trials and the real-world drug usage, since drugs often do not perform as well in routine clinical practice as in clinical trials. Clinical trials may not provide an accurate picture of drug effects. At the time of authorization, we have evidence from clinical trials which demonstrate efficacy, but only for a specific indication and only within the original test population. At this stage, we have evidence of adverse reactions, but only the most common ones (Black, 1996; Strom, 2005a).

The known limitations of clinical trials (e.g. selected study population, defined by strict inclusion and exclusion criteria; short duration of time; small sample size; conducted in selected sites which are typically better equipped than routine care facilities) have led to a number of well-described "unknowns" - primarily the effectiveness of the medicine in normal clinical practice and the full safety profile (Roher, 2008; Montori *et al*, 2005; Zimmerman *et al*, 2002).

The current regulatory process creates an evidence-free zone at the time of launch of new medicines and often decisions are taken under conditions of uncertainty. It is important to note that uncertainty about safety may be more common, as most studies for regulatory approval are powered on demonstrating efficacy rather than safety (Eichler *et al*, 2008; van Staa *et al*, 2008).

Eichler and colleagues argued that this efficacy-effectiveness gap is, in most cases, a problem of variability in drug response and described both biological and behavioural as sources of variability in the real-world environment (Eichler *et al*, 2011). The first source of variability is related to genetics factors and other intrinsic (e.g. sex, age, body weight, co-morbidities or baseline disease severity) and extrinsic (e.g. environmental influences, such as pollution, co-medication or influences of food on pharmacokinetics) factors. The second one is linked with prescribing and drug handling (e.g. inappropriate or off-label prescribing, sometimes encouraged by sponsors and promotion efforts) and patient adherence and utilization.

Due to this variety of factors that can influence exposure and patient response to drug treatment, an evolution in the current regulatory model, from a single pre-marketing authorization to a life-cycle approach, is required (Eichler *et al*, 2008). Society demands a transparent and an integrated assessment of benefits and risks, under real life conditions, as the next logical step after clinical trials (Garattini & Chalmers, 2009). The regulatory pathway will have to mirror real-world data for safety, effectiveness and patterns of drug utilization.

Over the last decade, the role of payers has become more prominent, and time-to-market no longer means time-to-authorization but time to reimbursement (Eichler *et al*, 2011b). General speaking, governments and payers are making health policy decisions, regarding access and reimbursement that should answer the three core questions of evidence-based technology evaluation, as defined by Archie Cochrane: "Can it work?", "Will it work" and "Is it worth it?" (Haynes, 1999). In heath technology assessment, external validity should not be neglected and real-world data is clearly a key issue in this context. It is essential that health technology assessments move from evaluating cost-efficacy in ideal populations with ideal interventions to evaluating cost-effectiveness in real-world populations with real interventions, since findings between these two worlds are clearly different, as markedly exemplified by van Staa and colleagues with the selective cox-2 inhibitors. In this study, it was highlighted that the published cost-effectiveness analyses of coxibs lacked external validity, did not represent patients in clinical practice and should not have been used to inform prescribing policies. They demonstrated that the cost effectiveness of coxibs was far worse when the analyses were based on data from clinical practice rather than RCT (van Staa *et al*, 2009).

One of the main issues of knowledge, on the effectiveness, safety and economics of drug usage, is the data sources available for analysis. It often takes more than scientific expertise and ambition to effectively bridge the gap between clinical trials and clinical daily practice. Frequently, several preconditions, mainly at the managerial level, need to be fulfilled which often requires an automated system that is constantly refined and kept up to date.

The last two decades have witnessed the development of key data resources along with the associated knowledge and methodology that have allowed landmark studies to be conducted. Large practice based and/or record-linked databases often meet the need for a cost-effective and efficient means of conducting post-authorization studies and have significantly fuelled pharmacoepidemiology research.

Despite the increased availability of databases, their use as a research tool may be a complex task (Harpe, 2009). The implementation of studies through databases requires a clear and comprehensive understanding of the strengths and weaknesses of pharmacoepidemiological methods, of how the data were collected, enrollment and coverage factors, and other factors that might have affected data quality and validity.

Moreover, an understanding of social, political, cultural and historical settings is crucial (Shatin, 2001). Lack of awareness of the limitations and failures to understand methodological challenges arising in the use of these databases can lead to the selection of inappropriate study methods and hinder the interpretation of results. Unequivocally, when conducting pharmacoepidemiology research through databases, we should bear in mind Brian Strom's quote: "Databases should not distract us from sound methodological and clinical thinking" (Strom, 2004).

To sum up, to get the complete picture and to (try to) understand everything about a drug, we must do both clinical trials and observational studies. Over time, this was clearly a lesson learned (Vandenbroucke, 2008) but we should do it with rigor and humility (Avorn, 2007).

2. Automated databases in pharmacoepidemiology research

Identifying a good research question is arguably the most important step in the research process. It must be clearly and precisely defined prior to the design and implementation of a study as it forms the foundation for the entire project (Harpe, 2009; Vanderbrouke, 2002; Hulley, 2007). After the research question and study design are careful constructed, a framework should be put in place which includes: selecting the database of interest, selecting the outcome, exposure and other variables of interest, understanding the limitations of the data source, and quality assessment methodology (Harpe, 2009).

Pharmacoepidemiology research studies may involve either data collected prospectively for the purpose of the particular study (*de novo* data collection), i.e. primary data, or data that were already collected for another purpose - as part of administrative records or patient health care -, which is called secondary data (Harpe, 2011).

Although pharmacoepidemiology uses all epidemiological study designs and sources, in recent decades there has been an enormous growth in the use of secondary data. 'So called' automated large healthcare databases, especially in North America and Europe, have proven to be a rich resource for pharmacoepidemiology and health services research (Hemmerlgarn *et al*, 1994; Arana *et al*, 2004).

These automated databases are regularly used in a variety of settings to study the use and outcomes of therapeutics and often meet the need for a cost-effective and efficient means of conducting post-authorization surveillance studies. Their size allows the study of infrequent drug effects and their longer follow-up times and representativeness, in terms of routine clinical practice, make it possible to study real-world effectiveness, safety and utilization patterns.

According to Brian Strom, to meet the needs of pharmacoepidemiology an ideal database would include records from all inpatient and outpatient care, emergency care, all laboratory and radiological tests, all both prescribed and non-prescribed medications. The population covered would be large enough to detect rare events and would be stable over its lifetime, from birth to death. Moreover, it would be kept updated and have information on potential confounders variables, such as smoking status, alcohol consumption, etc. (Strom, 2005b).

However, no single existing database is ideal. The information necessary for a study is often stored in separate databases. In order to gather all the information, it is often necessary to identify the same participants across databases, which can be complex (Florentinus *et al*, 2006). In 1946, Dunn stated that in some way, each person in the world creates a book of their life, which starts with birth and ends with death, and has pages that are records that represent the principal events during the course of each person's life. Record linkage was the name given by Dunn to the process of assembling the pages of this book into a volume (Dunn, 1946). Applying this concept to the field of pharmacoepidemiology, record linkage can be defined *"as a method for bringing together the information contained in two or more records – e.g., in different sets of medical charts, and in vital records such as birth and death certificates – and a procedure that each individual is identified and counted only once. This procedure incorporates a unique identifying system such as a personal identification number"* (Porta *et al*, 2008).

Although, this concept of assembling unique health information about individuals from various sources is far from new - it has been around for more than 150 years (Rawson & Shatin, 2008), this is not an easy task. It requires high qualified human resources, such as system engineers and data managers, who should have the capacity, flexibility and familiarity with the knowledge in this demanding medical field (Takahashi *et al*, 2011).

On the other hand, in the process of analyzing the data source, a number of factors must be taken into consideration, including the extensiveness and depth of data, the quality of database, the population covered, and the duration of information contained in the databases (Berger *et al*, 2009). It is important to be aware of the drawbacks and limitations of databases discussed below.

Databases can be broadly divided into two general categories: administrative databases, which include transactions primarily to achieve administrative purposes, such as claims for reimbursement from insurance companies; and electronic health medical records, which include records maintained for the management of patients' clinical care (Strom, 2005b).

- Administrative databases

  In U.S.A. and Canada, administrative health databases were initially developed to administer payments to healthcare providers in nationally funded healthcare systems or managed care organizations (Suissa & Garbe, 2007). They were designed for billing and record-keeping purposes, where information is recorded as a by-product of financial transactions, and not for research. Limited information is required for billing, including type of insurance coverage, dates of medical service and associated diagnoses (ambulatory and hospitalizations information), tests performed and prescriptions dispensed by community pharmacies. These databases usually consist of patient-level information from two or more separate files that can be linked via a unique patient identifier (Hennessy, 2006; Rawson, 2009). Typically, researchers have to submit a protocol to an ethics review committee and they receive only the specific data to investigate a particular research question in exchange for a fee charged for time needed to extract data from the database.

  Group Health Cooperative (U.S.A.), Medicaid databases (U.S.A.) and Health Services Databases in Saskatchewan (Canada) are just few examples of this type of database. Detailed information about these and other administrative health databases has been described previously (Strom, 2005a).

- Electronic health medical records and linkage systems (non-administrative)

  In contrast to administrative databases, in electronic medical records, data are recorded as part of clinical patient care and not for billing purposes. These type of databases normally consist of data entered by general practitioners (GP) (often the gatekeeper of the healthcare system) into their practice computers and are maintained primarily for documenting the patient's conditions and treatments. As medical practices increasingly became electronic (over time computers are replacing paper medical records as the primary medical record), a unique opportunity for pharmacoepidemiology research was opened (Strom, 2005b). In practical terms, physicians maintain records of all visits and events: diagnoses (outpatient conditions and procedures diagnosed and performed by GP, respectively; conditions diagnosed by outpatient specialist, information pertaining hospital admissions, including hospital diagnoses), medical history, prescriptions issued, laboratory tests (ordered and their results). In comparison to administrative databases, medical records databases usually include much more detailed information on their patient files, such as alcohol consumption, smoking status, height and weight, although this may be missing in many patients. It is worth noting here that the existence of these types of databases is more frequent in Europe.

  The General Practice Research Database (GPRD) is generally considered to be the largest medical records database in routine use for medical investigation (it is representative of the United Kingdom (UK) and has population-based data on over 9 million patients, with over 44 million years of follow-up time) and the one which has been used most extensively for published research in the pharmacoepidemiology field (Gelfand *et al*, 2005). This database was created in June 1987 as the Value Added Medical Products (VAMP) research databank. The salient feature of GPRD is its comprehensive nature, since it collects information on demographics, medical diagnoses, prescriptions, referrals to hospitals, smoking status, immunizations, weight and height, and for a growing number of patients also laboratory results (Walley & Mantgani, 1997).

  A 'proof of concept' of the feasibility and utility of implementing cluster randomized trials utilizing electronic patient records in GPRD was recently provided. An application of electronic patient records to the evaluation of health interventions, including their health impacts and effectiveness, was developed and will be tested on antibiotic prescribing for acute respiratory infection. Results from this study will provide guidance and methodological evidence concerning the use of electronic patient records and databases for implementing cluster randomized trials in primary care (Gulliford *et al*, 2011).

  There are few published examples of randomized database studies, but this design could become more common in the near future, since they attempt to combine the advantages of randomization and observational studies (Sturkenboom, 2008).

  GPRD is derived from medical records whereas other medical record databases are often derived from pharmacy dispensing records. In the Netherlands, there is an automated pharmacy record linkage called PHARMO that was developed in the early

1990s by Herings and Stricker. The PHARMO medical record linkage system is a population-based data system that includes the drug-dispensing records from community pharmacies and hospital discharge records of community-dwelling inhabitants in the Netherlands. The drug-dispensing histories are linked to the hospital discharge records of the same patient, using a probabilistic algorithm (based on characteristics such as date of birth, gender, and a code for the GP) that is comparable to unique personal identifier system (Goettsch *et al*, 2004; Pouwels *et al*, 2011). The Dutch health care system has strong regulatory and reimbursement incentives for Dutch patients to frequent a single GP (gate keeper system) and a single pharmacy which constitutes an important feature (Leufkens & Urquhart, 2005).

Access to data must comply with certain rules and conditions. For example, to access GPRD adequate computer software and hardware are required, as well as experienced data managers. Moreover, access to data is often not free of charge and the study protocol's approval by the Scientific and Ethical Advisory Board is mandatory (Gelfand *et al*, 2005).

Detailed overviews with comprehensive description of strengths and weaknesses of these and similar databases are available elsewhere (Strom, 2005a).

Health care databases throughout the world diverge noticeably with regard to their representativeness of population, the range and detail of information they contain, their data quality and completeness and their capability to link with other sources (Schneeweiss & Avorn, 2005), as discussed below. Indeed, the minimum requirement for drug utilization research is the availability of a pharmacy dispensing database, which allows at least a descriptive analysis of drug use (Geleedst-De *et al*, 2010; Elseviers *et al*, 2007). Additionally, in specific situations, even without diagnostic information, it can be used to assess the association between drug use and adverse effects in a prescription symmetry design (Hallas, 2005). One example of such a database is the Portuguese pharmacy sales (medicines, health products and pharmacy services) database of the National Association of Pharmacies, which is a nationwide database with representative drug dispensing data from ambulatory care (79% of pharmacies) at a regional level (hmR/CEFAR Pharmacy Sales Information System) (Torre *et al*, 2011).

In terms of complexity, combining databases from different countries, although a challenging task, is also possible. Both Food and Drug Administration (FDA) and European Medicines Agency (EMA) have issued similarity initiatives to develop innovative methodologies for drug safety monitoring based on analysis of large databases. Recently, in Europe, under the EU-ADR umbrella project, a methodology was developed and tested that enabled the combining of data from electronic health record databases of various countries and types (medical records, administrative registries, record-linkage databases). This represents an enormous step in large-scale drug monitoring, namely an early-detection of safety signals field (Colomba *et al*, 2011) and on detection of rare drug-associated outcomes (García Rodriguez *et al*, 2010). In this area of cooperation, formal collaborative networks of centres active in pharmacoepidemiology and pharmacovigilance are rapidly changing the landscape of drug post-authorization studies in Europe and will have promising results in the near future (Blake *et al*, 2011; ENCePP, 2011).

2.1 Exposure and outcome: Definition and measurement

Once the research question is defined, it is necessary to consider what information is required to answer it.

Outcomes of interest in pharmacoepidemiology can include diseases or conditions, medical procedures, laboratory tests results, or the use of particular medication, including medication adherence and persistence (Harpe, 2011).

The use of databases, either administrative or electronic medical records, to record diagnosis information usually requires the diagnosis to be transferred using a formalized coding system, frequently the International Classification of Diseases, Injuries and Causes of Death (ICD) or other classification system (e.g. OXMIS). First of all, however, it should be noted that the process of diagnose is fundamentally probabilistic and it is usually a matter of making choices amongst alternatives in the face of uncertainty (Rawson & Shatin, 2008).

Once more, with respect to ICD classification, it is important to note that ICD was primarily designed to record mortality and morbidity information, therefore, often signs, symptoms and less specific diagnoses are poorly recorded. When researchers use databases without detailed access to medical data, some diseases are impossible to study (outcomes poorly defined by ICD-9-CM), such as Stevens-Johnson Syndrome (Strom, 2001).

If hospitalization occurs, the discharge diagnosis is the primary source of information of a particular disease. One of the most basic outcomes of interest in pharmacoepidemiology is mortality. From the inpatient viewpoint, this can be easily identified from the discharge files. Nonetheless, from the outpatient standpoint, identifying mortality may require more effort;patient identity must be known and cross-checked with vital records (Harpe, 2009).

The number of diagnoses may diverge from institution to institution, with one code being identified as primary or principal diagnosis and all the other diagnoses (if extant) identified as secondary diagnosis. Because payments and reimbursements are linked to diagnosis codes, there may be a predisposition to include codes, within certain boundaries, that could increase the amount of money paid or reimbursed for a given diagnosis. Researchers should be aware that conditions that are likely to get a higher reimbursement or payment are more likely to be included as a discharge diagnosis (Harpe, 2011).

Here it is important to emphasize a crucial difference between the quality of outpatient diagnoses and inpatients diagnoses. With respect to claims data, if a patient goes to a hospital, the hospital charges for the care using an ICD (ICD-9-CM) code but also a Diagnosis Related Group (DGR). Hospitals employ people to code diagnosis for reimbursement and inpatient diagnosis are scrutinized for errors. Conversely, outpatient diagnoses are assigned by the practitioners themselves. In this case reimbursement does not depend on actual diagnosis, but on procedure codes used. Since there is no incentive to use ICD-9-CM diagnosis codes or to be careful and comprehensive - data are not audited in respect to this issue - outpatient diagnoses are the weakest link in claims databases (Strom, 2001; West *et al*, 2005). Other questions regarding data quality will be discussed later.

Procedures (e.g. inpatient procedures or those that are billed through the hospital or facility) and the utilization of services (e.g. counting the number of days in the hospital) may be also outcomes of interest.

Finally, results of laboratory tests may be surrogates of the outcome of interest. For example, low-density lipoprotein cholesterol and glycated hemoglobin (HbA1c) are surrogate measures for effectiveness of high cholesterol treatment and diabetes, respectively (Cox *et al*, 2009). The availability of these results varies from source to source, being more frequently recorded in electronic medical records. Administrative claims data usually have information about whether a laboratory test was ordered or not and not typically its results, unless both sources are properly linked. More commonly, administrative databases can identify final endpoints such as stroke, myocardial infraction or fractures.

In pharmacoepidemiology research, the primary exposure of interest is often the drug exposure. It must be noted however, that diseases, conditions or procedures may also be exposures of interest.

Drug use information in databases is not susceptible to recall and interviewer bias. Nevertheless, amongst databases we can find several degrees of accuracy. The most frequently used and the most accurate measurement of drug exposure is outpatient claims prescription/pharmacy records (Cox *et al*, 2009). When a patient goes to a pharmacy and gets a drug dispensed, the pharmacy bills the insurance carrier for the cost of that drug, and has to identify which medication was dispensed and all drug attributes (milligrams per tablet, number of tablets, etc.). Since this process involves reimbursement, claims are often audited which results in a high level of data quality (Strom, 2005b). This level of quality is also true for pharmacy records. Pharmacy records in the Netherlands can provide high quality data because there is universal computerization of pharmacy records and there have been strong regulatory and reimbursement incentives, over time, for Dutch patients to frequent a single pharmacy (and also a single GP). This enables the gathering of complete drug histories and therefore enhances the longitudinal nature of the medication data (Leufkens & Urquart, 2005).

In the case of prescription/pharmacy records, the uncertainty about whether a patient actually fills a prescription does not exist (unlike GPRD data), however the uncertainty still remains about whether the patient, after filling a prescription, actually takes the drug as prescribed. Studies based on prescription and dispensing records assume that most people who receive a prescription for a drug actually take it (Jick *et al*, 1991), because uncertainty would presumably be to a lesser degree.

Electronic medical records are another data source that may be used to identify drug exposure; recording whether the physician prescribed medication for the patient, the dose and the intended regimen. It is, however, much less accurate than claims/pharmacy records. In the U.S.A., it should be noted that FDA does not accept electronic medical records as a source for measuring drug exposure with respects to effectiveness assessment (Cox *et al*, 2009). Even so, prescription data in the GPRD are known to be well documented, since GPs use the computer to generate prescriptions and these are automatically recorded in the database (Herrett *et al*, 2010). It is also noteworthy that unlike medical records (where information about drug is often derived only from the GP and specialist-prescribed data are often not available), prescription claims from administrative databases (or pharmacy records) are derived from pharmacy billing records, regardless the prescriber (as long as the drug is dispensed by a pharmacy that submits a bill to the administrative system), and thus reflect all drugs dispensed.

Just like diseases, drugs are assigned codes in secondary databases. There is a clear need for a standardized classification system for drugs that can be used as a common language for describing and quantifying drug use. National Drug Code (NDC) and Anatomic Therapeutic Chemical Classification System (ATC) developed by World Health Organization are commonly used as drug classification systems. Even though these coding schemes can be used to measure categorical drug exposure (exposed *vs* non-exposed) it is also important to quantify drug exposure. We can use information available in prescription claims, pharmacy records or potentially in electronic medical records, and the amount of drug over the study period can be calculated for a given patient (total exposure) or transformed into a daily dose (average amount of drug per day). The identification of exposure date is essential and this is especially true when the outcome must be determined to have occurred after the exposure (Harper, 2011).

The ATC/DDD (defined daily dose) system is of paramount importance to drug utilization research in order to improve quality of drug use. The DDD is a stable drug utilization metric that enables comparisons of drug consumption between healthcare systems, regions and countries and therefore makes it possible to examine trends in drug use over time and in different contexts. This is the purpose for which the system was developed and it is with this purpose in mind that all decisions about ATC/DDD classification are made. Advantages and limitations of ATC/DDD system are presented elsewhere (Lee & Bergman, 2005; Wettermark *et al*, 2008).

2.2 Advantages and limitations of automated databases

The process of using databases for research involves careful selection and definition of research questions, using appropriate methods for analysis and interpretation of results, and selection of appropriate data sources. A thorough understanding of the advantages and limitations of data sources and methods is essential.

There are a number of clear advantages to using databases for pharmacoepidemiology research. These include allowing research to be conducted in a real-life setting, which permits the analysis of populations that are often excluded from clinical trials, particularly elderly people and women (Gurwitz *et al*, 1992; Lee, 2001). Databases can also help to enhance the representativeness of research. Some databases provide population-based data which cover the entire population of a region and are fully representative of the population (Assimes *et al*, 2009). Moreover, their large sample size (patient number ranging from several hundred thousand to several million) allows the study of drugs that are used relatively infrequently and rare effects in large population (Suissa, 2004).

Their computerized longitudinal data of routine clinical care facilitates drug utilization studies as well as the study of effectiveness and safety (including rare and late events, and also events from chronic exposure) in a real-world (Takahashi *et al*, 2011). Data are already collected and stored in computerized format in automated databases which means that research can be undertaken at a relatively low cost and the amount of time required to complete a study is reduced. Databases do not require informed patient consent and are therefore, less prone to bias from nonresponse (Suissa & Garbe, 2007).

Another advantage of databases is that they can demonstrate precise drug dispensing patterns since they avoid recall and interviewer bias, as they do not rely on patient recall or interviewers to obtain their data, a typical concern with primary data collection (Brenda *et al*, 1994).

Finally, as secondary databases may include a wide variety of data since they can link together various forms of healthcare information (Harpe, 2009) their applications vary broadly, including relative (comparative) effectiveness, cost-effectiveness, drug utilization, active safety surveillance, healthcare costs and resource use, among others (Takahashi *et al*, 2011).

Automated databases are not, however, without limitations. As mentioned above, administrative databases are typically designed for billing and record-keeping purposes and not for research. Even electronic medical records data are recorded as part of clinical patient care and again not for research purposes. The potential errors that may occur at many points during the record-keeping process were described by Schneeweiss and Avorn (Schneeweiss & Avorn, 2005).

The major weakness of automated databases is related to the quality of data inputted into them; the validity of diagnostic information contained in the database is often uncertain. This is especially true for administrative/claims databases (where diseases are primarily coded for "billing" and not for research purposes), particularly for outpatient data. However, it is less problematical for inpatient diagnosis and for health medical records (Strom, 2005b), as discussed below.

Databases, particularly administrative databases, lack information on some potential confounding variables, namely data on smoking, alcohol consumption, date of menopause/menarche and reproductive history in women, physical activity, occupation, etc. In addition, information about disease severity is frequently lacking and therefore it may not be possible to exclude confounding by disease severity (Strom *et al*, 1991). All these variables can be of great importance to investigate specific research questions (Park & Stergachis, 2008).

Obtaining medical records to evaluate the validity of diagnosis data (especially when the outcome is poorly defined by the diagnostic coding system) can be essential. However, it is not always easy to get access to primary medical records to collect this data, or other data related to patient's clinical care, due to privacy and legal issues (Mackenzie *et al*, 2011), or simply because it is not available. Even when it is available, this is a time-consuming and an expensive process (Rawson & Shattin, 2008).

Databases often do not include data on medications obtained without a prescription (e.g. Over-the-Counter (OTC)) which may be responsible for drawbacks in the assessment of associations between non-prescription medicines and diseases (Ilkhanoff *et al*, 2005) or lacking as a confounder variable. Similarly, medication obtained outside of a particular insurance carrier's prescription plan, for example in U.S.A., represents also a limitation (Strom, 2005b).

Finally, high membership turnover at Health Maintenance Organization can lead to population instability over time (Schneeweiss & Avorn, 2005). This means that data might not be representative of the population being studied (some databases cover the entire population, while others, for example cover the elderly or low-income or those who have higher educational achievements). These are limitations that should be taken into consideration particularly when using administrative databases for pharmacoepidemiological research.

2.3 Evaluation of the quality of automated databases for pharmacoepidemiology research: An emphasis on validity and completeness

As research becomes increasingly focused on real-world data, including automated databases, it is imperative to know how to evaluate the quality of these data sources.

In order to assess the association between drug use and outcome (adverse or beneficial effects) throughout databases, two fundamental concerns should guide the evaluation of data sources: validity and completeness. Deep awareness of these issues is crucial, as emphasized by van Staa's critique of a recent validation study of a database (van Staa & Parkinson, 2008).

Errors in estimation are conventionally classified as either random or systematic. Both types of errors can occur in measuring exposure and outcome. Systematic errors are commonly referred as bias; the opposite of bias is validity, hence a valid estimate has little systematic error. In the same way, an estimate with little random error is considered precise, thus the opposite of random error is precision. Validity and precision are both components of accuracy. Furthermore, validity is usually broadly divided in two components: internal validity (*the validity of the inferences drawn as they pertain to the member of study population)* and external validity or generalizability (*the validity of inferences as they pertain to people outside the population)* (Rothman *et al*, 2008). These key definitions should always be considered when assessing the quality of databases.

Misclassification of drug exposure and outcomes can occur and lead to bias (misclassification bias) with the magnitude and direction of bias depending on the mechanism of the misclassification (Csizmadi & Collet, 2005). The validity of drug exposure and outcomes, as well as covariates, can be measured by their sensitivity and specificity. Sensitivity of exposure or outcome information is defined as the proportion of all drug exposures or health outcomes - that are truly exposed or truly have the health outcome - in the covered population that appear in the database and therefore are classified as exposed or are positive for the health outcome. The specificity of a database with respect to drug exposure or to health outcome refers to its capability in ensuring that patients classified as unexposed or negative for the outcome are done so correctly (Rothman *et al*, 2008; Park & Stergachis, 2008).

A way to measure the validity of outcomes and exposures using databases is to compare it with a gold standard. In terms of outcome measures in administrative databases, the gold standard is often the medical record or patient self-report, these contain a high level of specificity but a great deal of variability in sensitivity across diagnoses (Strom, 2001; Wilchesky *et al*, 2004). However, Schneeweiss & Avorn have argued that a lack of specificity in the outcome measurement is worse than a lack of sensitivity in most situations and highlighted the fact that if specificity of the outcome assessment is 100% then relative risk estimates are therefore unbiased (Schneeweiss & Avorn, 2005). This brings up the idea that, for certain conditions, outpatient diagnosis derived from administrative databases are not of such poor quality. One the other hand, generally speaking, it is important to note that the validity of diagnosis data amongst medical records data is better than in claims databases, as these data are being used for medical care and not just for billing purposes.

Missing subjects, exposures or events could also introduce bias in the study results. As an illustration, a bias may be introduced in the association between a serious adverse drug reaction if hospitalizations due to that adverse reaction are missing from the database (Hartzema *et al*, 2011). Another example is connected to potentially stigmatizing diagnoses which often may be more likely written in free text data, to avoid occurrence in summary records (false negative). Evans and colleagues have estimated that only 50% of HIV patients have their diagnosis coded in their primary care records (Evans *et al*, 2009).

For reason previously mentioned in this chapter, prescription claims/pharmacy records provide some of the best data in pharmacoepidemiology. A Dutch study investigated the validity of medicine exposure measurement based on pharmacy records compared with home inventory and concluded that pharmacy records can be a reliable source of the true medicine exposure when adequate attention is given to the definition time window and when these records are comprehensive with regard to prescription drugs (Lau *et al*, 1997). However, as mentioned before, since there is no information about compliance with therapy, uncertainty arises about true drug consumption.

Another issue that should be considered when interpreting results derived from studies conducted through databases is the importance of evaluating testing bias. Laboratory testing in clinical practice is never a random process (physicians selectively request tests for patients with a high probability of abnormalities and *vice versa*) which means results obtained from databases may be biased due to testing bias and, therefore, in certain circumstances need careful interpretation. A study conducted by Velthove and colleagues demonstrated that requests for neutrophil counts in the Utrecht Patient Oriented Database were associated with the underlying disease and particularly with cardiovascular disease, emphasizing the importance of evaluating this type of bias in databases studies' context (Velthove *et al*, 2010). Moreover, when analyzing trends over time, we need to be aware of certain issues regarding laboratory test result recording, particularly the availability of laboratory tests' recording codes and its results in the database (Dial *et al*, 2005).

The generalizability (external validity) of a database can be defined as the degree to which the population covered by the database is representative of the total population. At a glance, generalizability of a database can be assessed by: 1) statistical comparison of socio-demographic information (age, gender, education level, occupation, among others) between the population covered by the database and the external target population or 2) evaluation of eligibility criteria for enrollment defined by the organizations' owners. Little hard evidence is available about generalizability, however, concern has been raised about the applicability of data from Health Maintenance Organization plans in U.S.A. to the broader population (Park & Stergachis, 2008; (Strom, 2005b). As a result, careful interpretation of different results derived from different databases should be given, since like for like comparisons may not be possible considering the different populations with different attributes.

Taking into consideration the diversity of characteristics in databases, Park and Stergachis have defined completeness of data coverage as the extent to which all filled prescriptions, all coded diagnoses for outpatient visits and hospitalizations, exposure to non-prescription medications, and potential confounding patient factors appear as variables in the database (Park & Stergachis, 2008). In other words, completeness can be defined as the proportion of all cases (exposures and outcomes) that occurred in the population covered by the database that is recorded.

Finally, it should be noted that given the importance of this matter, the International Society of Pharmacoepidemiology has developed guidelines for conduct in database research in pharmacoepidemiology in order to assist researchers in the selection and use of databases, highlighting limitations and quality and validation procedures (Hall *et al*, 2011). Nevertheless, given its utility in the field and the number of promising databases developments that are in the horizon, ongoing updates should be put in place (Rothman & Poole, 2007).

3. Use of automated databases: Pitfalls and methodological challenges

The nonrandomized world of research on drug effects is complex, certainly more complex than the world of randomized trials (Schneeweiss, 2009). Methods and strategies employed to evaluate intended and unintended drug effects in a real-life context require rigorous epidemiology. Contrary to any preconceptions, the use of databases for pharmacoepidemiology research is challenging - "*It is not a simple process of get some data and do some statistics*" (Harpe, 2009). Challenges of conducting studies throughout databases include concerns about study design, careful understanding of the underlying health care system in which the data were generated, data quality, limited ability to control confounding in the absence of randomization and to handle bias, and data analysis, among others (Berger *et al*, 2009).

For over two decades ago, the growing enthusiasm for automated databases went together with harsh criticism. In 1989, Samuel Shapiro criticized several studies that had been published in the 1980s without adequate appraisal of data, study design and epidemiologic methods which had, in turn, led to spurious conclusions (Shapiro, 1989a). At that time, Shapiro claimed that the basic concepts of pharmacoepidemiology should not be abandoned as a result of using the so-called "modern" automated databases and argued that the basics (e.g. use of proper definitions of outcome an exposure, addressing bias and confounding, etc.) should be kept in mind when using those sources of information. This publication raised a lot of controversy and an extensive methodological soap opera about this issue was set in place (Strom, 1989; Faich & Stadel, 1989; Strom & Carson, 1989; Shapiro, 1989b; Tilson *et al*, 1989; Jick & Walker, 1989).

Advances in both epidemiology and biostatistics, over the past 20 years, including sophisticated software for analysis, have allowed novel methods for addressing confounding and bias to develop and despite the known limitations of databases, poor quality in conducting and reporting pharmacoepidemiologic studies still exits and there is definitely room for improvement. There are several examples of poorly conducted database studies that were published, even in the top journals with the highest impact factors (Suissa, 2007).

In the first decade of this century, observational studies showed surprising results associated with the use of statins. Statins were a kind of nonspecific miracle drug, reducing: fracture rate by 50% (Meier *et al*, 2000), rate of dementia by 71%(Jick *et al*, 2000), rate of depression by 60% and rate of suicidal behavior by 50%(Yang *et al*, 2003), all causes of mortality in patients with chronic obstructive pulmonary disease (COPD) (Søyseth *et al*, 2007), amongst others miracles - statin treatment was good for everything! A lot of interesting theories were developed to explain these associations, leaving often basic clinical pharmacology and epidemiologic principles behind. In addition to the classic example of statins, several other studies conducted through health-care databases have reported impressive results for commonly used drugs, for example, in reducing all–cause mortality (Hippisley-Cox & Coupland, 2005). The problem has appeared when discordance in the results of pharmacoepidemiology studies were revealed, either in studies that use different sources of information (different databases) or even in those that are conducted in the same database! For example, various studies have used the UK General Practice Research Database (GPRD) to evaluate the same side effects of drugs, often arriving at opposite conclusions. Associations between statins and fracture (de Vries *et al*, 2006); and oral bisphosphonates and cancer (de Vries F, 2010), are just a few examples, but there are several other, whether conducted with different or with the same database.

On which study is drug-therapy decision making based? (Etminan *et al*, 2006). How can investigator choices that may change results (investigator bias) be dealt with? The existence of guidelines and forms by themselves probably will not change this picture. Although sometimes neglected, understanding methodological issues and training basic epidemiology are essential.

Pharmacoepidemiology database research is challenging for researchers, peer- reviewers, editors and readers of medical journals (Suissa, 2007). Some pitfalls and methodological challenges are illustrated below.

- Immortal time bias

  Immortal time in epidemiology refers to a period of follow-up during which, by design, death or the outcome of the study cannot occur (Rothman & Greenland, 2008). This bias was first identified in the 70s in the context of heart transplantation research (survival benefit of heart transplantation) and recently reappeared in pharmacoepidemiology, particularly in studies conducted through databases, reporting that several drugs can be extremely effective at reducing morbidity and mortality (Suissa, 2008).

  Several poorly analyzed studies employed a time-fixed definition of exposure to emulate an intention-to-treat analysis used by clinical trials. This principle assumes that subjects are exposed to the drug under study immediately at the start of follow-up, which cannot occur in the real-world and, in fact, it is unknown in databases studies. Immortal time can arise when the period between cohort entry and date of first exposure, e.g., to a drug, during which death/outcome has not occurred, is either classified or excluded and therefore not accounted for in the analysis. As a result, immortal time bias is particularly problematic because it necessarily biases the results in favour of treatment under study by conferring a spurious survival advantage to the study group (Lévesque *et al*, 2010). The appropriate approach to data analysis requires that all immortal time be accounted for fully, including that before the start of exposure, and therefore it will be correctly classified in terms of exposure. The extent of the bias will depend directly on the amount of total person-time misclassified or excluded. Consequently, the longer the exposure window, the larger the bias (Suissa, 2007).

  Although these biases have been typically approached in cohort studies conducted using databases, they can occur also in case-control studies, since most of case-control studies in pharmacoepidemiology are conducted using databases as well, and subsequently it is essential to ensure an equal time-window to measure exposure for cases and for controls (Suissa *et al*, 2011). In these studies, if time is not properly considered in selection of controls, an artificial appearance of effectiveness for the drug will be generated.

Recently, Samy Suissa has illustrated time-related biases in 20 published studies – most of them in several respected journals and claimed for a re-assessment of all those studies for immortal time bias (Suissa, 2007).

- Confounding (by indication bias)

  Confounding is a challenging threat to validity in nonrandomized studies of drug effects. Automated databases, especially administrative databases, have been criticized for the incompleteness of their information on potential confounders (OTC medication, life-style habits, smoking status, body mass index, markers of clinical disease severity, among others).

  Moreover, such factors may lead to selective prescribing of drugs, which may, in turn, result in biased estimates of the association between drugs and outcomes - confounding by indication (Walker, 1996). Thus, the prescription of a drug is based on diagnostic and prognostic information available at the time of prescribing and also other factors such as behavioral characteristics from both physician and patient. Generally speaking, a drug is more likely to be prescribed to a patient with more severe diseases who, in turn, is more likely to experience an adverse outcome of the disease. The problem of confounding by indication can be illustrated in a way that is very similar to selection bias. The basic idea is that subjects who receive a certain drug are intrinsically different from those patients not receiving the drug.

  Strategies to adjust such confounding vary depending on whether the potential confounders are measured in a certain database. If confounders are measured in a certain database, then the usually strategies for controlling confounding can be applied: restriction, stratification, matching, and multivariable modeling (Schneeweiss & Avorn, 2005).

  On the other hand, confounding by indication is extremely difficult to control, even when the reason for prescribing is straightforward, mainly because the precise reason to prescribe is rarely measured. That is because "indication" is a complex and a multifactorial phenomenon, as described above (Csizmadi & Collet, 2005). Thus, control for confounding for indication, if possible, should be tackled at the design level (e.g. by restricting the study to a group of patients homogeneous with respect to disease severity or by comparing two drugs only for the same indication).

  Studies with potential confounding by indication can benefit from other appropriate analytic methods, explained below, including separating the effects of a drug taken at different times, sensitivity analysis for unmeasured confounders and instrumental variables.

  Sensitivity analysis is defined as a quantitative analysis of the potential for systematic error (Csizmadi & Collet, 2005). Basic sensitivity analyses of residual confounding (unmeasured confounders) try to determine how strong and how imbalanced a confounder would have to be among drug categories to explained the observed effect

(Schneeweiss & Avorn, 2005). Schneeweiss provided a systematic approach to sensitivity analyses to investigate the impact of residual confounding in studies conducted through databases and argued for a more frequent application of sensitivity analyses and external adjustments, substituting qualitative discussions of residual confounding (Schneeweiss, 2006).

Propensity scores and instrumental variables can be used to approximate the random allocation process. Propensity score is defined as the conditional probability of being treated, given an individual's covariates, the objective of propensity score is to simulate RCT treatment groups in order to estimate a causal treatment effect (Csizmadi & Collet, 2005). The purpose of propensity scores is to create groups that are similar with respect to all measured characteristics except treatment status (Wang & Donnan, 2001). The propensity score analyses, however, cannot address the issue of bias when there are important variables not included in the propensity score estimation (Johnson *et al,* 2009). If several conditions are fulfilled, instrumental variables (IV) have the potential to estimate unbiased estimates in databases studies (Brookhart, 2010). IV have the potential to adjust for all confounders, whether observed or not. The idea is that the causal effect of exposure on outcome can be captured by using the relationship between the exposure and another variable, the IV (Martens *et al*, 2006).

The use of all these methods is complex and requires extensive training, careful implementation, and appropriate balanced interpretation of findings (Murray, 2010; Johnson *et al,* 2009).

4. Conclusion

Bradford-Hill said that "*all scientific work is incomplete – whether it be observational or experimental. All scientific work is liable to be upset or modified by advancing knowledge. That does not confer upon us a freedom to ignore the knowledge we already have, or to postpone the action that it appears to demand at a given time*". This is especially true in the context of medicines' assessment. Society demands an answer to bridge the gap between clinical trials and real-world.

The increasing availability of large automated healthcare databases represents a unique opportunity to study the landscape of drug use patterns and both beneficial and adverse drug effects in routine clinical practice. But, research on the assessment of medicines under real-life conditions is methodologically complex and can be challenging. It will not infrequently result in biased drug effects estimates if epidemiological principles are not followed.

In recent decades, we have already learned much more about healthcare databases appropriate role in pharmacoepidemiology research. A clear and comprehensive understanding of the strengths and weaknesses of pharmacoepidemiological methods, of how the data were collected, enrollment and coverage factors, approaches to minimize confounding in the absence of randomization, the specificity of clinical outcome assessment amongst other factors that might have affected data quality and validity is essential.

The trend of utilization of healthcare databases for pharmacoepidemiology will continue to increase in coming years. But this must be unquestionably accompanied with high capacity building in this field.

There have been lessons learned, but there are challenges ahead. Knowing what those numbers mean for practice and communicating their meaning effectively will be ultimately one of the biggest real life challenges.

5. Acknowledgements

We would like to gratefully acknowledge Adam Standring and Sarah Fernandes for the linguistic revision of this chapter.

6. Disclosures

The views and opinions expressed in this chapter reflect the personal opinions of the authors and not necessarily the views of institutions or organizations with which they are affiliated with.

7. References

Arana A, Rivero E, Egberts TCG. (2004). What do we show and who does so? An analyses of the abstracts presented at the 19th ICPE. Proceedings of the 20th International Conference on Pharmacoepidemiology & Therapeutic Risk Management, Bordeaux, 22-25 August 2004. *Pharmacoepidemiol Drug Saf*, Vol 13:S330-1 (August 2004).

Assimes TL & Suissa S. (2009). Age at incident treatment of hypertension and risk of cancer: a population study. *Cancer Causes Control*, Vol. 20, No.10, (December 2009), pp. 1811-20.

Berger ML, Mamdani M, Atkins D & Johnson ML. (2009). Good research practices for comparative effectiveness research: defining, reporting and interpreting nonrandomized studies of treatment effects using secondary data sources: the ISPOR Good Research Practices for Retrospective Database Analysis Task Force Report--Part I. *Value Health*, Vol. 12, N° 8, (November-December 2009), pp. 1044-52.

Black N. (1996). Why we need observational studies to evaluate the effectiveness of health care. *BMJ*, Vol. 11, No. 312 (7040), (May 1996), pp. 1215-8.

Blake KV, Prilla S, Accadebled S, Guimier M, Biscaro M, Persson I, Arlett P, Blackburn S & Fitt H. (2011). European Medicines Agency review of post-authorisation studies with implications for the European Network of Centres for Pharmacoepidemiology and Pharmacovigilance. *Pharmacoepidemiol Drug Saf*, Vol. 20, No. 10, (October 2011), pp. 1021-9.

Brookhart MA, Rassen JA & Schneeweiss S. (2010). Instrumental variable methods in comparative safety and effectiveness research. *Pharmacoepidemiol Drug Saf*, Vol. 19, No. 6, (June 2010 Jun), pp. 537-54.

Bourbeau J, Ernst P, Cockcoft D & Suissa S. (2003). Inhaled corticosteroids and hospitalisation due to exacerbation of COPD. *Eur Respir J*, Vol. 22, No. 2, (August 2003), pp. 286-9.

Csizmadi I & Collet JP. (2005). Bias and confounding in Pharmacoepidemiology. *In Pharmacoepidemiology*, Strom, BL, pp. 791-809. John Wiley & Sons, ISBN 13 978-0-470-86681-8, Chichester, UK.

Coloma PM, Schuemie MJ, Trifirò G, Gini R, Herings R, Hippisley-Cox J, Mazzaglia G, Giaquinto C, Corrao G, Pedersen L, van der Lei J & Sturkenboom M; EU-ADR Consortium. (2011). Combining electronic healthcare databases in Europe to allow for large-scale drug safety monitoring: the EU-ADR Project. *Pharmacoepidemiol Drug Saf*, Vol. 20, No. 1, pp. 1-11.

Cox E, Martin BC, Van Staa T, Garbe E, Siebert U & Johnson ML. (2009) Good research practices for comparative effectiveness research: approaches to mitigate bias and confounding in the design of nonrandomized studies of treatment effects using secondary data sources: the International Society for Pharmacoeconomics and Outcomes Research Good Research Practices for Retrospective Database Analysis Task Force Report--Part II. *Value Health*, Vol. 12, No. 8, (November-December 2009) pp. 1053-61.

de Vries F. (2010). Bisphosphonates and cancer. Two studies, same data source, two answers. *BMJ*, (October 2010), 341: doi: 10.1136/bmj.c5980.

de Vries F, de Vries C, Cooper C, Leufkens B & van Staa TP. (2006). Reanalysis of two studies with contrasting results on the association between statin use and fracture risk: the General Practice Research Database. *Int J Epidemiol*, Vol. 35, No. 5, (October 2006), pp. 1301-8.

Dial S, Delaney JA, Barkun AN & Suissa S. (2005). Use of gastric acid-suppressive agents and the risk of community-acquired Clostridium difficile-associated disease. *JAMA*, Vol. 294, No. 23, (December 2005), pp. 2989-95.

Dreyer NA, Garner S. Registries for robust evidence. (2009). *JAMA*, Vol. 302, No. 7, (August 2009), pp. 790-1.

Dunn HL (1946). Record linkage. *Am J Public Health Nations Health*, Vol. 36, No. 12, (December 1946), pp. 1412-6.

Eichler HG, Abadie E, Breckenridge A, Flamion B, Gustafsson LL, Leufkens H, Rowland M, Schneider CK & Bloechl-Daum B. (2011). Bridging the efficacy-effectiveness gap: a regulator's perspective on addressing variability of drug response. *Nat Rev Drug Discov*. Vol. 10, No. 7, (July 2011), pp. 495-506.

Eichler HG, Bloechl-Daum B, Abadie E, Barnett D, König F & Pearson S. (2010). Relative efficacy of drugs: an emerging issue between regulatory agencies and third-party payers. *Nat Rev Drug Discov*, Vol. 9, No. 4, (April 2010), pp. 277-91.

Eichler HG, Pignatti F, Flamion B, Leufkens H & Breckenridge A. (2008). Balancing early market access to new drugs with the need for benefit/risk data: a mounting dilemma. *Nat Rev Drug Discov*. Vol. 7, No 10, (October 2008), pp. 818-26.

Elseviers MM, Ferech M, Vander Stichele RH & Goossens H: ESAC project group. (2007). Antibiotic use in ambulatory care in Europe (ESAC data 1997-2002): trends, regional differences and seasonal fluctuations. *Pharmacoepidemiol Drug Saf*, Vol. 16, No. 1, (January 2007), pp. 115-23.

Etminan M, Gill S, Fitzgerald M & Samii A. (2006). Challenges and opportunities for pharmacoepidemiology in drug-therapy decision making. *J Clin Pharmacol*, Vol. 46, No. 1, (January 2006), pp. 6-9.

European Network of Centres for Pharmacoepidemiology and Pharmacovigilance (ENCePP). (2011). *Guide on Methodological Standards in Pharmacoepidemiology*, European Medicines Agency. Retrieved from: http://www.encepp.eu/standards_and_guidances/documents/ENCePPGuideofMethStandardsinPE.pdf.

Evans HE, Mercer CH, Rait G, Hamill M, Delpech V, Hughes G, Brook MG, Williams T, Johnson AM, Singh S, Petersen I, Chadborn T & Cassell JA. (2009). Trends in HIV testing and recording of HIV status in the UK primary care setting: a retrospective cohort study 1995-2005. *Sex Transm Infect*, Vol. 85, No. 7, (December 2009), pp. 520-6.

Faich GA & Stadel BV. (1989). The future of automated record linkage for postmarketing surveillance: a response to Shapiro. *Clin Pharmacol Ther.* Vol. 46, No. 4, (October 1989), pp. 387-9.

Florentinus SR, Souverein PC, Griens FA, Groenewegen PP, Leufkens HG & Heerdink ER. (2006). Linking community pharmacy dispensing data to prescribing data of general practitioners. *BMC Med Inform Decis Mak*, Vol. 6, No. 18, (April 2006), doi:10.1186/1472-6947-6-18

Garattini S & Chalmers I. (2009). Patients and the public deserve big changes in evaluation of drugs. *BMJ*, Vol. 338, (April 2009), pp. 804-806.

García Rodríguez LA, Herings R & Johansson S. (2010). Use of multiple international healthcare databases for the detection of rare drug-associated outcomes: a pharmacoepidemiological programme comparing rosuvastatin with other marketed statins. *Pharmacoepidemiol Drug Saf*, Vol. 19, No. 12, (December 2010), pp. 1218-24.

Geleedst-De Vooght M, Maitland-van der Zee AH, Schalekamp T, Mantel-Teeuwisse A & Jansen P. (2010). Statin prescribing in the elderly in the Netherlands: a pharmacy database time trend study. *Drugs Aging*. Vol. 27, No. 7, (July 2010), pp. 589-96.

Gelfand J, Margolis J & Dattani H. (2005). The UK General Practice Research Database. In *Pharmacoepidemiology*, Strom, B.L, pp 337-346. John Wiley & Sons, ISBN 13 978-0-470-86681-8, Chichester, UK.

Goettsch WG, Janknegt R & Herings RM. (2004). Increased treatment failure after 3-days' courses of nitrofurantoin and trimethoprim for urinary tract infections in women: a population-based retrospective cohort study using the PHARMO database. *Br J Clin Pharmacol*, Vol. 58, No. 2, (August 2004), pp. 184-9.

Gulliford MC, van Staa T, McDermott L, Dregan A, McCann G, Ashworth M, Charlton J, Grieve AP, Little P, Moore MV & Yardley L; electronic Cluster Randomised Trial Research Team eCRT Research Team. (2011). Cluster randomised trial in the General Practice Research Database: 1. Electronic decision support to reduce antibiotic prescribing in primary care (eCRT study). *Trials*, Vol. 12, No. 115 (May 2011).

Gurwitz JH, Col NF & Avorn J. (1992). The exclusion of the elderly and women from clinical trials in acute myocardial infarction. *JAMA*, Vol. 268, No. 11, (September 1992), pp. 1417-22.

Hall GC, Sauer B, Bourke A, Jeffrey SB, Reynolds MW & LoCasale R. (2011). Guidelines for quality conduct in database research in pharmacoepidemiology. International Society of Pharmacoepidemiology. Available from: http://www.pharmacoepi.org/ resources/Quality_Database_Conduct_2-28-11.pdf.

Hallas J. (2005). Drug utilization statistics for individual-level pharmacy dispensing data. *Pharmacoepidemiol Drug Saf,* Vol. 14, No. 7, (July 2005), pp. 455-63.

Harpe SE. (2011). Using Secondary Data in Pharmacoepidemiology. In *Understanding Pharmacoepidemiology,* Yang Y & West-Strum D, pp. 55-77. McGrraw-Hill, ISBN 978-0-07-163500-4, USA.

Harpe SE. (2009). Using secondary data sources for pharmacoepidemiology and outcomes research. *Pharmacotherapy,* Vol. 29, No. 2, (February 2009), pp. 138-53.

Hartzema, A.G., Tilson, H.H. & Chan KA (Eds.) (2008). *Pharmacoepidemiology and Therapeutic Management.* (1st edition), Harvey Whitney Books, ISBN 978-0929375-30-4, Cincinnati, OH, USA.

Haynes B. (1999). Can it work? Does it work? Is it worth it? The testing of healthcare interventions is evolving. *BMJ,* Vol. 379, No. 7211, (September 1999), pp. 652-3.

Hennessy S. (2006). Use of health care databases in pharmacoepidemiology. *Basic Clin Pharmacol Toxicol,* Vol. 98, No. 3, (March 2006), pp. 311-3.

Hemmelgarn B, Blais L, Collet JP, Ernst JP & Suissa S (1994). Automated databases and the need for fielwork in Pharmacoepidemiology. *Pharmacoepidemiol Drug Saf,* Vol. 3, No.4, (July 1994), pp. 275-82.

Herrett E, Thomas SL, Schoonen WM, Smeeth L & Hall AJ. (2010). Validation and validity of diagnoses in the General Practice Research Database: a systematic review. *Br J Clin Pharmacol,* Vol. 69, No. 1, (January 2010), pp. 4-14.

Hippisley-Cox J & Coupland C. (2005) Effect of combinations of drugs on all cause mortality in patients with ischaemic heart disease: nested case-control analysis. *BMJ,* Vol. 330, No. 7499, (May 2005), pp. 1059-63.

Hulley S, Cummings S, Browner W, Grady D, Newman T. (2007). *Designing Clinical Research.* (3rd edition), Lippincott Williams&Wilkins, ISBN-13: 978-0-7817-8210-4, Philadelphia, USA.

Ilkhanoff L, Lewis JD, Hennessy S, Berlin JA & Kimmel SE. (2005). Potential limitations of electronic database studies of prescription non-aspirin non-steroidal anti-inflammatory drugs (NANSAIDs) and risk of myocardial infarction (MI). *Pharmacoepidemiol Drug Saf,* Vol. 14, No. 8, (August 2005), pp. 513-22.

Jick H, Zornberg GL, Jick SS, Seshadri S & Drachman DA. (2000). Statins and the risk of dementia. *Lancet,* Vol. 356, No. 9242, (November 2000), pp. 1627-31.

Jick H, Jick SS & Derby LE. Validation of information recorded on general practitioner based computerised data resource in the United Kingdom. *BMJ,* Vol. 302, No. 6779, (March 1991), pp. 766-8.

Jick H & Walker AM. (1989). Uninformed criticism of automated record linkage. *Clin Pharmacol Ther,* Vol. 46, No. 4, (October 1989), pp. 478-9.

Johnson ML, Crown W, Martin BC, Dormuth CR & Siebert U. (2009). Good research practices for comparative effectiveness research: analytic methods to improve causal inference from nonrandomized studies of treatment effects using secondary data sources: the ISPOR Good Research Practices for Retrospective Database Analysis Task Force Report--Part III. *Value Health,* Vol. 12, No. 8, (November-December 2009), pp. 1062-73.

Lau HS, de Boer A, Beuning KS & Porsius A. (1997). Validation of pharmacy records in drug exposure assessment. *J Clin Epidemiol,* Vol. 50, No. 5, (May 1997), pp. 619-25.

Lee D & Bergman U. (2005). Studies of drug utilization. In *Pharmacoepidemiology*, Strom, BL, pp. 401-417. John Wiley & Sons, ISBN 13 978-0-470-86681-8, Chichester, UK.

Lee PY, Alexander KP, Hammill BG, Pasquali SK & Peterson ED. (2001). Representation of elderly persons and women in published randomized trials of acute coronary syndromes. *JAMA*, Vol. 286, No. 6, (August 2001), pp. 708-13.

Leufkens HG & Urquart J. (2005). Automated Pharmacy Record Linkage in The Netherlands. In *Pharmacoepidemiology*, Strom, BL, pp. 311-322. John Wiley & Sons, ISBN 13 978-0-470-86681-8, Chichester, UK.

Lévesque LE, Hanley JA, Kezouh A & Suissa S. (2010). Problem of immortal time bias in cohort studies: example using statins for preventing progression of diabetes. *BMJ*, Vol. 340, No. b5087, (March 2010), pp. 907-911.

Mackenzie IS, Mantay BJ, McDonnell PG, Wei L & MacDonald TM. (2011). Managing security and privacy concerns over data storage in healthcare research. *Pharmacoepidemiol Drug Saf.* Vol. 20, No. 8, (August 2011), pp. 885-93.

Martens EP, Pestman WR, de Boer A, Belitser SV, Klungel OH. (2006). Instrumental variables: application and limitations. *Epidemiology*, Vol.17, No 3, (May 2006), pp. 260-7.

Meier CR, Schlienger RG, Kraenzlin ME, Schlegel B & Jick H. (2000). HMG-CoA reductase inhibitors and the risk of fractures. *JAMA*, Vol. 283, No. 24, (June 2000), pp. 3205-10.

Montori VM, Devereaux PJ, Adhikari NK, Burns KE, Eggert CH, Briel M, Lacchetti C, Leung TW, Darling E, Bryant DM, Bucher HC, Schünemann HJ, Meade MO, Cook DJ, Erwin PJ, Sood A, Sood R, Lo B, Thompson CA, Zhou Q, Mills E & Guyatt GH. (2005) Randomized trials stopped early for benefit: a systematic review. *JAMA*, Vol. 294, No. 17, (November 2005), pp. 2203-9.

Murray MD. (2011). Curricular considerations for pharmaceutical comparative effectiveness research. *Pharmacoepidemiol Drug Saf*, Vol. 20, No. 8, (August 2011), pp. 797-804.

Park BJ & Stergachis A. (2008). Automated databases in Pharmacoepidemiologic studies. In *Pharmacoepidemiology and Therapeutic Management*, Hartzema, AG, Tilson, HH, Chan KA (Eds.). Harvey Whitney Books, ISBN 978-0929375-30-4, Cincinnati, OH, USA.

Porta, M , Greenland S & Last M (Ed.). (2008). A Dictionary of Epidemiology (5th edition), Oxford Universuty Press, ISBN 978-0-19-531449-6, New York, USA.

Pouwels S, Lalmohamed A, Souverein P, Cooper C, Veldt BJ, Leufkens HG, de Boer A, van Staa T & de Vries F. (2011). Use of proton pump inhibitors and risk of hip/femur fracture: a population-based case-control study. *Osteoporos Int*, Vol. 22, No. 3, (March 2011), pp. 903-10.

Rawson N. (2009). Access to linked administrative healthcare utilization data for pharmacoepidemiology and pharmacoeconomics research in Canada: anti-viral drugs as an example. *Pharmacoepidemiol Drug Saf*, Vol. 18, No. 11, (November 2009), pp. 1072-9.

Rawson N & Shatin D. (2008). Assessing the validity of diagnostic data in large administrative healthcare utilization databases. In *Pharmacoepidemiology and Therapeutic Management*, Hartzema, AG, Tilson, HH, Chan KA (Eds.), pp 495-518. Harvey Whitney Books, ISBN 978-0929375-30-4, Cincinnati, OH, USA.

Roehr B. (2008). Trial participants need to be more representative of patients. *BMJ*, Vol. 336: 737.1, (April 2008).

Rothman KJ, Greenland S & Lash Timothy. (2008). Validity in Epidemiologic Studies. In *Modern Epidemiology* (3rd edition), Rothman KJ, Greenland S, Lash Timothy (Eds.), pp 128-147. Lippincott Williams & Wilkins, ISBN: 978-0-7817-5564-1, Philadelphia, USA.

Rothman KJ & Greenland S. (2008). Cohort Studies. In *Modern Epidemiology* (3rd edition), Rothman KJ, Greenland S, Lash Timothy (Eds.), pp 100-110. Lippincott Williams & Wilkins, ISBN: 978-0-7817-5564-1, Philadelphia, USA.

Rothman KJ & Poole C. (2007). Some guidelines on guidelines: they should come with expiration dates. *Epidemiology*, Vol. 18, No. 6, (November 2007), pp. 794-6.

Shatin D. (2001). Organizational context and taxonomy of health care databases. *Pharmacoepidemiol Drug Saf*, Vol. 10, No. 5, (August-September 2001), pp. 367-71.

Schneeweiss S. (2009). On guidelines for comparative effectiveness research using nonrandomized studies in secondary data sources. *Value Health*, Vol. 12, No. 8, (November-December 2009), pp. 1041.

Schneeweiss S. (2006). Sensitivity analysis and external adjustment for unmeasured confounders in epidemiologic database studies of therapeutics. *Pharmacoepidemiol Drug Saf*. Vol. 15, No. 5, (May 2006), pp. 291-303.

Schneeweiss S & Avorn J. (2005). A review of uses of health care utilization databases for epidemiologic research on therapeutics. *J Clin Epidemiol*, Vol. 58, No. 4, (April 2005), pp. 323-37.

Shapiro S. (1989a) The role of automated record linkage in the postmarketing surveillance of drug safety: a critique. *Clin Pharmacol Ther*, Vol. 46, No. 4, (October 1989), pp. 371-86.

Shapiro S. (1989b) Automated record linkage: a response to the commentary and letters to the editor. *Clin Pharmacol Ther*, Vol. 46, No. 4, (October 1989), pp. 395-8.

Søyseth V, Brekke PH, Smith P & Omland T. (2003). Statin use is associated with reduced mortality in COPD. *Eur Respir J*, Vol. 29, No. 2, (February 2007), pp. 279-83.

Strom, BL. (Ed.). (2005a). *Pharmacoepidemiology* (4th edition), John Wiley & Sons, ISBN 13 978-0-470-86681-8, Chichester, UK.

Strom, BL. (2005b). Overview of Automated Databases in Pharmacoepidemiology. In *Pharmacoepidemiology*, Strom BL, pp 219-222. John Wiley & Sons, ISBN 13 978-0-470-86681-8, Chichester, UK.

Strom, BL. Keynote Address. 20th International Conference on Pharmacoepidemiology & Therapeutic Risk Management, Bordeaux, France, August 22-25, 2004.

Strom BL. (2001). Data validity issues in using claims data. *Pharmacoepidemiol Drug Saf*, Vol. 10, No. 5, (August-September 2001), pp. 389-92.

Strom BL, Carson JL, Halpern AC, Schinnar R, Snyder ES, Stolley PD, Shaw M, Tilson HH, Joseph M, Dai WS, *et al.* (1991). Using a claims database to investigate drug-induced Stevens-Johnson syndrome. *Stat Med*, Vol. 10, No. 4, (April 1991), pp. 565-76.

Strom BL & Carson JL. (1989). Automated data bases used for pharmacoepidemiology research. *Clin Pharmacol Ther*, Vol. 46, No. 4, (October 1989), pp. 390-4.

Sturkenboom M. (2008). Randomized studies in General Practice Databases. In *Pharmacoepidemiology and Therapeutic Management*, Hartzema, AG, Tilson, HH, Chan KA (Eds.), pp 477-93. Harvey Whitney Books, ISBN 978-0929375-30-4, Cincinnati, OH, USA.

Suissa S, Dell'aniello S, Vahey S & Renoux C. (2011). Time-window bias in case-control studies: statins and lung cancer. *Epidemiology*, Vol. 22, No. 2, (March 2011), pp. 228-31.

Suissa S. (2008). Immeasurable time bias in observational studies of drug effects on mortality. *Am J Epidemiol*. 2008 Aug 1;168(3):329-35.

Suissa S & Garbe E. (2007) Primer: administrative health databases in observational studies of drug effects--advantages and disadvantages. *Nat Clin Pract Rheumatol*, Vol. 3, No. 12, (December 2007), pp. 725-32.

Suissa S. (2007). Immortal time bias in observational studies of drug effects. *Pharmacoepidemiol Drug Saf*, Vol. 16, No. 3, (March 2007), pp. 241-9.

Suissa S, Ernst P, Hudson M, Bitton A & Kezouh A. (2004). Newer disease-modifying antirheumatic drugs and the risk of serious hepatic adverse events in patients with rheumatoid arthritis. *Am J Med*, Vol. 117, No. 2, (July 2004), pp. 87-92.

Takahashi Y, Nishida Y & Asai S. (2011). Utilization of health care databases for pharmacoepidemiology. *Eur J Clin Pharmacol*, (August 2011), (*in press*).

Tilson HH. (1989). Pharmacoepidemiology: the lessons learned; the challenges ahead. *Clin Pharmacol Ther*. Vol. 46, No. 4, (October 1989), pp. 480.

Torre C, Guerreiro J & Costa S. (2011). Trends in the consumption of antidepressants, anxiolytics, hypnotics and sedatives in Portugal, over the National Health Plan period (2004-2010). Proceedings of the 27th International Conference on Pharmacoepidemiology & Therapeutic Risk Management, Chicago, 14-17 August 2011. Pharmacoepidemiol Drug Saf. 2011, Vol. 20:S112, (August 2011).

van Staa TP, Leufkens HG, Zhang B & Smeeth L. (2009). A comparison of cost effectiveness using data from randomized trials or actual clinical practice: selective cox-2 inhibitors as an example. *PLoS Med*. Vol. 6, No. 12, (December 2009), e1000194.

van Staa TP, Smeeth L, Persson I, Parkinson J & Leufkens HG. (2008). What is the harm-benefit ratio of Cox-2 inhibitors? *Int J Epidemiol*, Vol. 37, No. 2, (April 2008), pp. 405-13.

van Staa TP & Parkinson J. (2008). Response to: Validation studies of the health improvement network (THIN) database for pharmacoepidemiology research by Lewis *et al*. *Pharmacoepidemiol Drug Saf*. Vol. 17, No. 1, (January 2008), pp. 103-4.

Vandenbroucke JP. (2008). Observational research, randomised trials, and two views of medical science. *PLoS Med*. Vol. 5, No. 3, (March 2008), e67.

Vandenbroucke JP. (2002). Alvan Feinstein and the art of consulting: how to define a research question. *J Clin Epidemiol*, Vol. 55, No. 12, (December 2002), pp. 1176-7.

Velthove KJ, Leufkens HG, Souverein PC, Schweizer RC & van Solinge WW. (2010). Testing bias in clinical databases: methodological considerations. *Emerg Themes Epidemiol*, Vol. 7, No. 2, (May 2010).

Walley T & Mantgani A. (1997). The UK General Practice Research Database. *Lancet*, Vol. 350, No. 9084, (October 1997), pp. 1097-9.

Walker AM. (1996). Confounding by indication. Epidemiology. Vol. 7, No. 4, (July 1996), pp. 335-6.

Wang J & Donnan PT. (2001). Propensity score methods in drug safety studies: practice, strengths and limitations. *Pharmacoepidemiol Drug Saf*, Vol. 10, No. 4, (June-July 2001), pp. 341-4.

West S, Strom BL & Poole C. (2005). Validity of Pharmacoepidemiologic drug and diagnosis data. In *Pharmacoepidemiology*, Strom, BL, pp 709-765. John Wiley & Sons, ISBN 13 978-0-470-86681-8, Chichester, UK.

Wettermark B, Vlahovic-Palcevski V, Blix HS, Rønning & Stichele R. (2008). Drug Utilization Research. In *Pharmacoepidemiology and Therapeutic Management*, Hartzema, AG, Tilson, HH, Chan KA (Eds.), pp 159-195. Harvey Whitney Books, ISBN 978-0929375-30-4, Cincinnati, OH, USA.

Wilchesky M, Tamblyn RM & Huang A. (2004). Validation of diagnostic codes within medical services claims. J Clin Epidemiol. Vol. 57, No. 2, (February 2004), pp. 131-41.

Yang Y & West-Strum D (Ed.). (2011). *Understanding Pharmacoepidemiology* (1th edition), McGrraw-Hill, ISBN 978-0-07-163500-4, USA.

Yang CC, Jick SS & Jick H. (2003). Lipid-lowering drugs and the risk of depression and suicidal behavior. *Arch Intern Med*, Vol. 163, No. 16, (September 2003), pp. 1926-32.

Zimmerman M, Mattia JI & Posternak MA. (2002). Are subjects in pharmacological treatment trials of depression representative of patients in routine clinical practice? *Am J Psychiatry*, Vol. 159, No. 3, (March 2002), pp. 469-73.

9

Role of Epidemiological Data Within the Drug Development Lifecycle: A Chronic Migraine Case Study

Aubrey Manack, Catherine C. Turkel and Haley Kaplowitz
Allergan, Inc.
USA

1. Introduction

By definition, pharmacoepidemiology is the study of the use and the effects of drugs, medical devices or vaccines in large numbers of people (Strom, 1994). Epidemiologists working in the pharmaceutical and biotechnology industry use the principles of descriptive epidemiology in addition to analytical and clinical epidemiological applied concepts and methods to assess the impact, use and effects of these products in the population and in clinical trial settings. As an evolving field, the influence of pharmacoepidemiology continues to be broadened with increasing demands for a comprehensive understanding of the patient population within the development and post-authorization phases of a product's lifecycle.

Before exploring the role of epidemiology within the drug lifecycle, some familiarity with the phases of drug development is necessary. Herein, a brief overview of the drug development lifecycle is provided. The intent is not to present a detailed outline of the regulatory process by which a new drug is brought to market, but rather a selective review to offer context for the potential clinical and scientific contributions of the field of epidemiology. The established framework of a drug's lifecycle includes four phases: discovery and research (pre-clinical phase), clinical development, regulatory review and approval, and post-authorization (Table 1). Typically, discovery begins with industry or academic researchers testing tens of thousands of compounds to determine potential therapeutic benefit. Few compounds proceed to the next stage, which involves testing candidate drugs in animals to ensure there is no development of limiting toxic effects. It is estimated that only 1 out of 50 candidate drugs will move past the discovery phase and into clinical development trials in humans (phases I, II and III). Clinical trials in humans represent the most expensive phase of development. Cost estimates range in the hundreds of millions, and for every five drugs entering late-phase clinical trials, only one will eventually make it to market and generate revenue for the manufacturer (Tufts, 2001). Additionally, during this time, there is ongoing parallel work related to drug substance manufacturing (e.g., formulation activities, analytical and microbiological methods development and validation) to support development activities.

Phase	Title	Timing	Brief Description
Preclinical	Discovery and research	1 to 6 years	Preclinical testing - initiation for synthesis, purification and formulation of the drug; for conducting biology/pharmacology, pharmacokinetics and metabolism evaluations; for conducting GLP toxicity/safety evaluations including toxicology, pathology, mechanistic toxicology and bioanalytical support; for identification of potential drug-drug interactions.
Phases I-III	Clinical development	6 to 11 years	Phase I – The "safety" phase. Smaller clinical trials using healthy volunteers to determine the drug's basic pharmacokinetic and pharmacologic properties and safety profile in humans. Phase II - The "learn" phase. These trials are focused on evaluating effective and safe doses in persons with the target disease/disorder under consideration. Phase III - The "confirm" phase. These trials are usually the most extensive and most expensive part of drug development. These trials often are controlled (usually with placebo) and are designed to verify the safety and efficacy of a drug in large numbers, typically several hundred to several thousand persons, within the target population.
Peri-approval	Regulatory review and approval	0.6 to 2 years	After completing phases I-III, the manufacturer submits a registration dossier containing all non-clinical (eg, toxicology, pharmacology), efficacy and safety data in addition to manufacturing quality data for review by regulatory agencies (eg, FDA – United States Food and Drug Administration, EMA – European Medicines Agency). The agency evaluates the drug's safety, efficacy and labeling with specific emphasis on public health impact and the benefit-risk profile of the drug.
Phase IV	Post-authorization/ Post-market surveillance	11 to 14 years	Conditioned on the regulatory approval of the drug and involves ongoing safety evaluation of the drug (through periodic spontaneous reports, which may also be supplemented with observational studies) once it is used within the real-world setting with the emphasis of maintaining the benefit-risk profile.

Adapted from FDA review.org. http://www.fdareview.org/approval_process.shtml and Hartzema et al., 1998.

Table 1. Description of drug development lifecycle.

Epidemiological data and methods are utilized during each phase presented above; however, the degree of involvement is dependent on the current knowledge base and interactions between factors that are specific to the molecule (eg, biologic vs. drug; oral vs. injectable), the disease (eg, hypertension vs. cancer), other inventions (eg, competitive and/or complimentary products) and the patient (eg, males in their mid-40s vs. adolescent females) (Figure 1). Furthermore, underlying these interactions is the impact of patient's knowledge, attitude and behaviors about the study drug or disease as well as interactions with the geographical and social environment.

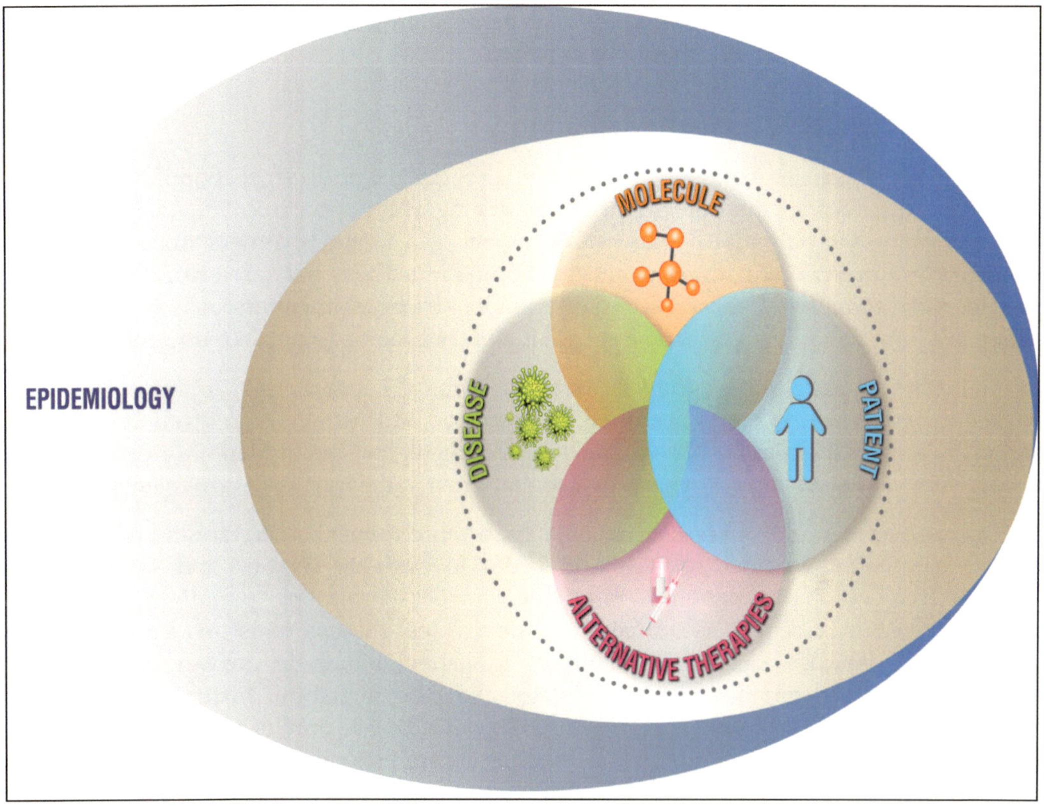

Fig. 1. Conceptual framework for the potential impacts for epidemiological data and methods within the clinical development phase

As there is a wide spectrum of data needs and requirements during any drug's lifecycle, a summary, including a real-world example, of the epidemiological data and methods utilized specifically during clinical development phase is helpful. To illustrate how epidemiologists can facilitate clinical development, this review provides a practical overview of the type of research questions addressed with epidemiological data and methods. In addition, a case study describing how epidemiological data was used to support the registration of onabotulinumtoxinA (BOTOX®, Allergan, Inc., Irvine, CA, USA) for treatment of headaches in adults with chronic migraine is presented. Using this framework, data generation is focused on the population epidemiology, treated natural history and burden of chronic migraine. The review is not meant to be a guidance document, but rather an illustration highlighting the importance of an evidence-based understanding of the patient population in order to adequately measure efficacy, to evaluate and maintain the safety of a drug during development and to prepare for post-registration activities once the product is available in the market. Although not the focus of this chapter, the role of pharmacoepidemiologists does not end at approval. In the post-authorization environment, the need shifts more toward understanding the patient population actually exposed to the drug, under what conditions, and with what outcomes, in the "real world" setting. For example, is the drug being used in patients not included in clinical trials? Is there compliance with the labeling? Is the safety and effectiveness similar to what was observed in clinical trials? If not, why not? To respond to these types of research questions, designs such as drug utilization studies, post-authorization safety and effectiveness studies should be explored.

2. Defining the target patient population

Epidemiology data can be used to estimate the size of the target population and its geographic distribution, quantify and describe demographic and clinical characteristics, and help determine the potential public health impact of a target treatment once the drug is marketed and prescribed within the general population. These data are critically important to help guide commercial and clinical development strategies; therefore, it is most useful to obtain this information starting early in phase II and continuing, as needed, through phase III.

By the time a drug enters clinical development, a sponsor (e.g. pharmaceutical or biotechnology company) has typically already assessed, at least at a high level, the incidence and prevalence of disease, the unmet needs for treatment, and the burden of disease, in order to have some understanding of where the drug might fit in the treatment armamentarium.

During the phase II and phase III clinical trials, a more robust understanding of the target patient population becomes necessary in order to evaluate efficacy and safety and to consider the optimal position within the current treatment paradigm. Therefore, epidemiologists rely on observational study design (eg, disease registries, cohort studies, cross-sectional studies, case-control studies) to generate data to answer more specific questions about the population epidemiology and disease natural history. (Strom, 1994; Hartzema et al., 1998) The population epidemiology of a disease provides estimates of the total number of people currently impacted as well as future estimates by utilizing current and projected prevalence and incidence rates. Aiming to stratify prevalence and incidence rates by country or geographic region, age, gender and, when appropriate, factors such as race or seasonal variation can provide a more complete picture of the demographic profile of the target population. Additionally, the symptom profile, disease-related morbidity and mortality, should be detailed in this context. The disease natural history refers to the progression of a disease from onset until either recovery or death. It encompasses factors related to the behavior of a disease so that the clinical course including the disease onset, disease duration, progression, and disease outcomes are well documented. Available treatment practices should be evaluated, as this often alters disease progression. Risk factors, including biological, genetic or environmental, should be discussed in terms of disease outcomes or progression rather than onset. It is worth noting that because typical drug development, with the exception of vaccine development, is not focused on disease prevention, but rather remission or recovery, then the focus is on understanding factors that alter disease duration and endpoints rather than disease onset and is referred to as the treated natural history.

Observational studies are used to generate data describing the target patient population in the "real world" rather than in the controlled "clinical trials" environment. Multiple observational approaches can be utilized, depending on research objectives. Cross-sectional studies collect data on various characteristics, experiences and behaviors in relation to exposure, outcomes and/or other variables of interest at the same time point. These studies can be either population-based or represent a select population, such as those in a clinic or those who have access to the internet. Cohort studies can be conducted prospectively or retrospectively, and identify and follow subjects according to either exposure or disease occurrence to assess multiple outcomes. Commonly utilized examples cohort studies include retrospective electronic health care database analyses and disease registries. Case-control studies are typically hypothesis testing, in that the design aims to quantify the odds of having an exposure given an outcome or the reverse depending on what is known. Subjects are predefined as either case or controls based on whether the patient has the disease or outcome of interest, and then patients' histories are compared for differences in exposure or other potential risk factors. When evaluating which study design is most appropriate, pharmacoepidemiologists assess and select study designs based on the particular research question, urgency of the data request, availability of data sources, concerns of internal and external validity, and feasibility and practicality, and cost (Hartzema et al., 1998).

It is not feasible to discuss every situation for which epidemiological data can be utilized in a single chapter; however, one of the key drivers of research is the need to put into context the clinical trial findings, for example, when monitoring safety within double-blind, placebo-controlled trials. In order for safety physicians to effectively monitor safety without unblinding patients in clinical trials, outcomes that are associated with natural disease course should be distinguished from adverse outcomes that are potentially drug-related, referred to as adverse drug reactions. This situation encompasses the potential for confounding by indication and reflects the importance in adequately "teasing apart" adverse events caused by the disease itself versus adverse events caused by the drug, or even a potential disease-drug interaction or when the adverse event may occur in the disease background but be exacerbated or prolonged by the drug. To clarify with examples, confounding is when a variable (e.g., adverse event such as weight gain) is a risk factor for a disorder (e.g., CM) among nonexposed persons (e.g., those not on study drug) and is associated with the exposure of interest (e.g., study drug) in the population from which the cases derive, without being an intermediate step in the causal pathway between the exposure and the disorder (Salas M et al., 1999). Given the potential complexity of natural clinical course of a disease, it is evident that if background rates within the target population unexposed to the drug are adequately quantified, then the determination of drug- or disease-related outcomes can be strengthened beyond the clinical assessment of treatment causality.

By answering questions in Table 2, row 1, epidemiologists support clinical development by providing strategic insight into defining the appropriate target patient profile and the predicted public health benefit. Defining diagnostic criteria and properly characterizing the target patient population will help in understanding the disease outside the clinical trial environment to ensure that clinical trials are evaluating treatments in the most appropriate target patient population. Epidemiological data can also help physicians monitor the safety without unblinding patients in clinical trials, and if a potential risk is identified, can help to estimate the impact in actual clinical practice.

Category	Description	Key Research Questions
Population Epidemiology	An overview of the condition for which the product is being developed, including incidence rate (rate of new cases in a population within a specified time frame), prevalence rate (number of existing cases) stratified by geography, patient demographics in a population within a specified time frame, clinical characteristics, trends over time and recommendations relating to studies needed to address data gaps	• What are the disease rates (eg, age-, gender-stratified)? More specifically, which populations are most affected both currently and prospectively by the disease? • What is the disease severity in relation to morbidity and mortality? • What is the disease duration? • What is the severity of the disease symptoms in relation to disease duration? • What are the characteristics (eg, age, correlated clinical deficiencies) of the disease onset? • What are the key drivers (eg, comorbidity profile, health care access) with regard to disease progression?

Treated Natural History	An overview of clinical course of the condition for which the product is being developed. Focused on detailing disease progression, defining a patient profile, quantifying rates of common comorbidities, treatments and treatment practices, disease outcome rates (e.g. morbidity, mortality, survival) and rates of potential drug-related adverse events. This report provides information to understand the types of adverse events that are associated with the planned indication and with its common therapies and to quantify the frequency (ie, risk) of these adverse events within the general population and to estimate the potential benefit of the product under development.	• What are the characteristics of the disease onset?
		  • Age
		  • Correlated deficiencies
		  • Potential covariates (eg, stress, environmental triggers)
		• What are the characteristics of the disease window?
		  • How long does the average person have the disease?
		  • What occurs in extreme cases?
		  • What are the common comorbidities?
		  • Understand differences with regard to factors such as:
		    • Nutrition
		    • Psychology
		    • Health care
		    • Socioeconomic status (SES)
		• What are the characteristics of the disease endpoint?
		  • Does disease endpoint depend on disease severity?
		  • Outline major and minor effects of the disease:
		    • Are there any permanent losses of ability?
		    • Correlate that loss of ability to quality of life

Category	Description	Key Research Questions

		• Understand the percentage of reoccurrence of disease after initial onset
		• What is the disease profile, combining genetic, environmental and cultural factors that may contribute to disease?
		  • Who is most likely to be diagnosed with the disease?
		  • Who is most likely to have severe progression of the disease?
		  • Are there cultural biases in relation to treatment and/or disease?

Burden of Disease	An overview focused on the negative disease-related impact for the individual suffering and his or her social network, as well as the associated direct and indirect costs in the real-world setting.	• What is the humanistic burden associated with the disease?
		  • Health-related quality of life assessments
		  • Disability assessments
		  • Disease-related impacts (eg, depression, anxiety, sleep)
		• What is the societal burden associated with the disease?
		  • Associated family and social burden
		  • Lost employment/education (ie, absenteeism)
		  • Suboptimal work productivity (ie, presenteeism)
		  • Caregiver burden
		• What is the economic burden associated with the disease?
		  • What are the direct costs associated with the disease?
		    • Healthcare encounters (eg, emergency room (ER) visits, hospitalizations, office visits)
		    • Over-the-counter and prescription medications
		    • Treatment-related procedures
		    • Diagnostic evaluations
		    • Patient co-payments
		• What are the indirect costs associated with the disease?
		  • Monetized assessment of work- or school-related impact
		    • Absenteeism and presenteeism

Table 2. Overview of epidemiology support for clinical development.

Real-world application can provide significant insights when discussing the role of epidemiology within the pharmaceutical or biotechnology development industry. When the onabotulinumtoxinA development program for chronic migraine was initiated, the International Headache Society had not standardized diagnostic criteria for chronic migraine, which had broadly been defined as those with migraine and 15 or more headache days per month. In subsequent years, and in parallel to the phase II and phase III trials, multiple diagnostic criteria were proposed to the clinical community and it proved difficult to create criteria applicable to clinical practice, clinical trials and population-based studies. As a consequence, a wide range of terms with a multiplicity of definitions were applied to persons with what is now defined as chronic migraine (Manack et al., 2009, 2010; Olesen 2006; Olesen et al., 2006). Due to the timing of this evolution relative to when the onabotulinumtoxinA trials were completed, the chronic migraine diagnostic criteria utilized in the phase III studies were in alignment, but were not identical to the most recent criteria proposed by the International Headache Classification Committee within the International Classification of Headache Disorders (ICHD) guidelines.

To ensure that the safety and efficacy trial findings were representative of findings for those diagnosed under the most recent ICHD criteria (ICHD-2R), profile concordance between criteria was evaluated within a large patient population that physicians identified as having chronic migraine. Epidemiological assessments of daily diary data were completed to compare the demographic and headache symptom profiles for the several of the proposed chronic migraine diagnostic criteria (Silberstein et al., 2011; Lipton et al., 2011). Within the test database, the ICHD-2R definition was set as the gold standard and sensitivity and specificity analyses against the onabotulinumtoxinA phase III diagnostic criteria were conducted. Assessments supported that the patient profiles of the chronic migraine diagnostic groups were similar across demographic profiles and headache characteristics. Results from the epidemiological assessments all supported the initial hypothesis that the chronic migraine population evaluated in the phase III clinical studies was not identical to, but was clinically representative of, the target population of patients currently defined by the ICHD-2R criteria and fully representative of patients who would be receiving onabotulinumtoxinA treatment.

Additionally, due to the chronic migraine classification variability, it was difficult to determine the disease prevalence during the time of the development program. To gain a better understanding of the actual number of people suffering from chronic migraine, a systematic literature search was conducted to summarize population-based studies reporting prevalence and incidence of chronic migraine and to explore variation across studies. Sixteen publications representing 12 studies were accepted as having a relevant study design and population. None presented data on chronic migraine incidence. The prevalence of chronic migraine ranged between 0 and 5.1%, with estimates typically in the range of 1.4–2.2% (Natoli et al., 2010). Prevalence varied by World Health Organization region and gender. Heterogeneity across studies and lack of data from certain regions left an incomplete picture; however, the review offered a comprehensive overview of the current knowledge base and provided direction for future research (Natoli et al., 2010).

Expanding beyond the assessments of drug safety and efficacy, the onabotulinumtoxinA development program incorporated a significant amount of epidemiological research to generate data that established the clinical course of chronic migraine and distinguished it from episodic migraine (migraine with less than 15 days of headache per month). Three robust epidemiological studies were utilized as data sources (Table 3). Of note, and emphasizing the collaboration between academia and industry, only one of these studies was initiated and completely sponsored by the manufacturer.

Study	Design	Duration	Sponsorship
American Migraine Prevalence and Prevention (AMPP) Study (Buse et al., 2010; Lipton et al., 2007)	Longitudinal, prospective, population-based, mailed survey identified individuals by screening 120,000 US households representative of the US population, resulting in a pool of 24,000 respondents with severe headache who have been followed annually.	5 years	Study initially funded by an unrestricted grant to the National Headache Foundation by Ortho-McNeil Neurologics, Inc., Titusville, NJ, USA. Additional analyses and data collection focused on chronic migraine epidemiology funded by Allergan Inc., Irvine, CA.
German Headache Consortium (GHC) Study (Katsarava et al., 2011)	Longitudinal, prospective, population-based, mailed/telephone survey used questionnaires sent annually to a random sample of 18,000 individuals aged 18-65 residing in demographically diverse regions, including a large and midsize city and a rural area of Germany.	3 years	Study funded by the German Research Council (DFG), German Ministry of Education and Research (BMBF), and European Union and conducted through the Department of Neurology in Essen. Additional analyses focusing on chronic migraine epidemiology supported by Allergan, Inc., Irvine, CA, USA.
International Burden of Migraine Study (IBMS) (Blumenfeld et al., 2011; Payne et al., 2011)	Cross-sectional web-based survey identified panelists through respondents who had previously reported suffering from headaches or migraine. Nine countries surveyed: United States, Canada, Germany, United Kingdom, France, Italy, Spain, Australia and Taiwan.	1 year	Study funded by Allergan, Inc., Irvine, CA, USA.

Table 3. Summary of chronic migraine epidemiological studies

Data from the three independent studies (AMPP study, GHC study, IBMS) concluded that the two headache disorders (chronic migraine and episodic migraine) differ with regard to clinical definitions, prevalence, symptom profiles, functional consequences and disabilities, indirect and direct costs, patterns of consultation and treatment, rates of comorbidities and risk factors (Manack et al., 2010, 2011; Bigal et al., 2008, Buse et al., 2010, 2011 in press; Blumenfeld et al., 2011; Katsarava et al., 2011; Stewart et al., 2010; Munakata et al., 2009). Data confirmed what had been previously hypothesized by the headache community: that chronic and episodic forms of migraine exist along a clinical spectrum with remission and progression between the two, but the disorders are distinct and differ in degree and kind (Lipton, 2009; Lipton and Chu, 2009) (Table 4).

Variable	Chronic Migraine	Episodic Migraine
Clinical description	ICHD-2 criteria for migraine and average ≥15 headache days/month	ICHD-2 criteria for migraine and average <15 headache days/month
Prevalence, %**	1.4-2.2	11
Age, mean (SD)	47.7 (14.0)	46.0 (13.8)
Race, % Caucasian	78.6	80.0
BMI, mean (SD)	29.8 (8.3)	29.2 (7.9)
Cutaneous allodynia, %	68.2	63.2
Headache duration with medication (average in hours) mean SD	24.1 (46.8)	12.8 (25.0)
Headache duration without medication (average in hours) mean SD	65.1 (62.2)	38.8 (39.9)
Headache pain intensity, % severe	92.4	78.1
Comorbid conditions	More likely to report or meet criteria for psychiatric, pain, respiratory and cardiovascular comorbid conditions	Less likely to report or meet criteria for psychiatric, pain, respiratory and cardiovascular comorbid conditions

*Significantly different finding reported in published AMPP study and IBMS data (Bigal et al., 2008; Buse et al., 2010; Blumenfeld et al., 2011; Buse et al., 2011 in press)
**Sources: Natoli et al., 2010; Lipton et al., 2007.

Table 4. Examples of differences* between chronic migraine and episodic migraine

3. Defining the burden

Due to high healthcare costs, manufacturers are under increasing scrutiny by regulators, policy-makers, employers and consumers to demonstrate the clinical and economic value of a new drug being brought to market. Given this environment, there is an evolving view that the drug approval process is expanding beyond the determination of a drug's safety and efficacy to include data on comparative effectiveness of a new drug to one or more available therapies. Comparative effectiveness is defined by the Institution of Medicine as "the comparison of effective interventions among patients in typical patient care settings with decisions tailored to individual patient needs" (Doyle, 2011; Sox & Greenfield, 2009). According to global regulations, demonstrating comparative effectiveness is not required for commercial license; however, it is often required for reimbursement by national and/or private insurance providers. Specifically, health technology assessments (HTAs) are the appraisal process by which public and private payers evaluate economic value (Doyle, 2011). In effect, establishing a positive economic value impact has become a milestone within the *regulatory review and approval* of a drug's lifecycle. By addressing research questions highlighted in Table 2, row 3, epidemiologists support industry health economists and outcomes researchers in the development of the economic value story by providing strategic insight into real-world disease-related burden and resource utilization.

In order to evaluate the real-world value of a drug, many factors and modeling techniques that are beyond the scope of epidemiology are employed (Gold et al., 1996; Briggs et al., 2006). However, epidemiological data and methods can support health economists in determining strategy and inputs into economic impact models. A key component when assessing the potential value impact of a new drug is to establish the current humanistic, societal and economic burden for the disease of interest within the real world. Phase III clinical trials are often designed to assess impacts on disease-related burden and economic consequences, which include but are not limited to data to evaluate health-related quality of life, disability, healthcare encounters and/or workplace impact. However, as burden and economic outcomes within a clinical trial setting may not represent outcomes in the real world, there is a recognized benefit to supporting the clinical trial data with population-based assessments that quantify burden and resource utilization (Doyle, 2011; Murray & McElwee, 2010; Conway & Clancy, 2010).

Through leveraging epidemiological data, the humanistic, economic and societal burden associated with chronic migraine was established during the development program. Specifically, data from the AMPP study, GHC study, and IBMS (Table 3 for study designs) was utilized to quantify the burden that frequent migraine attacks pose on patients, their families and employers, and healthcare systems.

In summary, chronic migraine was determined to be a disabling, underdiagnosed and costly disorder (Bigal et al., 2008; Blumenfeld et al., 2011; Manack et al., 2011), particularly when compared to episodic migraine. Those with chronic migraine often spend at least half their days suffering from debilitating pain and associated symptoms of nausea, vomiting, photophobia and phonophobia (Bigal et al., 2008; Manack et al., 2011). Data support the substantial direct and indirect treatment-associated costs as well as significantly increased interference on normal life activities, such as the ability to work or perform routine chores and build and maintain functional family, social and community relationships, for those with chronic migraine when compared to episodic migraine (Table 5).

Variable	Chronic Migraine	Episodic Migraine
Depression, % meeting criteria for clinical depression	25.2	10
Headache Impact Test (HIT-6), % in "severe" category	72.9	42.3
Headache-related treatment costs, mean US dollars	$1036 per 3 months	$383 per 3 months
Employment, % on disability	20 (1 in 5)	10 (1 in 10)
Headache-related Lost Productive Time (LPT)*	50% of sufferers lost more than 2 hours per 2 weeks	16%‡ of sufferers lost more than 2 hours per 2 weeks
LPT associated cost, US dollars per week	Women aged 25-64 years: $61.51-$118.64 per week per person	Women aged 25-64 years: $30.80-$46.49 per week per person
	Men aged 25-64 years: $62.13-$287.12 per week per person	Men aged 25-64 years: $53.15-$86.82 per week per person

*LPT is the sum of self-reported absenteeism and presenteeism during a 2-week period.
†Significantly different findings were reported in the AMPP study and IBMS (Bigal et al., 2008; Stewart et al., 2010; Blumenfeld et al., 2011; Buse et al., 2011 in press; Stokes et al., 2011; Manack et al., 2012; Serrano et al., 2011, in progress)
‡Based on those with fewer than 10 headache days per month.

Table 5. Examples of burden of chronic migraine compared to episodic migraine†

4. Post-approval pharmacoepidemiology plan

The approval to market a drug, device or vaccine depends primarily on the results of the clinical trial program which includes investigational trials with a variety of potential designs; generally, randomized, double-blind placebo-controlled studies are considered the gold standard. However, even these studies are not without limitations, including relatively small sample sizes, selective populations, short follow-up, use of intermediate (surrogate) endpoints and limited generalizability (Glasser et al., 2007). Furthermore, problems seen after product approval has placed demands on manufacturers, regulators and policy makers to more effectively monitor and expand the knowledge of safety in the post-authorization period. This requires a proactive plan, including an assessment of research gaps and appropriate study designs, beginning in the clinical development phase so that strategies can be initiated upon drug approval.

Post-marketing research, or more specifically phase IV studies, can either be interventional or non-interventional by design, with epidemiologists typically focusing on those that are non-interventional. Again, descriptive or observational designs are used to evaluate drug utilization patterns; additionally, with a study design that allows for exposure in a broader range of patients, more real-world information about the drug's safety and effectiveness can be captured (Wise, 2011; Glasser et al., 2007). Analytical epidemiology or the design, execution and analysis of studies to evaluate potential associations between exposure and outcome, has a defined role within pharmacovigilance, which deals with the detection, assessment, understanding and prevention of adverse effects or other drug-related problems (Wise, 2011; Glasser, et al., 2007). To this end, post-marketing research has become an integral part of the drug's lifecycle (Wise, 2011; Glasser et al., 2007)

5. Conclusion

Epidemiologists provide data, methods and strategic direction to optimize product development and commercialization. Key deliverables within the clinical development teams include describing and quantifying disease incidence and prevalence, clinical course, real-world treatment practices, adverse events rates, patient exposure, and the design, analysis and reporting of observational studies. Although an important contribution, data from epidemiological studies should not be viewed in isolation, as evaluation of safety and efficacy includes data from multiple sources including clinical studies, spontaneous adverse event reports and preclinical datasets, and all offer important context.

6. References

Bigal, M.E., Serrano, D., Reed, M., & Lipton, R.B. 2008. Chronic migraine in the population: burden, diagnosis, and satisfaction with treatment. *Neurology*, Vol. 71, No. 8, pp. 559-566.

Blumenfeld, A., Varon, S., Wilcox, T.K., Buse, D., Kawata, A.K., Manack, A., Goadsby, P.J., & Lipton, R.B. 2011. Disability, HRQoL and resource use among chronic and episodic migraineurs: Results from the International Burden of Migraine Study (IBMS). *Cephalalgia*, Vol. 31, No. 3, pp. 301-315.

Briggs, A., Claxton, K., & Sculpher, M. 2006. *Decision Modelling for Health Economic Evaluation (Handbooks in Health Economic Evaluation)*. Oxford University Press, ISBN 9780198526629, New York, New York, USA.

Buse, D.C., Manack, A., Serrano, D., Turkel, C., & Lipton, R.B. 2010. Sociodemographic and comorbidity profiles of chronic migraine and episodic migraine sufferers. *J Neurol Neurosurg Psychiatry*, Vol. 81, No. 4, pp. 428-432.

Buse, D.C., Manack, A.N., Serrano, D., Varon, S.F., Turkel, C.C., & Lipton, R.B. 2011. Headache impact of chronic and episodic migraine: Predictors of impact from the American Migraine Prevalence and Prevention (AMPP) study. *Headache*, in press.

Conway, P.H., & Clancy, C. 2010. Charting a path from comparative effectiveness funding to improved patient-centered health care. *JAMA*, Vol. 303, No. 10, pp. 985-986.

Doyle, J.J. 2011. *The effect of Comparative Effectiveness Research on Drug Development Innovation: A 360° Value Appraisal*, Dove Press, Retrieved from www.dovepress.com/the-effect-of-comparative-effectiveness-research-on-drug-development-i-a6837

FDA review.org. n.d. *The Drug Development and Approval Process.* Retrieved from www.fdareview.org/approval_process.shtml

Glasser, S.P., Salas, M., & Delzell, E. 2007. Importance and challenges of studying marketed drugs: What is a phase IV study? Common clinical research designs, registries, and self-reporting systems. *J Clin Pharmacol,* Vol. 47, No. 9, pp. 1074-1086.

Gold, M.R., Siegel, J.E., Russell, L.B., & Weinstein, M.C. (Eds.) 1996. *Cost-Effectiveness in Health and Medicine,* Oxford University Press, ISBN 9780195108248, New York, New York, USA.

Hartzema, A.G., Porta, M., & Tilson, H.H. (Eds.) 1998. *Pharmacoepidemiology: An Introduction* (3rd edition), Harvey Whitney Books, ISBN 978-0929375182, Cincinnati, OH, USA.

Katsarava, Z., Manack, A., Yoon, M.-S., Obermann, M., Becker, H., Dommes, P., Turkel, C., Lipton, R.B., & Diener, H.C. 2011. Chronic migraine: Classification and comparisons. *Cephalalgia,* Vol. 31, No. 5, pp. 520-529.

Lipton, R.B., Bigal, M.E., Diamond, M., Freitag, F., Reed, M.L., & Stewart, W.F. 2007. Migraine prevalence, disease burden, and the need for preventive therapy. *Neurology,* Vol. 68. No. 5, pp. 343-349.

Lipton, R.B. 2009. Tracing transformation: chronic migraine classification, progression, and epidemiology. *Neurology,* Vol. 72, No. 5 Suppl., pp. S3-S7.

Lipton, R.B., & Chu, M.K. 2009. Conceptualizing the relationship between chronic migraine and episodic migraine. *Expert Rev Neurother,* Vol. 9, No. 10, pp. 1451-1454.

Lipton, R.B., Silberstein, S.D., Diener, H.C., Dodick, D.W., Aurora, S.K., Manack, A., DeGryse, R.E., & Turkel, C.C. 2011. Field testing chronic migraine diagnostic criteria: Assessment of sensitivity and specificity. Abstract and poster presented at the 15th Congress of the International Headache Society, Berlin, Germany, June 23-26, 2011.

Manack, A., Turkel, C., & Silberstein, S. 2009. The evolution of chronic migraine: Classification and nomenclature. *Headache,* Vol. 49, No. 8, pp. 1206-1213.

Manack, A.N., Buse, D.C., & Lipton, R.B. 2010. Chronic migraine: Epidemiology and disease burden. *Curr Pain Headache Rep,* Vol. 15, No. 1, pp. 70-78.

Manack, A., Buse, D.C., Serrano, D., Turkel, C.C., Lipton, R.B. 2011. Rates, predictors, and consequences of remission from chronic migraine to episodic migraine. *Neurology,* Vol. 76. No. 8, pp. 711-718.

Manack, A.N., Buse, D.C., Serrano, D., Turkel, C., & Lipton, R.B. 2012. Lost productive time and cost due to headache in chronic migraine and episodic migraine: Results from the American Migraine Prevalence and Prevention (AMPP) study. Abstract submitted to the 54th Annual Scientific Meeting of the America Headache Society, Los Angeles, CA, USA June 21-24, 2012.

Munakata, J., Hazard, E., Serrano, D., Klingman, D., Rupnow, M.F., Tierce, J., Reed, M., & Lipton, R.B. Economic burden of transformed migraine: Results from the American Migraine Prevalence and Prevention (AMPP) study. *Headache* 2009, Vol. 49, No. 4, pp. 498-508.

Murray, R.K, & McElwee, N.E. 2010. Comparative effectiveness research: critically intertwined with healthcare reform and the future of biomedical innovation. *Arch Intern Med*, Vol. 170, No. 7, pp. 596–599.

Natoli, J., Manack, A., Dean, B., Butler, Q., Turkel, C., Stovner, L., & Lipton, R. 2010. Global prevalence of chronic migraine: a systematic review. *Cephalalgia*, Vol. 30, No. 5, pp. 599-609.

Olesen J. 2006. International Classification of Headache Disorders, Second Edition (ICHD-2): current status and future revisions. *Cephalalgia*, Vol. 26, No. 12, pp. 1409-1410.

Olesen, J., Bousser, M.G., Diener, H.C., Dodick, D., First, M., Goadsby, P.J., Gobel, H., Lainez, M.J., Lance, J.W., Lipton, R.B., Nappi, G., Sakai, F., Schoenen, J., Silberstein, S.D., & Steiner, T.J. 2006. New appendix criteria open for a broader concept of chronic migraine. *Cephalalgia*, Vol. 26, No. 6, pp. 742-746.

Payne, K.A., Varon, S.F., Kawata, A.K., Yeomans, K., Wilcox, T.K,, Manack, A., Buse, D.C., Lipton, R.B., Goadsby, P.J., & Blumenfeld, A.M. 2011. The International Burden of Migraine Study (IBMS): Study design, methodology and baseline cohort characteristics. *Cephalalgia*, Vol. 31, No. 10, pp. 1116-1130.

Salas M, Hofman A, Stricker BH. Confounding by indication: an example of variation in the use of epidemiologic terminology. *Am J Epidemiol* 1999 1;149(11):981-983.

Serrano, D., Manack, A.N., Reed, M.L., Buse, D.C., Varon, S., & Lipton, R.B. 2011. Cost of lost productive time in chronic migraine and episodic migraine: Results from the American Migraine Prevalence and Prevention (AMPP) study. In progress.

Silberstein, S.D., Lipton, R.B., Diener, H.C., Dodick, D.W., Aurora, S.K., Manack, A., DeGryse, R.E., & Turkel, C.C. 2011. Field testing chronic migraine (CM) diagnostic criteria: Assessments of demographic and headache profiles. Abstract and poster presented at the 15th Congress of the International Headache Society, Berlin, Germany, June 23-26, 2011.

Sox, H.C., & Greenfield, S. 2009. Comparative effectiveness research: a report from the Institute of Medicine. *Ann Intern Med*, Vol. 15, No. 3, pp. 203-205.

Stewart, W.F., Wood, G.C., Manack, A., Varon, S.F., Buse, D.C., & Lipton, R.B. Employment and work impact of chronic migraine and episodic migraine. *J Occup Environ Med*, Vol. 52, No. 1, pp. 8-14.

Stokes, M., Becker, W.J., Lipton, R.B., Sullivan, S.D., Wilcox, T.K., Wells, L., Manack, A., Proskorovsky, I., Gladstone, J., Buse, D.C., Varon, S.F., Goadsby, P.J., & Blumenfeld, A.M. 2011. Cost of health care among patients with chronic and episodic migraine in Canada and the USA: Results from the International Burden of Migraine Study (IBMS). *Headache*, Vol. 51, No. 7, pp. 1058-1077.

Strom, B.L. (Ed.) 1994. *Pharmacoepidemiology* (2nd edition), John Wiley & Sons, ISBN 9780471940586, Chichester, UK.

Tufts 2001 report. Retrieved from www.cptech.org/ip/health/econ/rndcosts.html

Wise, L. Risks and benefits of (pharmaco)epidemiology. *Ther Adv in Drug Saf*, Vol. 2, No. 3, pp. 95-102.

10

Clinical Epidemiology: Principles Revisited in an Approach to Study Heart Failure

Ana Azevedo
University of Porto Medical School & Institute of Public Health of the University of Porto
Portugal

1. Introduction

Clinical research studies in general aim to help answer questions that patients most frequently ask their physicians (or these ask themselves): What is wrong with me (diagnosis)? What can you do for me (treatment)? Will I get better (prognosis)?

Diagnosis, prognosis and treatment are obviously related, although not so simply as might be thought at first sight, with prognosis and treatment being dependent on a previously established diagnosis. In fact, the information produced in any of these three activities of clinical practice influences the others and they are much interdependent. For example, prognostic information provides the final confirmation of the diagnosis in some cases, and response to treatment can be used as evidence in favor of a suspected diagnosis. Also, a diagnosis is often immediately connoted with a certain prognosis and the need for certain treatments, and these may be more important to the patient than the diagnosis itself. A good example of this is cancer, with its expected ominous outcomes and fearful treatments.

Another type of concern raised in clinical practice, but of more general interest, is usually addressed in more wide scope epidemiological studies (What caused my illness (etiology)?) and will not be approached in this chapter.

The purpose of this chapter is to review the essentials of clinical epidemiology as a bridging discipline that provides information useful to care for individual patients. The approach to the theme is based on an overview of the modern probabilistic approach to diagnosis, prognosis and assessment of disease management in heart failure.

Heart failure is a complex syndrome with a large and increasing burden that poses interesting and at times unresolved challenges in all the issues that are to be technically discussed. We aim at providing the concepts and guiding the development of competencies necessary for using the medical literature and making clinical decisions.

2. Diagnosis

As Edmond A. Murphy put in his claim for the need for a theory of Medicine, "There is probably no more important field in Medicine than diagnosis and none more difficult to teach. It seems astonishing that it is not attracting hundreds of theorists. We have a crisis of medical care on our hands, and the need to optimize the efficiency of diagnosis is obvious.

What work has been done on diagnosis and by whom? Some statisticians have developed algebraic models; but since they have never seen the diagnostician at work, the models are hopelessly unrealistic. Some few clinicians have accepted the idea that diagnosis is a straightforward application of Bayes' theorem. (…) These imported approaches will not do because they do not start from, and attempt to refine, how the process works in clinical practice. The diagnostic process is a sequential strategy in which the facts are nonindependently and nonidentically distributed, usually collected not singly but in groups, and with an end point constrained by urgency, compassion, cost and redundancy. No useful solution to that challenge is likely to be successful unless the first goal is to specify what the clinician is trying to do" (Murphy, 1997).

The clinical diagnosis of heart failure is unreliable and current recommendations for diagnosis warrant the objective demonstration of cardiac structural or functional abnormalities, usually by echocardiogram (Dickstein et al., 2008). However, its syndromic nature implies that symptoms and signs are the fundamental basis of diagnosis and echocardiographic measurements are also susceptible to measurement error and are strongly observer-dependent. To complicate things further, objective evidence of diastolic dysfunction of some form is currently recommended for the diagnosis of heart failure with preserved ejection fraction (Paulus et al., 2007), which used to be an exclusion diagnosis. This contrasts with the past reliance mainly on left ventricular systolic dysfunction as the underlying cardiac functional abnormality to explain a clinical picture of heart failure, with the exception of valvular heart disease. Diastolic function is technically more difficult to characterize by echocardiogram. Symptoms and signs of heart failure and objective evidence of cardiac dysfunction must both be present for a diagnosis of heart failure to be established, and in case of doubt response to treatment can be considered (Dickstein et al., 2008).

There is no consensual gold standard for the diagnosis of heart failure and the current best reference is an expert's opinion based on clinical, laboratorial and functional data.

Plasma concentrations of natriuretic peptides are useful biomarkers in the diagnosis of heart failure. B-type natriuretic peptide (BNP) and N-terminal pro-BNP (NT-proBNP) rise in response to an increase in myocardial wall stress. Evidence exists supporting their use for diagnosing, staging, making hospitalization/discharge decisions, and identifying patients at risk for clinical events. The evidence for their use in monitoring and adjusting drug therapy is less clearly established. There is no definitive cut-off value recognized for either of the two natriuretic peptides for the diagnosis of HF. A normal concentration in an untreated patient has a high negative predictive value and makes HF an unlikely cause of symptoms (Bettencourt, 2005; Dickstein et al., 2008).

2.1 Concordance

Diagnosis starts with clinical history collection and registration.

To assess the relative completeness and validity of data sources for evaluating the quality of care, 1270 patients with at least one of a set of chronic diseases were sampled from 39 American medical organizations and surveyed. Self-reported information and ambulatory care record data were compared to assess concordance (Tisnado et al., 2006).

In this study, the prevalence of previous diagnosis of heart failure was 13% according to the medical record, 9% according to patient's self-report and 18% according to one or both sources. The proportion of cases in which medical records and patient's self-report agreed regarding previous history of heart failure was 86%, which might seem high. However, if the data in medical records and patient's self-report were truly independent, that is if having a diagnosis of heart failure registered in the medical record was in no way related with the probability of the patient reporting such diagnosis (the extreme, and for this matter absurd, situation of independence, the null hypothesis), then by chance alone agreement could be observed in some cases. This effect of chance is usually the most difficult to understand, but the point is in the concept of statistical independence.

Consider the raw data presented in the following table:

		Medical record		
		Heart failure	No heart failure	Total
Patient's self-report	Heart failure	50 [a]	64 [b]	114
	No heart failure	115 [c]	1041 [d]	1156
	Total	165 [g]	1105 [g]	1270

Table 1. Cross-classification of diagnosis of heart failure according to data source. In concordance tables, paired data are presented so the number of observations is the number of subjects but for each subject two variables are being presented at the same time; for instance, in the first cell 50 cases are counted with heart failure registered in the medical record and also reported by the patient. (Note: the data presented in this table were derived for the purpose of presentation but were not published as such in the original paper (Tisnado et al., 2006) and it is possible they are not real.)

Under independence, one would expect to observe a distribution of heart failure *versus* no heart failure that was the same by strata of what was observed in the other data source. Specifically, if 165/1270, that is 13%, of patients are considered to have heart failure according to the medical record, this distribution would be 13% with heart failure among the 114 who self-reported heart failure (n=14.82) and 13% with heart failure among the 1156 who did not (n=150.28). Thus, the expected number of cases in cell "a" would be 14.82 and the expected number of cases in cell "d" would be 1005.81, and the agreement would be 100x(14.82+1005.81)/1270=80%.

Given the low prevalence of heart failure, even in this sample of patients with chronic diseases, the probability of no heart failure is so high that the agreement expected by chance becomes very high. In other words, regardless of the other data source, in any data source the likelihood of no heart failure is so high that the probability of both data sources reporting no heart failure is also high.

The kappa coefficient aims at quantifying concordance beyond that expected by chance alone, to avoid overestimation of true concordance when looking at absolute agreement. The underlying idea is that concordance varies from 0 to 100% (no cases concordant to all cases concordant). The absolute agreement is the proportion of concordant cases directly observed (in this case 86%). If it was true that the information registered in both data sources was independent of each other, by chance alone one would expect to have observed concordant classification in 80% of cases. So, 86% is only 6% higher than expected by chance under independence. Departing from the expected agreement due to chance, the maximum increase in agreement up to perfect concordance is 20% and kappa expresses the 6% increase as a proportion of this maximum possible: 6/20=0.3 (Fig. 1).

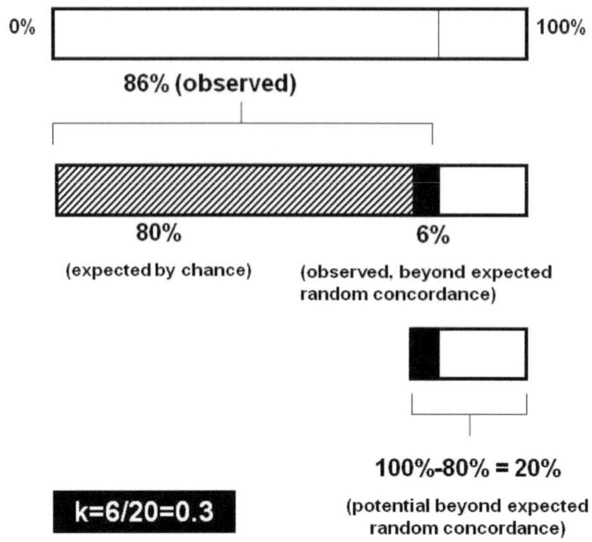

Fig. 1. Interpretation of kappa coefficient.

Assuming the meaning and interpretation of the kappa coefficient is now clear, its definition is: k=(absolute agreement - expected agreement) / (100 - expected agreement). In our example, k=(86-80)/(100-80)=0.3.

It is clear that kappa is zero when the absolute agreement is equal to that expected by chance and its maximal value is 1, when the absolute agreement is 100%, that is, perfect concordance. In theory it can take up negative values if the observed absolute agreement is lower than that expected by chance, but if this happens in situations where you expect some agreement, check for errors in coding of variables in your database before you accept the result.

There are suggestions of ranges of values for kappa to be interpreted as excellent, good, fair or poor agreement but no universal solution exists. The same value might be considered excellent if we are assessing the concordance between scales to measure a subjective and imprecise phenomenon, while it may be unacceptably low when assessing for example the concordance between two laboratory methods to measure the same protein.

Many software packages are available to calculate kappa coefficients, along with confidence intervals estimation, and for more complex scenarios than a two-rater or two-method classification of a dichotomous variable.

Obviously, the kappa coefficient is adequate to assess the concordance in categorical variables that are expected to have the same value. It can be used to quantify the inter- or intra-observer reproducibility (between observers that rate the same subjects or repeated measurements by the same observer), an instrument's precision, or, as in the case presented, the agreement between different methods of assessing the same construct.

The agreement between two observers/methods in assessing a continuous variable cannot be approached with the calculation of a kappa coefficient, unless the results are categorized, resulting in loss of information. The correlation coefficient between two continuous variables, such as for example two measurements of the same phenomenon by different methods or different observers, measures the extent to which they are linearly related, and concordant observations are obviously expected to be strongly correlated. However, very high correlations do not necessarily reflect agreement. An extreme example illustrates this clearly: the correlation between x and $2x$ is perfect, yet for no subject will they be equal except when $x=0$.

Over 20 years ago, Bland and Altman proposed a graphical method to assess agreement between methods of clinical measurement (Bland & Altman, 1986). This method is based on the graphical display of the difference between the two raters/methods (Y axis) against the average of both values for each subject (X axis).

Let us see how this applies with an example. A frequently raised question in clinical practice that has important implications on therapeutic decisions in the management of heart failure is that estimates of ejection fraction vary between alternative methods of assessing it, namely standard two-dimensional echocardiogram, nuclear imaging perfusion studies and magnetic resonance.

Mistry et al. determined left ventricular ejection fraction and end-diastolic volumes in 150 patients treated for acute ST-elevation myocardial infarction using four imaging studies - standard echocardiography (standard echo), contrast echocardiography (contrast echo), single-photon emission computed tomography (SPECT), and magnetic resonance imaging (MRI) (Mistry et al., 2010). Fig. 2 depicts a sample of Bland-Altman plots for left ventricular ejection fraction and end-diastolic volume from this study.

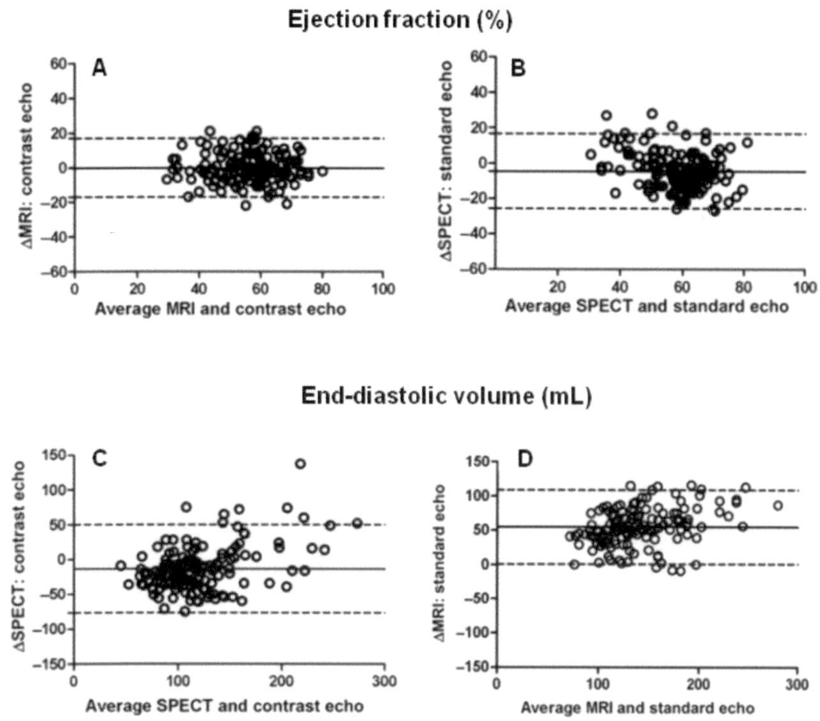

Fig. 2. Agreement in estimation of left ventricular ejection fraction and end-diastolic volume between standard echocardiography (standard echo), contrast echocardiography (contrast echo), single-photon emission computed tomography (SPECT), and magnetic resonance imaging (MRI). Adapted from (Mistry et al., 2010) with kind permission of Elsevier.

With the graph and a few simple calculations, one can extract several informations. Firstly, is the mean difference close to zero? Under perfect concordance, not only would the mean of individual differences be zero but all differences (for all subjects) should be zero. Secondly, is the distribution of differences symmetrical in relation to the horizontal line at the mean of differences? Such symmetry argues in favor of random variation explaining the dispersion. The correlation coefficient between measurements' difference and their mean tests for the presence of systematic error (bias), with higher values suggesting more severe bias. Thirdly, what are the boundaries for variation in differences? These are usually presented and quantified using 95% limits of agreement which are no more than the limits of the interval between 1.96 times the standard deviation of the difference above and below the mean difference. Of course that this works well if the width of variation of differences does not differ much by the average value from the two methods.

In some cases (Fig. 2, Panel C), the width of the variation in differences is larger for higher values of the variable and then it is best to use the logarithm of the initial variables which corresponds to assessing the relative instead of absolute differences.

Bland–Altman analysis of ejection fraction measured by all four imaging modalities showed generally low mean differences but wide limits of agreement. Left ventricular end-diastolic volume was systematically larger when assessed by MRI and, when assessed by SPECT in comparison with contrast echo, it was higher by SPECT only for severely dilated cavities (Fig. 2). While it is known that MRI is the most valid method, it is relevant to assess concordance of alternative methods with the standard since MRI is not always feasible.

The reproducibility of clinical findings in heart failure is important not only at the time of diagnosis but also to interpret changes or absence of change over time, namely because physical examination findings, specifically the jugular venous pressure coupled with biomarker trends, are useful in timing discharge planning or making therapeutic decisions. For example, in order to assess how large the variation between measurements of NT–pro-BNP can be in patients with clinically stable heart failure, we measured its plasma concentration at rest repeatedly at 3-week intervals, in 118 patients. The results supported the clinical use of NT–pro-BNP in the monitoring of patients with HF with high NT–pro-BNP levels (>1,300 pg/mL). In these patients, variations between around 30% more and 30% less than the baseline can be expected without clinical improvement or deterioration; therefore, only changes larger than these should be valued. In patients with lower mean values, the variability was even larger, but in those patients the answer to the appropriateness of monitoring the biomarker over time is not as relevant (Araújo et al., 2006).

Lack of concordance can result from lack of precision or systematic error. Its correct interpretation depends on judgment and familiarity with the question being studied. For example, in the study cited above where the relative completeness and validity of ambulatory medical record and patient's self-report as data sources for evaluating the quality of care setting was assessed (Tisnado et al., 2006), when data on echocardiogram as a delivered service were analyzed, that is, whether the patient had undergone an echocardiograhic examination, the concordance between medical record and patient's self-report was very low (absolute agreement 55%, kappa=0.1). This could have happened for several reasons, some representing systematic error in medical records, such as the absence of registration of ordered tests, the fact that an ordered test might not have been done, etc, systematic error in patient's self-report, such as the patient not knowing that the test performed was an echocardiogram, etc, or by lack of precision of both data sources. The point is that concordance is not a good measure of validity, even if one of the methods/observers can be considered the standard against which the other(s) is(are) being assessed. Measurement of validity particularly applied to diagnosis will be addressed in the next section of this chapter.

2.2 Validity

Validity of a piece of information for diagnosis, be it a fact collected by clinical history, a finding (or lack thereof) in physical examination or the result of an ancillary test, is assessed by confronting that information with the true state regarding presence or absence of a certain disease one is aiming to confirm or rule out.

The first challenge is that very often there is no good standard to define the true state. Sometimes, only the test of time or response to therapy can bring a definite conclusion regarding a hypothetical diagnosis, but these are affected by other factors, such as competitive risks, effectiveness of interventions, determinants of the treatment decisions and assessment of the patient's condition after some follow up time. Also, even if there is a standard with which to compare a test whose validity one aims to assess, if the standard is not perfect, and it seldom if ever is, apparent lack of sensitivity of the new test may result from mere lack of specificity of the standard (false positive cases in assessment with the standard are actually well classified as negative by the new test, but since the standard is our reference, we see the test result as false negative) and apparent lack of specificity of the test may result from lack of sensitivity of the standard.

In comparing with the standard, the accuracy of the test results is usually quantified with two measures of the proportion of correctly classified cases: sensitivity is the proportion of true cases that are considered positive by the test and specificity is the proportion of true non-cases that are considered negative by the test.

Specificity, like sensitivity, is often considered an intrinsic property of a test and therefore independent of the population under study. However, as specificity is determined by unaffected individuals who have positive results, it is in fact dependent on the characteristics (even subclinical) of this comparison population (Rutjes et al., 2005). It is critical to evaluate the study design from which the specificity of a test has been determined and to consider whether the test can be used more appropriately to distinguish one disease from another or to distinguish the presence or absence of disease. Also, sensitivity is vulnerable to variation depending on the spectrum of severity of the cases studied (Lunet et al., 2009; Ransohoff & Feinstein, 1978). For example, due to these spectrum effects and characteristics of the comparison population, published values for sensitivity and specificity of a long list of history, physical examination and ancillary tests for the diagnosis of heart failure as the cause of dyspnea in the emergency department (Wang et al., 2005) do not necessarily apply to the same clinical findings in primary care or in an epidemiologic study in the general population.

All clinicians understand that predictive value is critical for moving beyond the simplicity of sensitivity and specificity for interpretation of test results. In simple terms, the starting point of a clinical encounter immediately influences the probability of the patient being affected by a certain disease one may be trying to diagnose. Whether the patient came by his initiative due to a complaint or referred by another colleague or was actually called for a screening procedure, the clinician, more or less consciously depending on personal characteristics and the circumstances, immediately elaborates a list of possible diagnoses, ordered by the probability of being the right diagnosis for that case. He then works from there to gather additional information that will help reorder this list, hopefully bringing some hypotheses to become such remote possibilities that they are excluded and a few, preferably one, to such high probability that it is considered the final diagnosis.

In everyday clinical practice with individual patients, quantitative probability theory is usually not explicitly used. However, diagnostic reasoning, as described in the previous paragraph, involves a probabilistic approach and takes into account the validity of tests when incorporating their results in the process of diagnosis. To interpret any diagnostic test, one must have information not only about the test's characteristics but also about the patient (or a population with similar characteristics). Incomplete epidemiological information that facilitates estimation of pretest probability certainly contributes to the challenge (Bianchi & Alexander, 2006). Few tests are inherently accurate enough to "rule in" or "rule out" disease effectively in all cases. We should look at results as altering disease probability. This requires estimation of a pretest probability that will be adjusted up or down by the test results (Bianchi & Alexander, 2006). This is bayesian logic, which uses an adjustment factor called the likelihood ratio to convert a pretest probability into a posttest probability (Grimes & Schulz, 2005).

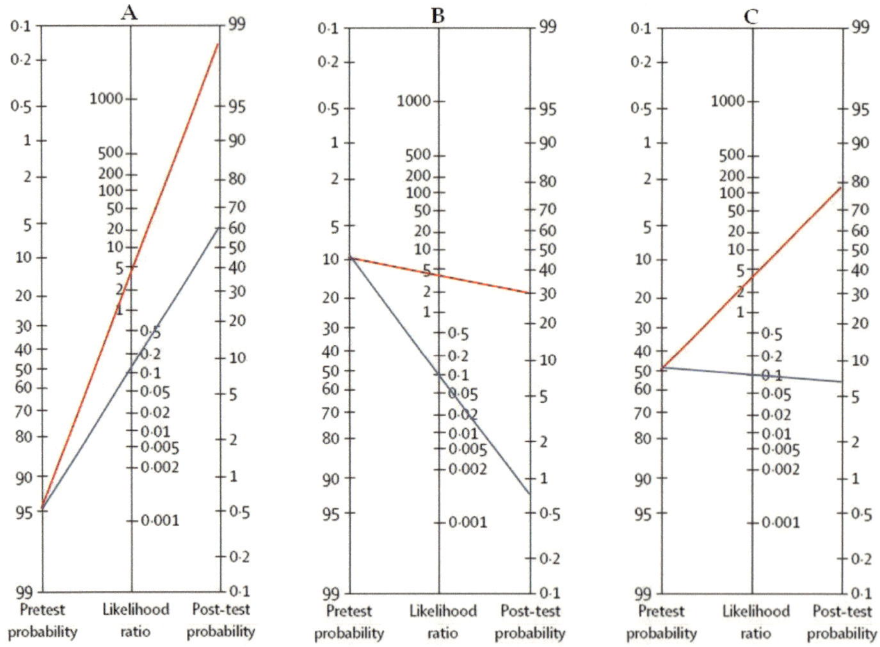

Fig. 3. Change from pre- to posttest probability, after a BNP test result is obtained, considering a positive (≥100pg/mL, red line) or negative (<100pg/mL, blue line) test result, with likelihood ratios of approximately 4 and 0.1, respectively (Wang, 2005), in three hypothetical scenarios in the emergency department: A – acute lung edema (pretest probability assumed to be 95%); B – unspecific malaise in an old patient without previous diagnosis of heart disease (pretest probability assumed to be 10%); C – aggravated dyspnea in a heavy smoker, with chronic obstructive lung disease and past history of myocardial infarction (pretest probability assumed to be 50%).

The key feature of the likelihood ratio is that, unlike traditional indices of validity, it incorporates all four cells of a 2-by-2 table (Grimes & Schulz, 2005). Likelihood ratios help clinicians to navigate zones of clinical uncertainty. Building on an accurate pretest probability of disease, likelihood ratios from ancillary tests can refine clinical judgment.

Clinicians should be wary of ordering tests when the pretest probability of disease is high or low. Tests are unlikely to alter disease probability and will only confuse the situation: unexpected results will usually be false-positives or false-negatives. Consider for example the scenarios represented in Fig. 3. In the case of an acute lung edema (Panel A), in which the clinical diagnosis is generally very accurate, a high BNP level will increase our certainty of the diagnosis from 95% to almost 99%, which is irrelevant. A low BNP value, on the other hand, does not exclude the diagnosis of heart failure and would still leave us thinking that the diagnosis is more likely (66%) to be heart failure than not. The correct clinical attitude would be to treat the acute lung edema immediately, avoiding the delay and cost of the test. If, on the contrary, the pretest probability is low (Panel B), then a low BNP value would only tell us what we already know and a high BNP would more likely be a false positive than represent heart failure. It is in the case of uncertainty (Panel C depicts equal probability of the diagnosis being heart failure or not, the maximum uncertainty) that the test is more able to change our thought: a high BNP value will yield a predictive value of 80%, which in the emergency department and for the hypothesis of heart failure is enough to decide treating as such, while a low BNP will practically exclude heart failure or at least lower its probability so much as to guide the diagnostic work-up in alternative directions.

Likelihood ratios enable clinicians to interpret and use the full range of diagnostic test results, not only dichotomous. For each test result, the likelihood ratio is the ratio between the probability of that result among cases to the probability of that same result among non-cases. Thus, test results with likelihood ratio close to 1, say between 0.5 and 2, are not informative because they are practically as likely to occur in cases as in non-cases and do not change the probability in the diagnostic reasoning. High likelihood ratios above 1 increase the probability of disease and low likelihood ratios below 1 decrease it. Going one step further from dichotomous test results, likelihood ratios can help deal with grey zones. For example, natriuretic peptides have a very low likelihood ratio for low plasma values, say <30 pg/mL, in untreated patients and reasonably high likelihood ratio for high values, say >250 pg/mL (Bettencourt, 2005; Wang, 2005). Between these two cut points, it is not such an informative test.

Ruling disease in or out (or considering subsequent decisions on management) depends on a comparison of posttest probability with thresholds for further action based on factors such as severity of disease, risks of further testing, or side effects of treatment. The posttest probability is the predictive value. Test results cannot be said to have predictive value; only a test result in a given patient (or population) has predictive value (Bianchi & Alexander, 2006).

Recognizing that most tests are imperfect and therefore do nothing more than adjust probability, which may or may not "rule in" or "rule out" the disease depending on the situation, protects against the misconception that a result can be interpreted without considering pretest probability.

The medical history and physical examination remain fundamentally important. Indeed, a precise assessment of the chance of disease can be far more important than the likelihood ratios of sophisticated, usually expensive and sometimes dangerous tests. Although clinical diagnosis might not necessarily be more accurate than ancillary testing, its accuracy has a striking effect on the interpretation of any test results that follow. An accurate pretest probability and subsequent testing can greatly improve clinical diagnosis.

Tests can build on each other in sequence as long as they are independent. Test independence means that the result from one test cannot bias the outcome of the next, such that the posttest probability after one test becomes the pretest probability of the subsequent test.

The purpose of diagnostic work-up is to assess whether the probability of disease is above or below the treatment threshold. Tests should only be used when they will affect management. If a clinician's pretest probability of disease securely rules in or out a diagnosis, further testing is unwarranted. More testing should be considered only in the murky middle zone of clinical uncertainty. The location of the decision thresholds along the continuum of diagnostic certainty needs to be determined before testing is done and should be tailored to the specific patient. Using a nomogram or a simple calculation, a clinician can estimate how high or low a likelihood ratio would have to be to shift the pretest probability down to exclude the diagnosis or up to begin treatment. If no test result would achieve this shift in probability, the test should not be done (Grimes & Schulz, 2005).

2.3 Early diagnosis (and screening?)

The increasingly deeper understanding of the pathophysiology of heart failure led to the definition of stages of heart failure (Hunt et al., 2001), considering asymptomatic cardiac dysfunction as an intermediate step to the development of overt heart failure. Long before this paradigm was established, the importance of asymptomatic left ventricular systolic dysfunction, one of the most important cardiac abnormalities underlying heart failure, was recognized. This recognition is related not only to its frequency, with a prevalence at least as high as that of symptomatic heart failure, but also to the fact that inhibition of the renin-angiotensin-aldosterone system could delay or prevent progression to symptomatic heart failure.

However, screening asymptomatic patients for heart failure remains controversial. In the Cardiovascular Health Study, only 9% of elderly patients who ultimately developed systolic heart failure had a reduced left ventricular ejection fraction on study enrollment, on average 5.5 years before (Gottdiener et al., 2000).

Biomarkers, such as the already mentioned natriuretic peptides, could potentially play this role; however, the cost-effectiveness and target populations for these strategies remain unsettled (Betti et al., 2009). For example, in the Olmsted County cohort, with a low prevalence of left ventricular systolic dysfunction (1.1%), 24% of the population would require an echocardiogram based on raised BNP concentrations and the vast majority of these echocardiograms (96%) would reveal an ejection fraction over 40%. The performance of BNP and NT-proBNP for the detection of left ventricular systolic dysfunction in the community is fair, mainly because of the low specificity, compromising the potential usefulness of the test as a screening procedure. Therefore, BNP testing for screening for left ventricular systolic dysfunction in the general population is not recommended (Bettencourt, 2005).

Effective primary and secondary prevention to decrease the burden of heart failure can be expected to be attained through adherence to existing guidelines and reduction of the financial and psychosocial barriers that impair adherence to prescribed medical therapy and lifestyle changes recommendations. In clinical practice, it is the practitioner's responsibility to search with clinical examination alone for latent structural heart disease and manifest heart failure, in a case-finding more than screening approach (Raffle & Muir Gray, 2007). Such screening can be accomplished by asking a simple series of questions related to the occurrence of such symptoms as easy fatigability, functional limitations, and development of lower extremity swelling (Ramani et al., 2010). This approach would contribute to better refine the pretest probability of ancillary tests which would no longer be done for screening but rather for diagnosis.

In general, the goodness of attempting an early diagnosis does not depend only on the existence of a valid test for identification of the altered state one is interested in identifying, but also on the ability to define an appropriate target population, that is, with a pretest probability upon which the test results can turn out to have acceptable predictive value. Moreover, early diagnosis should be considered only if effective treatment can be offered and the natural course of the disease changed by this intervention. Such effects on outcomes are best assessed using experimental approaches for complex interventions, that is, the intervention being tested should be the fact that early diagnosis is attempted and all consequences thereof. Obviously, such studies warrant a considerable investment of resources, adequate sample size and a favorable prior odds of successful long-term negative and positive predictive values. An interesting challenge is to create conditions in which these effects can be understood using observational or quasi-experimental research, namely using real-world data of actual practices and their relation with outcomes.

2.4 Utility of a diagnostic test

The rationale as to when a test should be applied requires a judgment that among patients to whom the test is administered, the costs of the illness, both monetary and physical, along with the cost of the test and the errors that arise when it does not classify patients accurately, will be exceeded by the costs of the illness, had the test not been done (Weiss, 2006).

The utility of a diagnostic test is multidimensional and its comprehensive assessment should take into account reproducibility, validity, feasibility, acceptability by subjects, costs and effects on decisions and clinical outcomes. This means that the answer may vary from place to place, institution to institution, physician to physician, and patient to patient.

Earlier sections of this chapter have reviewed issues of reproducibility and validity. We will now briefly address the effect of diagnostic tests on decisions and clinical outcomes, illustrating with an example.

The etiology of systolic heart failure affects prognosis and treatment. In newly diagnosed cardiomyopathy, the exclusion of underlying coronary artery disease and myocardium that might benefit from revascularization is critical. Patients with coronary artery disease and concomitant heart failure have a worse prognosis than those with nonischemic cardiomyopathy, but myocardial function may substantially improve after revascularization, highlighting the importance of making the appropriate diagnosis early and accurately.

Current European guidelines for the diagnostic work-up of acute and chronic heart failure recommend that coronary angiography should be considered in heart failure patients with a history of exertional angina or suspected ischemic left ventricular systolic dysfunction, following cardiac arrest, and in those with a strong risk factor profile for coronary heart disease, and may be urgently required in selected patients with severe heart failure (shock or acute pulmonary oedema) and in patients not responding adequately to treatment (Dickstein et al., 2008).

Angiographic evidence of atherosclerosis does not necessarily mean that revascularization will be beneficial. Left ventricular dysfunction in patients with coronary artery disease can improve substantially and even normalize after coronary artery bypass grafting (CABG) surgery, presumably due to recovery of function by hibernating myocardium, which is defined as myocardial tissue with abnormal function but maintained cellular function. The assessment of myocardial viability with the use of single-photon-emission computed tomography (SPECT) or low-dose dobutamine echocardiography is commonly performed to predict improvement in left ventricular function after CABG, and numerous studies have suggested that the identification of viable myocardium also predicts improved survival after CABG (Allman et al., 2002). However, studies that suggested an association between myocardial viability and outcome were retrospective in nature, and it is uncertain in most of these studies whether the decision to perform CABG may have been driven by the results of the tests, whether adjustment for key baseline variables was adequate, and whether patients who did not undergo CABG received aggressive medical therapy for heart failure. Therefore, the efficacy of this approach is uncertain.

The Surgical Treatment for Ischemic Heart Failure (STICH) trial was designed to compare the efficacy of medical therapy alone with that of medical therapy plus CABG in patients with angiographic documentation of coronary artery disease amenable to surgical revascularization and with left ventricular systolic dysfunction (ejection fraction ≤35%) (Velazquez et al., 2011). In the initial design of the trial, viability testing with SPECT was required for the enrollment of patients. However, due to unfeasibility of this requirement, the protocol was subsequently revised to make viability testing optional and to allow the use of either SPECT or dobutamine echocardiography for viability testing. Investigators at all study centers were strongly encouraged to perform viability testing in every patient, but the decision to perform the test was left up to the recruiting investigators. This resulted in only around half of patients in the trial undergoing viability testing. The differences in baseline characteristics between patients who underwent viability testing and those who did not undergo such testing suggest that at least some patients may have been selected for testing on the basis of clinical factors.

The risk of death was strongly and significantly lower in patients with than without viability (hazard ratio, 0.64; 95% confidence interval, 0.48–0.86), but after adjustment for other prognostic baseline variables the between-group difference was no longer significant (Bonow et al., 2011).

In patients without viability, the hazard ratio of all-cause death for CABG *versus* medical therapy alone was 0.70 (95% confidence interval: 0.41-1.18) and in patients with viability 0.86 (95% confidence interval: 0.64-1.16), p for interaction=0.53, which was interpreted as evidence that the effect of CABG does not depend on the existence of viability (Bonow et al., 2011). Since in the STICH trial there was overall no significant difference between medical therapy alone and medical therapy plus CABG with respect to this primary end point (Velazquez et al., 2011), this may not be the best endpoint to assess an interaction with viability. Patients assigned to CABG, as compared with those assigned to medical therapy alone, had lower rates of death from cardiovascular causes and of death from any cause or hospitalization for cardiovascular causes (Velazquez et al., 2011); the authors did not find a significant interaction between myocardial-viability status and medical *versus* surgical treatment with respect to the rates of death from any cause or from cardiovascular causes or the rate of death or hospitalization for cardiovascular causes either (Bonow et al., 2011).

Despite the strengths of the study described in comparison with the previous literature, the shortcomings acknowledged by the authors in the STICH trial leave some doubt regarding the effect of viability studies on clinical outcomes. The direct response to this question would warrant the randomization of patients to undergo viability testing or not. A pragmatic approach to estimate effectiveness would leave to the physicians' discretion the decision of management after knowing the result (or not).

Cost-effectiveness analyses are out of scope of this chapter.

3. (Evidence-based) Management

The fact that the decision to order a viability test, and then acting upon the observed result, is dependent on clinical characteristics and on the clinicians' impression of the benefit a particular patient may derive from that approach introduces confounding when comparing outcomes of patients managed this way with those of patients managed otherwise. This is called confounding by indication (the indication for the intervention being tested, or the clinical "hunch" that such indication exists).

Confounding by indication is one of the main reasons why a randomized controlled trial is the study design that creates best conditions for valid causal inferences in attributing an effect in outcomes to an intervention being tested, pharmacological or of other nature. The high position of randomized clinical trials in the hierarchy of study designs for intended effects of therapy derives from this requisite.

Jan Vandenbroucke argues that we may have been deluding ourselves about their unique superiority because they start with much higher prior odds than most observational research (Vandenbroucke, 2008). In fact, for obvious reasons, clinical trials are conducted only under conditions of high probability of success (benefit of the intervention), specifically 1:1, that is, "equipoise" (Djulbegovic et al., 2000) in the sense that it is at least as likely to be beneficial as not, which contributes to the much lower risk of not standing the test of time than observational research which is conducted under much lower prior odds (Vandenbroucke, 2008).

This is not to suggest that this hierarchy is senseless or useless. This author suggests that we need two different hierarchies, the hierarchy of discovery and explanation and that of evaluation, to assess the evidence of studies designed and conducted for different purposes. Etiologic researchers should pursue low probability hypotheses because these may lead to new insights, particularly if they are able to take advantage of detecting what was wrong when they go down the wrong way (Vandenbroucke, 2008).

In conclusion, the widely accepted hierarchy of levels of evidence in clinical research must be interpreted specifically for the context of evaluation of interventions, be them pharmacological or as "macro" as the organization of services.

It is not the purpose of this text to review extensively the principles and characteristics of clinical trials and several sources of literature can be found regarding this issue. I suggest introductory epidemiology books for a more rapid overview of the fundamental concepts and principles in study design, Haynes et al's Clinical Epidemiology for a thorough review from the clinical point of view with sensible calls of attention useful for interpretation (Haynes et al., 2006), and Friedman and DeMets' references for more applied approach based on case studies covering also execution issues (DeMets et al., 2006; Friedman et al., 2010).

In aiming to provide the concepts and develop competencies necessary for using the medical literature and making clinical decisions, as announced at the beginning of this chapter, we will briefly review an issue that is often misunderstood by clinicians, leading to misinterpretation of the results of trials, and which is intimately related with issues of precision and validity discussed in previous sections.

When, as is the case for most outcomes in heart failure, there are several interventions with well documented benefit and clearly recommended, alternative options for the same effect are tested under non-inferiority and equivalence hypotheses, raising the need to define minimally important differences, which must be established based on knowledge of the natural history of disease guided by clinical judgment. One major condition for credibility of trials is complete preplanning of every aspect of the trial and advance registration and documentation of everything that was preplanned (Laine et al., 2007), including the *a priori* definition of this threshold of effect (Moher et al., 2010).

If a study is designed to test whether a new treatment is significantly different from the control intervention at the 5% significance level, with the null hypothesis being no difference between groups (relative risk = 1 or difference = 0), the absence of a significant difference, that is, failure to reject the null hypothesis, is not synonymous with the interventions being clinically equivalent. Absence of proof of difference is not proof of absence of difference (Haynes et al., 2006). Minimally important differences from the clinical point of view must be defined beforehand and then the results must be interpreted in light of these thresholds and considering the whole width of the confidence interval of the effect estimate (Haynes et al., 2006).

Let us consider an example. In chronic heart failure, inhibition of the renin–angiotensin–aldosterone system by angiotensin-converting enzyme inhibitors improves survival and decreases morbidity, improving exercise capacity, quality of life, and left ventricular function and size (Konstam et al., 1993; Konstam et al., 1992). Although a cornerstone in the treatment of heart failure, angiotensin-converting enzyme inhibitors are underused, partly due to side effects. If proven at least similarly efficacious to angiotensin-converting enzyme inhibitors, angiotensin-receptor blockers could at least be considered an alternative due to their superior tolerability. The primary objective of the HEAVAN study was to test the hypothesis that valsartan, in comparison with enalapril, is at least as effective on exercise capacity, measured as distance walked during a 6-minute walk test, in heart failure patients stabilised on an angiotensin-converting enzyme inhibitor (Willenheimer et al., 2002).

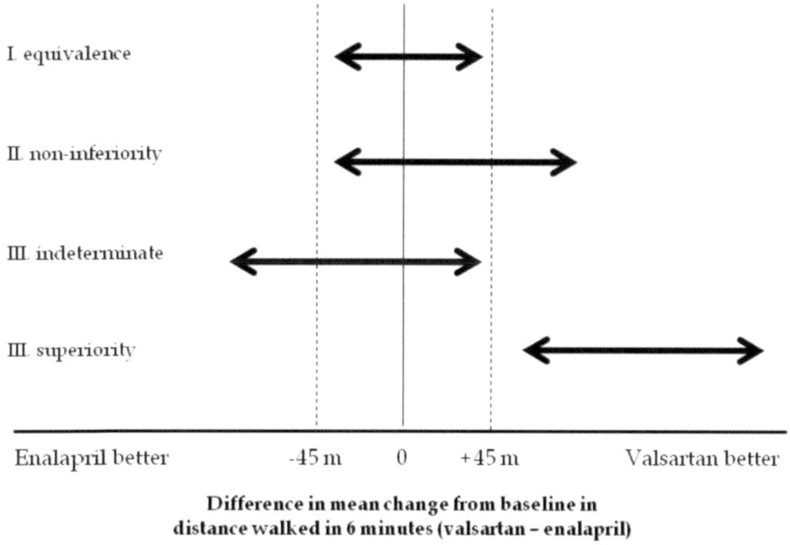

Fig. 4. Schematic representation and interpretation of 4 possible results of the HEAVAN study. The horizontal two-headed arrows represent the 95% confidence interval of the difference between the valsartan and enalapril treatment groups in the change, from baseline to after treatment, in distance walked in 6 minutes.

Non-inferiority was defined as a treatment effect of valsartan, with respect to mean change from baseline in the distance walked during the 6-minute walk test, better than 45 m less than that of enalapril.

A distance of 45 m was chosen based on an expected average baseline 6-min-walk test distance of 450 m, since a difference of 10% in this distance is not considered clinically relevant (Willenheimer et al., 2002). The 10% threshold must at least cover the imprecision of the outcome measurement, if not more, as long as there is fundament from previous data. For example, if one was to study the effect of some intervention on the change in NT-proBNP in chronic heart failure patients, only variations beyond 30% of baseline, upwards or downwards, should be considered clinically important, given the (apparently random) fluctuation of this biomarker under clinical stability, as described above (Araújo et al., 2006).

In the HEAVAN study, the null hypothesis under test is not that there is no difference between treatments. Rather, this is an example of a situation where a one-sided test best suits the underlying reasoning. Unilateral questions warrant one-sided answers (Haynes et al., 2006). The four hypothetic scenarios represented in Fig. 4 show a situation of equivalence (I), with the limits of the confidence interval of the difference between treatments not surpassing 45 m in either direction; non-inferiority (II), with the lower limit of the confidence interval excluding the possibility of enalapril being more than 45 m more beneficial than valsartan, that is, the data are compatible with valsartan being better than or equivalent to enalapril, but not inferior; scenario III is the most vulnerable to misinterpretation, since the fact that zero difference is not excluded from the range of the confidence interval does not mean that the two interventions are not different and in fact in the situation represented in the figure, the superiority of enalapril, beyond 45 m, cannot be excluded based on the data; superiority (IV) implies that the whole confidence interval is beyond the minimal clinically important difference of 45 m.

Reaching target doses of angiotensin-converting enzyme inhibitors was once the main (process) objective when treating systolic heart failure patients. Angiotensin receptor blockers were initially candidates to replace angiotensin-converting enzyme inhibitors in case of low tolerability, as described above, but there is now evidence that adding an angiotensin receptor blocker to angiotensin-converting enzyme inhibitor leads to a further clinically important reduction in relevant cardiovascular events in such patients (McMurray et al., 2003), possibly even when a beta-blocker and an aldosterone antagonist are concurrently prescribed (Weir et al., 2008). The current state-of-the-art management of heart failure involves use of multiple drugs, which are not free from side-effects particularly when used together and in high doses, with a lower benefit being generally obtained if the highest tolerated dose up to the target is not used. Moreover, patients in need of such care are old and with multiple comorbidities, but it is important to emphasize that the recommended schemes can be tolerated with benefit by a large proportion of patients under the care of experienced professionals.

The complexity of the heart failure syndrome, together with the increasingly recognized need for demonstration of cost-effectiveness of interventions, motivates research to assess the effect of specialized multidisciplinary heart failure management programmes. The heterogeneity of the content and organization of these programmes in large part justifies conflicting results (McDonagh et al., 2011). On the other hand, observational approaches to study the effect of such interventions have been threatened by serious selection bias and confounding by indication (Azevedo et al., 2002). However, experimental evidence has been accumulating supporting the benefit of a range of models of programmes and it is generally accepted that specialized teams of different kinds are more successful in achieving higher rates of patients under recommended prognosis modifying drug and device therapy, with drug doses closer to the recommended targets and overall benefit for patients namely in reducing hospitalizations. Consequently, heart failure management programmes are recommended for patients with HF recently hospitalized and for other high-risk patients (Dickstein et al., 2008).

4. Prognosis

Physicians need to counsel patients about prognosis to enable informed decisions about medications, devices, transplantation, and end-of-life care.

Heart failure has an ominous prognosis, particularly after an acute heart failure episode requiring hospitalization. Half of patients admitted with acute heart failure are readmitted within 6 months (Bettencourt et al., 2004; Jong et al., 2002). Analysis of 100 000 cases of acute decompensated heart failure in the United States revealed that in-hospital mortality after hospital admission ranges from 5% to 8%, with 1-year mortality averaging 40% to 60% (Adams Jr et al., 2005). It has been general practice to discharge patients according to improvement in symptoms, but, given the reproducibility and validity of clinical examination discussed above, it becomes clear that this decision threshold suffers from severe inter-observer variability. Some studies have tried to identify patients at higher risk of death and/or readmission who might benefit from more intensive therapy. Also for this prognosis issue, natriuretic peptides were good candidates for objective assessment of risk since they decrease in close correlation with falling wedge pressures, and correlate with functional capacity.

We followed a sample of 156 patients consecutively admitted to the hospital due to acute decompensated heart failure and discharged alive, excluding acute coronary syndromes, for the primary end-point of death or hospital readmission for 6 months. The plasma concentration of NT-proBNP at admission was not associated with the endpoint, in contrast with that at discharge, suggesting that it is the change in response to therapy during hospitalization, that matters most. Thus, to refine the risk stratification with the dynamic perspective of change in neuro-humoral activation, we studied the effect of the relative change in NT-proBNP from baseline to discharge. Categories of this new variable were defined according to a change of at least 30%, in agreement with the clinical meaning that can be attributed to the time variation discussed above. The results are depicted in Fig. 5 and clearly show an increase in risk that can be predicted from the change in NT-proBNP during hospitalization and which was independent of clinical signs of volume overload at discharge, thus confirming that new information is being obtained from this biomarker (Bettencourt et al., 2004).

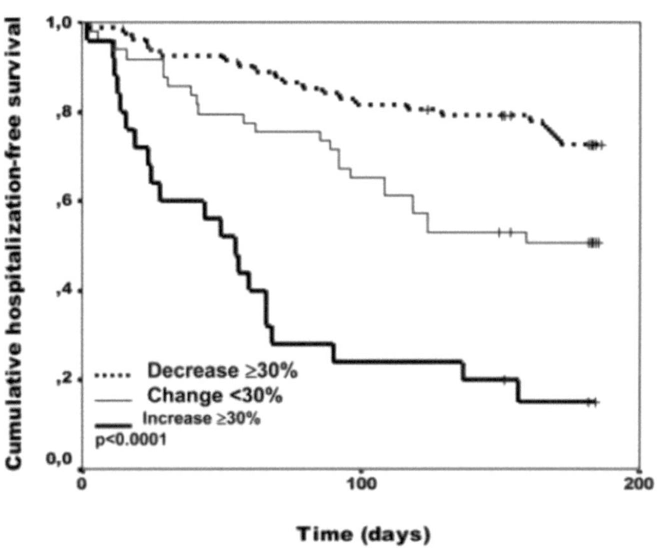

Fig. 5. Cumulative hospitalization-free survival according to patterns of response of NT-proBNP (decreased by ≥30% of baseline value, changed by <30%, increased by ≥30%). Reprinted from (Bettencourt et al., 2004) with kind permission of Wolters Kluwer Health.

Many clinical, laboratory and functional variables have been identified as associated with prognosis in chronic and acute heart failure patients. Clinical prediction rules include simultaneous consideration of several factors in predicting the prognosis of individual patients.

Evaluation of prediction models should consider two attributes. Discrimination is related to higher values of the predicted value of the outcome being obtained among those who actually develop the outcome. This is exactly what the area under a ROC curve represents, specifically the probability that a random person with the outcome has a higher value of the measurement than a random person without the outcome (Altman & Bland, 1994). Calibration goes a step forward and measures to which extent the model predicts well what will happen. This is usually done with a goodness-of-fit test such as the Hosmer-Lemeshow statistic (Lemeshow & Hosmer, 1982) or by simply comparing predicted and observed numbers of events, usually by deciles of predicted risk. Deviations in absolute risk prediction are important when applying a model for clinical decision-making and suggest that recalibration might be necessary, which consists in correcting the baseline risk function with data from the population in which the model is to be used while importing the coefficients (if discrimination is good).

Most existing models to predict the risk of death or urgent transplantation in heart failure have features that may limit their applicability. These models relied on either peak oxygen consumption or invasive measures of cardiac performance, and most have not been validated in another sample than the one used for its development. An exception is the Seattle Heart Failure Model (SHFM) which allows prediction of survival of heart failure patients with the use of easily obtained clinical characteristics. The model provides an accurate estimate of mean, 1-, 2-, and 3-year survival and is unique in allowing estimation of effects of adding medications or devices to a patient's regimen (Levy et al., 2006), potentially contributing to the better prediction of mortality than clinical characteristics alone, because medications and devices are critically altered by physicians to improve the chances of survival of their patients. The model was developed using previously collected data in a cohort of 1125 patients with predominantly left ventricular systolic heart failure [the Prospective Randomized Amlodipine Survival Evaluation (PRAISE)] and 9942 patients from other 5 cohorts were used to prospectively validate the model. PRAISE was a randomized trial of amlodipine *versus* placebo among patients in the United States and Canada with ejection fraction below 30% and New York Heart Association functional class IIIB to IV heart failure (Packer, 1996, as cited in (Levy et al., 2006)).

The SHFM and 3 other predictive models, namely Acute Decompensated Heart Failure National Registry (ADHERE), the American Heart Association Get With The Guidelines-Heart Failure score (GWTG-HF), and Association of Health Aging and Body Composition Heart Failure score (ABC), were all calculated in each of 2472 consecutive patients hospitalized with acute heart failure. The authors compared predicted and observed mortality and also compared the predicted mortality with the observed composite end point, including death, heart transplantation, or implantation of left ventricular assist device (Nakayama et al., 2011). For all the outcomes assessed, the SHFM had highest discrimination as indicated by a higher area under the receiver operating characteristic curve (Fig. 6).

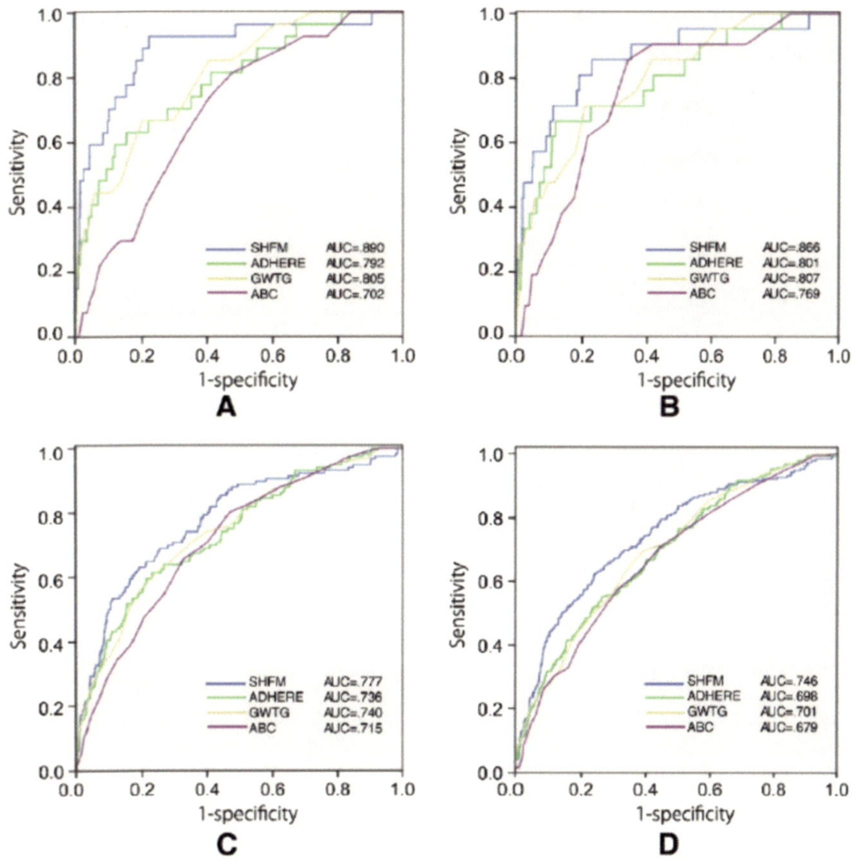

Fig. 6. Area under the receiver operating characteristic curves (AUC) for combined end point of death, heart transplantation, or left ventricular assist device implantation for Seattle Heart Failure Model (SHFM), Acute Decompensated Heart Failure National Registry (ADHERE), the American Heart Association Get With The Guidelines-Heart Failure score (GWTG-HF), and Association of Health Aging and Body Composition Heart Failure score (ABC), for *(A)* in-hospital death, and combined end points at *(B)* 30 days and *(C)* 1- and *(D)* 2 years of follow-up. Reprinted from (Nakayama et al., 2011) with kind permission of Elsevier.

Calibration analysis, presented in Fig. 7, shows absence of important or significant differences between predicted and observed events, supporting the validity of this prognostic model for populations quite different from those of the original study, and indicating that the SHFM is also an adequate risk prediction model in patients with milder heart failure.

Much of the accumulated evidence on the prognosis of heart failure resulted from the prospective assessment of outcomes in patients included in the negative control arm of randomized clinical trials in which a patient population might have been limited because of strict enrollment criteria, resulting in the exclusion of patients with severe conditions and comorbidities. With the development and generalization of access to informatic resources, large administrative databases and electronic medical records have increasingly been used to fit risk prediction models to assess prognosis. Major issues raised by these settings and data sources are the generalizability of results from randomized trials and completeness and accuracy of data from large administrative databases or electronic medical records.

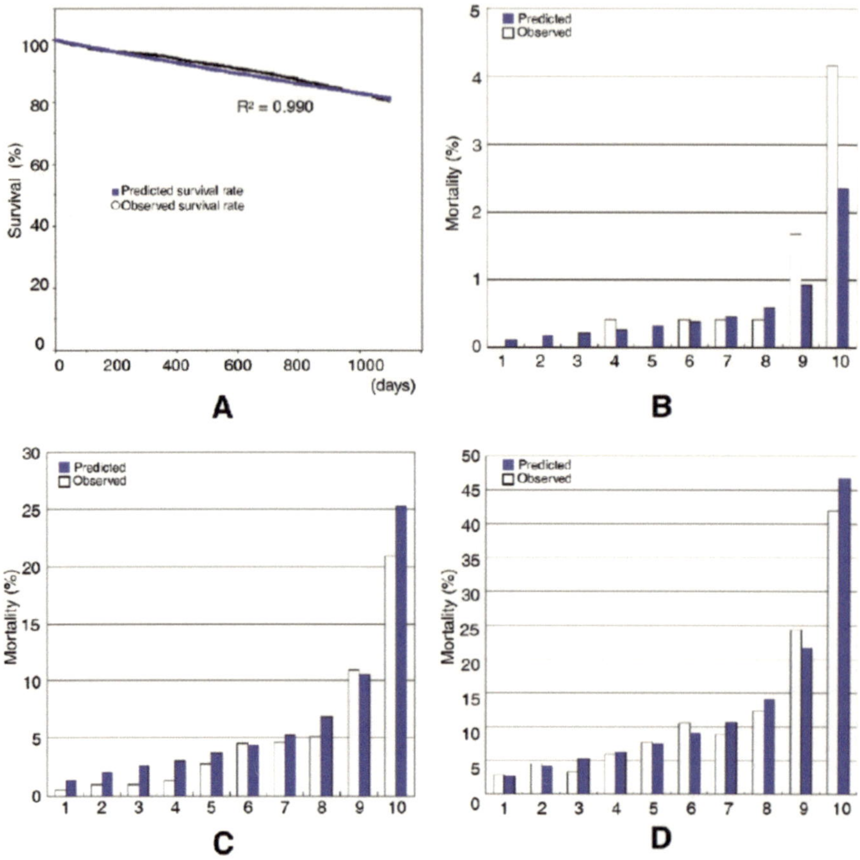

Fig. 7. (A) Comparison of predicted and observed survival for the Seattle Heart Failure Model (SHFM). Predicted (blue) *versus* observed (white) survival rate at each day plotted during follow-up period of ≤3 years. Calibration plots for composite outcome at (B) 30 days and (C) 1 and (D) 2 years for SHFM. Hosmer-Lemeshow chi-square was 7.21 (p = 0.51), 11.15 (p = 0.19), and 5.04 (p = 0.74) at 30 days and 1 and 2 years, respectively. Reprinted from (Nakayama et al., 2011) with kind permission of Elsevier.

Technological evolution led to the possibility of telemonitoring patients and continuously collecting physiological data through implanted devices. These large amounts of data, representing repeated measures over time, raise new challenges for the inclusion of all those time-varying data as independent variables in risk prediction models.

5. Conclusion

In contrast to other major cardiovascular diseases in developed countries, heart failure is a growing problem as the population ages and survivors of myocardial infarction live longer. The successful management of this population depends on risk factor reduction via lifestyle modification and application of currently established guidelines. During the past 3 decades, a combination of pharmacological, device-based and surgical treatment modalities has tremendously enhanced the survival and quality of life of patients with heart failure. Technological developments improve our capacities but also raise new challenges for their proper use.

The concepts and tools reviewed in this chapter help clinicians and researchers deal with uncertainty. Continued application of these principles in clinical practice and research is vital for optimal medical care for heart failure patients. These are, however, general principles that apply to clinical practice in other areas and heart failure was merely an example setting.

6. Acknowledgment

A project grant from the Portuguese Foundation for Science and Technology is gratefully acknowledged (PTDC/SAU-ESA/107940/2008).

7. References

Adams Jr, K. F.,Fonarow, G. C.,Emerman, C. L.,LeJemtel, T. H.,Costanzo, M. R.,Abraham, W. T.,Berkowitz, R. L.,Galvao, M. & Horton, D. P. (2005). Characteristics and outcomes of patients hospitalized for heart failure in the united states: Rationale, design, and preliminary observations from the first 100,000 cases in the acute decompensated heart failure national registry (ADHERE). *Am Heart J*, Vol.149, No.2, pp.209-216, 0002-8703.

Allman, K. C.,Shaw, L. J.,Hachamovitch, R. & Udelson, J. E. (2002). Myocardial viability testing and impact of revascularization on prognosis in patients with coronary artery disease and left ventricular dysfunction: A meta-analysis. *J Am Coll Cardiol*, Vol.39, No.7, pp.1151-1158, 0735-1097.

Altman, D. G. & Bland, J. M. (1994). Statistics notes: Diagnostic tests 3: Receiver operating characteristic plots. *BMJ*, Vol.309, No.6948, pp.188.

Araújo, J. P.,Azevedo, A.,Lourenço, P.,Rocha-Gonçalves, F.,Ferreira, A. & Bettencourt, P. (2006). Intraindividual variation of amino-terminal pro-b-type natriuretic peptide levels in patients with stable heart failure. *Am J Cardiol*, Vol.98, No.9, pp.1248-1250, 0002-9149.

Azevedo, A.,Pimenta, J.,Dias, P.,Bettencourt, P.,Ferreira, A. & Cerqueira-Gomes, M. (2002). Effect of a heart failure clinic on survival and hospital readmission in patients discharged from acute hospital care. *Eur J Heart Fail*, Vol.4, pp.353–359.

Bettencourt, P.,Azevedo, A.,Pimenta, J.,Friões, F.,Ferreira, S. & Ferreira, A. (2004). N-terminal–pro-brain natriuretic peptide predicts outcome after hospital discharge in heart failure patients. *Circulation*, Vol.110, No.15, pp.2168-2174.

Bettencourt, P. M. (2005). Clinical usefulness of B-type natriuretic peptide measurement: Present and future perspectives. *Heart*, Vol.91, No.11, pp.1489-1494.

Betti, I.,Castelli, G.,Barchielli, A.,Beligni, C.,Boscherini, V.,De Luca, L.,Messeri, G.,Gheorghiade, M.,Maisel, A. & Zuppiroli, A. (2009). The role of N-terminal pro-brain natriuretic peptide and echocardiography for screening asymptomatic left ventricular dysfunction in a population at high risk for heart failure. The PROBE-HF study. *J Card Fail*, Vol.15, No.5, pp.377-384, 1071-9164.

Bianchi, M. & Alexander, B. (2006). Evidence-based diagnosis: Does the language reflect the theory? *BMJ*, Vol.333, pp.442-445.

Bland, J. & Altman, D. (1986). Statistical methods for assessing agreement between two methods of clinical measurement. *Lancet*, Vol.1, No.8476, pp.307-310.

Bonow, R. O.,Maurer, G.,Lee, K. L.,Holly, T. A.,Binkley, P. F.,Desvigne-Nickens, P.,Drozdz, J.,Farsky, P. S.,Feldman, A. M.,Doenst, T.,Michler, R. E.,Berman, D. S.,Nicolau, J. C.,Pellikka, P. A.,Wrobel, K.,Alotti, N.,Asch, F. M.,Favaloro, L. E.,She, L.,Velazquez, E. J.,Jones, R. H. & Panza, J. A. (2011). Myocardial viability and survival in ischemic left ventricular dysfunction. *N Engl J Med*, Vol.364, No.17, pp.1617-1625.

DeMets, D.,Furberg, C. & Friedman, L. (2006). *Data monitoring in clinical trials: A case studies approach* Springer, ISBN 978-0387-20330-0, New York.

Dickstein, K.,Cohen-Solal, A.,Filippatos, G.,McMurray, J. J. V.,Ponikowski, P.,Poole-Wilson, P. A.,Strömberg, A.,van Veldhuisen, D. J.,Atar, D.,Hoes, A. W.,Keren, A.,Mebazaa, A.,Nieminen, M.,Priori, S. G. & Swedberg, K. (2008). ESC guidelines for the diagnosis and treatment of acute and chronic heart failure 2008. *Eur Heart J*, Vol.29, No.19, pp.2388-2442.

Djulbegovic, B.,Lacevic, M.,Cantor, A.,Fields, K.,Bennett, C. & al., e. (2000). The uncertainty principle and industry-sponsored research. *Lancet*, Vol.356, pp.635-638.

Friedman, L.,Furberg, C. & DeMets, D. (2010). *Fundamentals of clinical trials* (Fourth edition), Springer, ISBN 978-1441915856, New York.

Gottdiener, J. S.,Arnold, A. M.,Aurigemma, G. P.,Polak, J. F.,Tracy, R. P.,Kitzman, D. W.,Gardin, J. M.,Rutledge, J. E. & Boineau, R. C. (2000). Predictors of congestive heart failure in the elderly: The Cardiovascular Health Study. *J Am Coll Cardiol*, Vol.35, No.6, pp.1628-1637, 0735-1097.

Grimes, D. A. & Schulz, K. F. (2005). Refining clinical diagnosis with likelihood ratios. *Lancet*, Vol.365, No.9469, pp.1500-1505, ISSN 0140-6736.

Haynes, R.,Sackett, D.,Guyatt, G. & Tugwell, P. (2006). *Clinical epidemiology: How to do clinical practice research* (Third edition), Lippincott Williams & Wilkins, ISBN 0-7817-4524-1, Philadelphia.

Hunt, S. A.,Baker, D. W.,Chin, M. H.,Cinquegrani, M. P.,Feldmanmd, A. M.,Francis, G. S.,Ganiats, T. G.,Goldstein, S.,Gregoratos, G.,Jessup, M. L.,Noble, R. J.,Packer, M.,Silver, M. A.,Stevenson, L. W.,Gibbons, R. J.,Antman, E. M.,Alpert, J. S.,Faxon, D. P.,Fuster, V.,Jacobs, A. K.,Hiratzka, L. F.,Russell, R. O. & Smith, S. C. (2001). ACC/AHA guidelines for the evaluation and management of chronic heart failure in the adult: Executive summary a report of the American College of Cardiology/American Heart Association task force on practice guidelines (committee to revise the 1995 guidelines for the evaluation and management of heart failure). *Circulation*, Vol.104, No.24, pp.2996-3007.

Jong, P.,Vowinckel, E.,Liu, P. P.,Gong, Y. & Tu, J. V. (2002). Prognosis and determinants of survival in patients newly hospitalized for heart failure: A population-based study. *Arch Intern Med*, Vol.162, No.15, pp.1689-1694.

Konstam, M.,Kronenberg, M.,Rousseau, M.,Udelson, J.,Melin, J.,Stewart, D.,Dolan, N.,Edens, T.,Ahn, S. & Kinan, D. (1993). Effects of the angiotensin converting enzyme inhibitor enalapril on the long-term progression of left ventricular dilatation in patients with asymptomatic systolic dysfunction. SOLVD (Studies of Left Ventricular Dysfunction) investigators. *Circulation*, Vol.88, No.5, pp.2277-2283.

Konstam, M.,Rousseau, M.,Kronenberg, M.,Udelson, J.,Melin, J.,Stewart, D.,Dolan, N.,Edens, T.,Ahn, S. & Kinan, D. (1992). Effects of the angiotensin converting enzyme inhibitor enalapril on the long-term progression of left ventricular dysfunction in patients with heart failure. SOLVD investigators. *Circulation*, Vol.86, No.2, pp.431-438.

Laine, C.,Horton, R.,DeAngelis, C.,Drazen, J., Frizelle, F. A., Godlee, F., Haug, C., Hébert, P. C., Kotzin, S, Marusic, A, Sahni, P, Schroeder, T. V., Sox, H. C., Van der Weyden, M. B. & Verheugt, F. W. (2007). Clinical trial registration—looking back and moving ahead. *N Engl J Med*, Vol.356, pp.2734-2736.

Lemeshow, S. & Hosmer, D. J. (1982). A review of goodness of fit statistics for use in the development of logistic regression models. *Am J Epidemiol*, Vol.115, pp.92-106.

Levy, W. C.,Mozaffarian, D.,Linker, D. T.,Sutradhar, S. C.,Anker, S. D.,Cropp, A. B.,Anand, I.,Maggioni, A.,Burton, P.,Sullivan, M. D.,Pitt, B.,Poole-Wilson, P. A.,Mann, D. L. & Packer, M. (2006). The Seattle heart failure model. *Circulation*, Vol.113, No.11, pp.1424-1433.

Lunet, N.,Peleteiro, B.,Carrilho, C.,Figueiredo, C. & Azevedo, A. (2009). Sensitivity is not an intrinsic property of a diagnostic test: Empirical evidence from histological diagnosis of Helicobacter pylori infection. *BMC Gastroenterology*, Vol.9, No.1, pp.98, 1471-230X.

McDonagh, T. A.,Blue, L.,Clark, A. L.,Dahlström, U.,Ekman, I.,Lainscak, M.,McDonald, K.,Ryder, M.,Strömberg, A. & Jaarsma, T. (2011). European Society of Cardiology Heart Failure Association standards for delivering heart failure care. *Eur J Heart Fail*, Vol.13, No.3, pp.235-241.

McMurray, J. J. V.,Östergren, J.,Swedberg, K.,Granger, C. B.,Held, P.,Michelson, E. L.,Olofsson, B.,Yusuf, S. & Pfeffer, M. A. (2003). Effects of candesartan in patients with chronic heart failure and reduced left-ventricular systolic function taking angiotensin-converting-enzyme inhibitors: The CHARM-ADDED trial. *Lancet*, Vol.362, No.9386, pp.767-771, 0140-6736.

Mistry, N.,Halvorsen, S.,Hoffmann, P.,Müller, C.,Bøhmer, E.,Kjeldsen, S. E. & Bjørnerheim, R. (2010). Assessment of left ventricular function with magnetic resonance imaging vs. Echocardiography, contrast echocardiography, and single-photon emission computed tomography in patients with recent ST-elevation myocardial infarction. *Eur J Echocardiogr*, Vol.11, No.9, pp.793-800.

Moher, D.,Hopewell, S.,Schulz, K. F.,Montori, V.,Gøtzsche, P. C.,Devereaux, P. J.,Elbourne, D.,Egger, M. & Altman, D. G. (2010). Consort 2010 explanation and elaboration: Updated guidelines for reporting parallel group randomised trials. *J Clin Epidemiol*, Vol.63, No.8, pp.e1-e37, 0895-4356.

Murphy, E. (1997). *The logic of medicine.* (Second edition), The Johns Hopkins University Press, ISBN 0-8018-5538-1, Baltimore.

Nakayama, M.,Osaki, S. & Shimokawa, H. (2011). Validation of mortality risk stratification models for cardiovascular disease. *Am J Cardiol*, Vol.108, pp.391-396.

Paulus, W. J.,Tschöpe, C.,Sanderson, J. E.,Rusconi, C.,Flachskampf, F. A.,Rademakers, F. E.,Marino, P.,Smiseth, O. A.,De Keulenaer, G.,Leite-Moreira, A. F.,Borbély, A.,Édes, I.,Handoko, M. L.,Heymans, S.,Pezzali, N.,Pieske, B.,Dickstein, K.,Fraser, A. G. & Brutsaert, D. L. (2007). How to diagnose diastolic heart failure: A consensus statement on the diagnosis of heart failure with normal left ventricular ejection fraction by the heart failure and echocardiography associations of the European Society of Cardiology. *Eur Heart J*, Vol.28, No.20, pp.2539-2550.

Raffle, A. & Muir Gray, J. (2007). What screening is, and is not, In: *Screening: Evidence and practice*. A. Raffle and J. Muir Gray. pp. 33-57, Oxford University Press, ISBN 978-0-19-921449-5, New York.

Ramani, G. V.,Uber, P. A. & Mehra, M. R. (2010). Chronic heart failure: Contemporary diagnosis and management. *Mayo Clin Proc*, Vol.85, No.2, pp.180-195, ISSN 1942-5546.

Ransohoff, D. & Feinstein, A. (1978). Problems of spectrum and bias in evaluating the efficacy of diagnostic tests. *N Engl J Med*, Vol.299, pp.926 - 930.

Rutjes, A. W. S.,Reitsma, J. B.,Vandenbroucke, J. P.,Glas, A. S. & Bossuyt, P. M. M. (2005). Case-control and two-gate designs in diagnostic accuracy studies. *Clin Chem*, Vol.51, No.8, pp.1335-1341.

Tisnado, D. M.,Adams, J. L.,Liu, H.,Damberg, C. L.,Chen, W.-P.,Hu, F. A.,Carlisle, D. M.,Mangione, C. M. & Kahn, K. L. (2006). What is the concordance between the medical record and patient self-report as data sources for ambulatory care? *Med Care*, Vol.44, No.2, pp.132-140, 0025-7079.

Vandenbroucke, J. P. (2008). Observational research, randomised trials, and two views of medical science. *Plos Med*, Vol.5, No.3, pp.e67.

Velazquez, E. J.,Lee, K. L.,Deja, M. A.,Jain, A.,Sopko, G.,Marchenko, A.,Ali, I. S.,Pohost, G.,Gradinac, S.,Abraham, W. T.,Yii, M.,Prabhakaran, D.,Szwed, H.,Ferrazzi, P.,Petrie, M. C.,O'Connor, C. M.,Panchavinnin, P.,She, L.,Bonow, R. O.,Rankin, G. R.,Jones, R. H. & Rouleau, J.-L. (2011). Coronary-artery bypass surgery in patients with left ventricular dysfunction. *N Engl J Med*, Vol.364, No.17, pp.1607-1616.

Wang, C. S.,FitzGerald, J. M.,Schulzer, M.,Mak, E. & Ayas, N. T. (2005). Does this dyspneic patient in the emergency department have congestive heart failure? *JAMA*, Vol.294, No.15, pp.1944-1956.

Weir, R. A. P.,McMurray, J. J. V.,Puu, M.,Solomon, S. D.,Olofsson, B.,Granger, C. B.,Yusuf, S.,Michelson, E. L.,Swedberg, K.,Pfeffer, M. A. & Investigators, C. (2008). Efficacy and tolerability of adding an angiotensin receptor blocker in patients with heart failure already receiving an angiotensin-converting inhibitor plus aldosterone antagonist, with or without a beta blocker. Findings from the candesartan in heart failure: Assessment of reduction in mortality and morbidity (CHARM)-ADDED trial. *Eur J Heart Fail*, Vol.10, No.2, pp.157-163.

Weiss, N. (2006). *Clinical epidemiology. The study of the outcome of illness.* (Third edition), Oxford University Press, ISBN 978-0-19-530523-4, New York.

Willenheimer, R.,Helmers, C.,Pantev, E.,Rydberg, E.,Löfdahl, P. & Gordon, A. (2002). Safety and efficacy of valsartan versus enalapril in heart failure patients. *Int J Cardiol*, Vol.85, No.2-3, pp.261-270, 0167-5273.

11

The Use of Systematic Review and Meta-Analysis in Modern Epidemiology

Nuno Lunet
Department of Clinical Epidemiology, Predictive Medicine and Public Health,
University of Porto Medical School,
Institute of Public Health,
University of Porto (ISPUP)
Portugal

1. Introduction

The techniques for systematic review and meta-analysis provide tools for a standardized and sound assessment of the evidence available on different topics, and have gradually earned an important place in biomedical research [1], as well as in other scientific fields [2-3].

The extent to which systematic reviews/meta-analyses are used properly, their results interpreted correctly, and recognized as useful resources in biomedical research depends on the understanding of their methodological bases and on the pursuing of objectives compatible with the level of inference allowed by these methods and by the characteristics of the primary data sources. This comes ultimately from the comprehension of "the nature of meta-analysis" [4], which has been summarized beautifully as the "epidemiology of results of independent studies" [5] or "observational study of the evidence" [6], where the subjects are independent investigations, just as in ecological designs the group replaces the individual as the unit of analysis. In *Modern Epidemiology*, Greenland and O'Rourke [4] state that "meta-analysis can be viewed as the transference of good analytic practice from the single-study to the multiple-study context", and recognize that "the need to identify, abstract, and analyze data from multiple studies parallels the need of single studies to identify eligible subjects, abstract their information, and analyze the resulting data by summarizing information across subjects".

A corollary of this conceptual framework is that expertise in epidemiological methods in general and a deep understanding of the particular subjects under study, in addition to the proficient use of the specific techniques for literature search and synthesis, are essential for conducting sound and meaningful systematic reviews/meta-analyses. This chapter will address only concepts and methods specific or particularly important in this field, placing them in the context of epidemiological research in general. The detailed discussion of the resources that may be used to conduct systematic reviews and the statistical methods for meta-analysis is out of the scope of this chapter.

2. Systematic review/meta analysis vs. traditional reviews

The aims and scope of systematic reviews are clearly distinct from those of meta-analyses, and these methods can be used independently from each other, although both provide tools useful in the process of summarising information. These terms, however, are often used as synonyms, reflecting the fact that meta-analyses are seldom accomplished out of the context of a systematic review, although the opposite is not true.

While **systematic review** may be defined as "the application of strategies that limit bias in the assembly, critical appraisal, and synthesis of all relevant studies on a specific topic" [7], a **meta-analysis** is "a statistical analysis of the results from separate studies, examining sources of differences in results among studies, and leading to a quantitative summary of the results if the results are judged sufficiently similar to support such synthesis" [7]. To perform a meta-analysis we compute a weighted average of the results from each study, although some techniques involve statistical procedures with a degree of technical complexity much higher than the suggested by weighted averaging [8-10]. The weights vary with the method selected for meta-analysis, but the studies with more precise estimates are assigned higher weights [3].

Meta-analysis may be a valuable tool to summarize the evidence gathered in a systematic review, which is expected to yield an unbiased sample of the evidence available on a topic, and the quantitative synthesis therefore provide a summary estimate usually interpreted as the state of the art on that specific subject. However, in the context of a literature review, the results of meta-analyses conducted over biased samples of the evidence, which are more likely when a systematic approach is not adopted, are meaningless [3]. A large proportion of the published systematic reviews do not include a meta-analysis, either because the statistical synthesis of the results is not advisable, when studies are not considered similar enough or their results are heterogeneous, or possible, when the needed information is not available or is provided in different formats across the studies. A small number of studies use meta-analysis to summarize results not obtained from systematic reviews, which reflects the fact that these statistical techniques may be used in any set of individual studies considered "combinable", even if the units of analysis are not obtained from a literature review (*e.g.* meta-analyses of results from different centres of multicentre studies [11]).

In a sample of published systematic reviews/meta-analyses presented in Figure 1, less that 5% of the reports used meta-analysis on results that were not obtained from a systematic review and approximately one-third were systematic reviews that used meta-analysis for quantitative synthesis of the results; the remaining systematic reviews relied on other methods for data synthesis.

The systematic reviews, with or without meta-analysis, are expected to address a clearly defined research question and to present the methodological options and procedures with the necessary detail to make the review fully replicable by others, in addition to providing a thorough description and discussion of the characteristics of the studies and their results [12-14]. Although there is an element of subjectivity in the definition of the criteria to adopt in the different steps of the review and when drawing the conclusions, the mechanism by which the review achieves its final outcome is transparent, as long as all decisions are specified clearly, and it is possible to estimate the extent to which systematic reviews yield biased conclusions [3]. In contrast, it is often impossible to judge whether traditional or narrative reviews are trustworthy, as the definition of the objectives is often ambiguous and the materials and methods opaque [15].

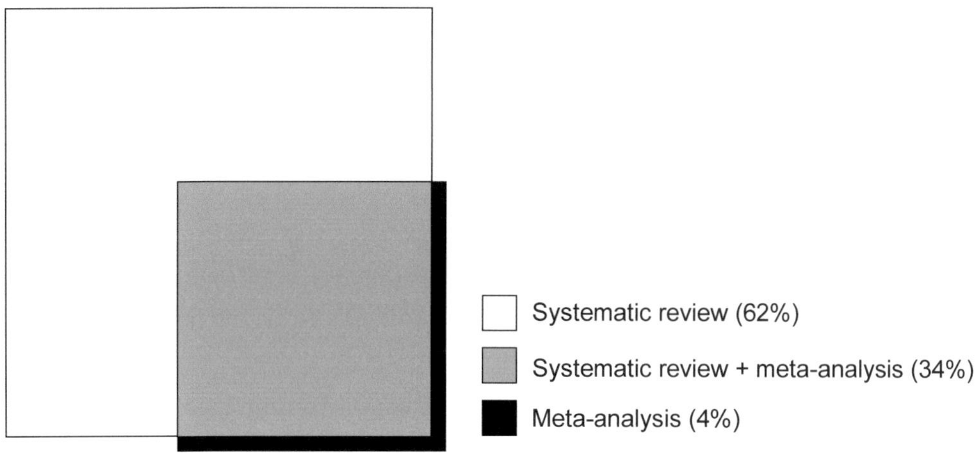

Fig. 1. Joint and independent use of systematic review and meta-analysis methods in published systematic reviews/meta-analyses*.

It should also be kept in mind that although the rigorous framework of a systematic review is expected to contribute to limit some of the biases that may affect literature searches, by itself it does not ensure the quality of the review, or the validity of its conclusions. On the one hand, the final result is dependent on the quality of the original studies that are evaluated, and the systematic review cannot be seen as a tool to improve the quality of primary sources that are methodologically flawed. On the other hand, as for any other epidemiological study design, the use of sound methodologies is not always the most appropriate; in fact, a relatively large proportion of systematic reviews has been reported to have suboptimal quality and caution is needed in their interpretation [16-20].

Despite the scope for improvement in the conduct and reporting of systematic reviews and meta-analysis, these remain the best option when the aim is a quantitative synthesis, or a transparent and reproducible qualitative assessment of the evidence. The latter is the most likely outcome when focusing on complex interventions/exposures or heterogeneous reports. There is also room for narrative reviews or essays addressing broader questions, providing essential information on relevant concepts or theory, or discussing key studies in detail, which may contribute to place the evidence into context and identify new directions for research. However, these should not be confused with unbiased systematic reviews regarding their appropriateness and potential for driving evidence-based decisions [21-22].

*Estimated from the analysis of abstracts (and full paper whenever necessary to obtain the required information) from the 50 systematic reviews (classified as such when at least the search strategy was described) or meta-analyses (classified as such when summary estimates were computed) published closest to the end of the first semester 2007, identified through a Pubmed search using the following expression: "meta-analysis" [Text Word] OR "meta-analysis" [Publication type] OR "systematic review"[Text Word] AND English [Language].

3. General structure and procedures for conducting a systematic review

The methodology and tools that have gradually been developed for systematic reviews are expected to limit the potential biases to which literature reviews are prone to. A protocol for the review, with the detailed description of the methods to be used, should be prepared in advance and, ideally, maintained unchanged until the study is finished. The detailed description of the whole process allows the assessment of the quality of the reviews and validity of their conclusions. Figure 2 provides an overview of the essential steps of a systematic review, and identifies the main determinants of its quality.

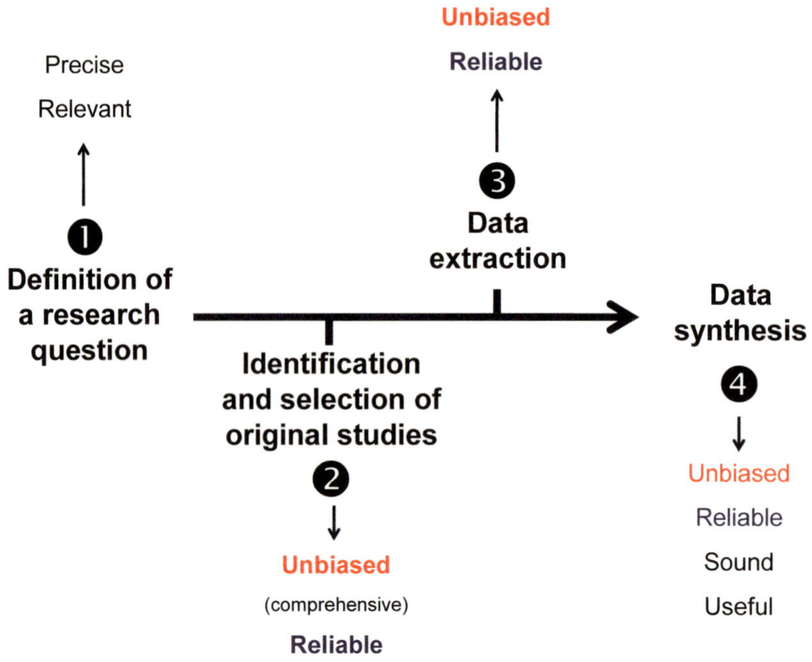

Fig. 2. Overview of the process that underlies a systematic review.

3.1 Definition of a research question

The whole review builds upon the research question being targeted, which largely determines the impact of the conclusions and how smooth the review process will be. We may identify two major determinants of accomplishing this step successfully. On the one hand, the setting up of a relevant research question depends primarily on how well the researchers know the topic under study, from the biological, clinical and epidemiological standpoints, as applicable. Thus, having in the research team people with a deep understanding of the issue at hand is highly recommended. On the other hand, the precision of the objectives defined for the review will influence the amount of work required and the external validity of the conclusions. Research questions with a broad scope are probably more appealing to a general audience and also more likely to generate conclusions that apply to different contexts or settings. However, these are also more likely to result in amounts of information that are unmanageable in a reasonable time if no substantial resources are available. For example, the largest ever report on how diet, physical activity and body fatness affect the risk of different cancers was published by the World Cancer Research Fund/American Institute for Cancer Research (WCRF/AICR) [23]. It included evidence from over 7000 papers, and involved research teams from nine different institutions and over 200 people worldwide [23]. When the available resources are more modest, which is usually the case, a much smaller number of exposures and outcomes need to be addressed (*e.g.* fruit and vegetables versus gastric cancer instead of diet and cancer) for the review to be feasible.

The number of systematic reviews and meta-analyses being published has increased substantially in the last years (Figure 3) and is not surprising that many interesting research questions have been addressed before by other authors. However, a new systematic review on a topic that has been previously addressed with these methods is not necessarily redundant, and frequently is necessary. For example, one of the key principles of the Cochrane Collaboration's work is "keeping up to date, by a commitment to ensure that Cochrane Reviews are maintained through identification and incorporation of new evidence" [24]. The WCRF global network is also committed to the updating of the evidence of the 1997 and 2007 Expert Reports on food, nutrition, physical activity and cancer [25]. Several strategies, techniques or statistical methods have been developed to support different aspects of the updating of systematic reviews/meta-analyses [26-29].

The use of the findings of the previous systematic reviews also needs to be taken into account, for fine-tuning of the objectives and/or a more efficient design of a new review on the same topic; the identification of systematic reviews/meta-analyses conducted before should probably be the first step of any new review on a given topic.

3.2 Identification and selection of original studies

The search for original studies needs to take into account the need to yield an unbiased sample of the eligible reports. This depends on the comprehensiveness of the search strategy, regarding the number and types of sources and the eligibility of different types of reports and languages of publication, as well as on the implementation of procedures to ensure the reliability of the selection procedures.

Ideally, systematic reviews would be based on the assessment of all the evidence available on a given topic. Although this may be possible, when the eligibility criteria restrict the search to a small number of investigations or when reviewing clinical trials, which may be identified in registries of this type of studies, it is virtually impossible otherwise, and an unbiased sample of the evidence is usually the aim to be targeted. The extent to which a systematic review approaches this objective depends on the type and number of data sources selected for a comprehensive search strategy, which should be defined taking into account the probability of studies with different characteristics being identified when searching each source.

The search strategy should be as comprehensive as necessary to achieve an unbiased sample of the evidence on the topic being studied. The decision on the number and type of the data sources to be included is influenced by the researchers understanding of the topic under study and the available time and resources.

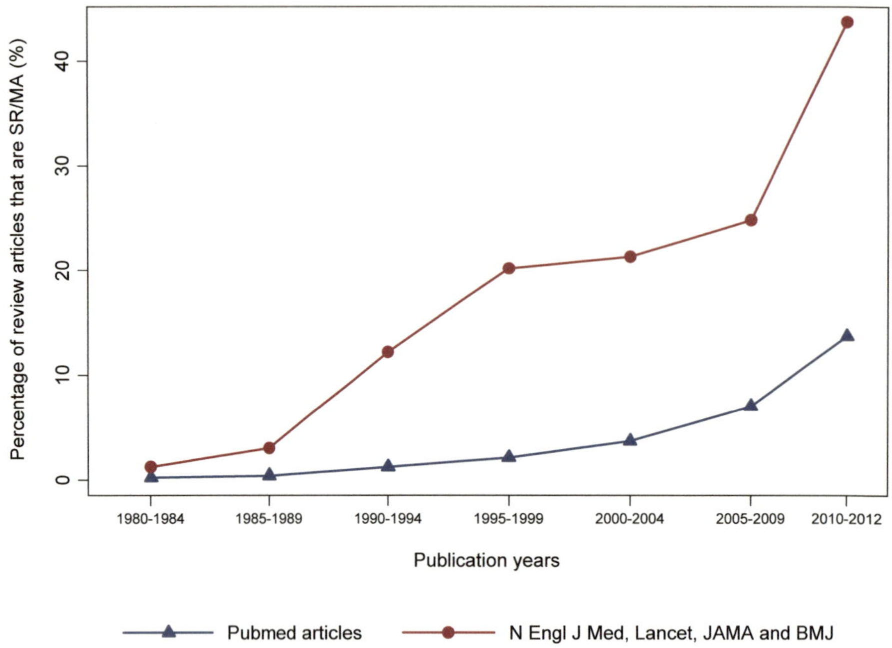

SR/MA - Systematic review/meta-analysis; N Engl J Med - The New England journal of medicine; JAMA - JAMA: the journal of the American Medical Association; BMJ - British Medical Journal.

Fig. 3. Percentage of review articles that are systematic reviews/meta-analyses (SR/MA), among those indexed in Pubmed and among those published in four general medical journals with a high impact factor†.

The main sources of data for reviews are presented in figure 4.; the publications from journals indexed in electronic databases such as MEDLINE are easily available, while unpublished material may only be obtained from the authors and therefore its retrieval tends to be a much more difficult and time-consuming task.

Electronic databases are the source of the largest number of articles included in any systematic review on health-related topics, which reflects both the easy access to these resources, and their wide coverage. However, the inclusion of data sources with different characteristics, namely those that include unpublished results or publications with a more limited circulation may be essential to overcome selection bias, as the probability of a study being published or the place where it is published may depend on the extent to which the results are in accordance with the nature of the results and their statistical significance (publication and related biases [30]).

† PeN Engl J Med, Lancet, JAMA and BMJ, in each of the periods represercentages were computed using the number of references retrieved in Pubmed (2012 March 10) using search expressions to identify all review articles (review [Publication Type] OR "meta-analysis" [Text Word] OR "meta-analysis" [Publication type] OR "systematic review"[Text Word]) or systematic reviews or meta-analyses ("meta-analysis" [Text Word] OR "meta-analysis" [Publication type] OR "systematic review"[Text Word]), among all articles indexed in Pubmed and among those published in the journals nted in the figure.

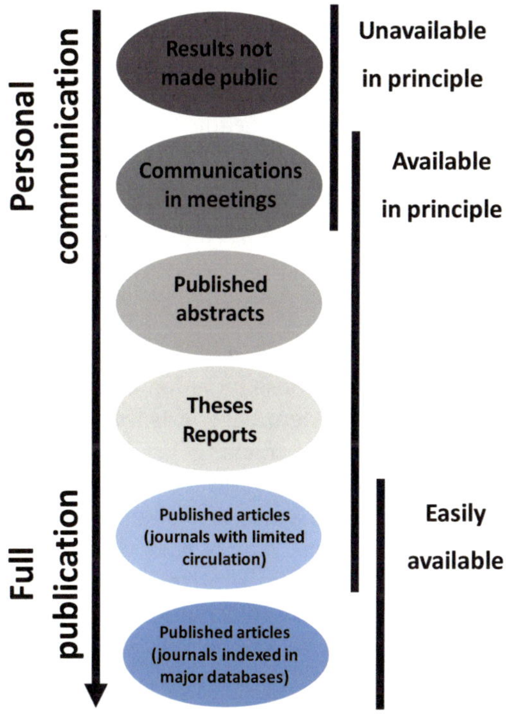

Fig. 4. Data sources that may be used in a systematic review.

Regardless of the sources of data selected, a decision has to be made on the eligibility of studies written in different languages; the impact of language restrictions in the comprehensiveness of the search and the potential for selection bias depends primarily on the subject of the review.

On the one hand, language restrictions may lead to the exclusion of a large proportion of the available studies when the outcomes or the exposures being studied have a geographical distribution that makes likely the publication of a large number of articles in a language other than English. For example, when addressing a topic related with the Chagas disease, which is found mainly in Latin America, it is important to consider articles written in Portuguese and in Spanish [31] while for a review on the treatment with hyperbaric oxygen for neonatal hypoxic-ischemic encephalopathy, which is frequent in China and used much less often in Western countries [32], articles written in Chinese should be included. Resources such as LILACS (http://lilacs.bvsalud.org/), which indexes specifically scientific and technical Latin American and Caribbean literature, and Chinese bibliographic databases [33], respectively, are likely to allow the identification of a large proportion of studies for reviews on the previous topics.

On the other hand, studies not published in English, predominantly in journals with a more limited circulation, are more likely to have non-statistically significant results or "negative" findings, and therefore language restrictions may contribute to biased samples of studies to be reviewed.

When conducting searches over several electronic database, it should be taken into account that each of them may have different search fields and key-words for indexation of the articles, which requires that the search expressions are adjusted to the specificities of each source. Therefore, a detailed description of the search expression used in each database is essential for the systematic review to be replicable by others. Unfortunately, that does not seem to be the rule in many published reviews.

The indexation of the articles in the electronic databases is known to be imperfect, and a hand-search may be used to increase the sensitivity of the search strategy. This strategy, however, is time consuming and its use is restricted to searches on specific topics that are addressed in a relatively small number of journals.

Citation searching is usually one of the components of any search strategy, namely through the identification of the articles cited by those included in the systematic review ("backward citation tracking"). It is also possible to identify reports that cited specific studies included in the systematic review ("forward citation tracking"), which may be useful when we may expect that a specific article is important enough to be cited by a large proportion of those that we aim to identify. This requires the use of resources that include citation databases, only available by subscription, such as the Web of Knowledge or Scopus. Citation searching may also be useful when defining the search strategy, as it may be used as an independent source of references that provides valuable information to estimate the completeness of the main database searches and to improve the search expressions and the overall search strategy.

The glossary of the Cochrane collaboration [34] refers to "grey literature" as "the kind of material that is not published in easily accessible journals or databases" and it is expected to include "things like conference proceedings that include the abstracts of the research presented at conferences, unpublished theses, and so on". A large number of internet resources may be used to locate the so called grey literature [35-36]. However, each of them has a different scope and relatively limited coverage, in addition to specific modes of functioning, which results in the need of using several of these resources to answer a specific research question.

It should be taken into account that the different sources of data may yield quite heterogeneous results regarding the quality of the investigations and the detail of the reporting. For example, when the investigations are reported solely in the form of abstract, often reflect preliminary analysis that will be improved in subsequent publications based on the same datasets and it is also less likely that the methods and results are described with the necessary detail [37]. A large number of reports that may be classified as "grey literature" are not peer reviewed, which may translate into a larger heterogeneity of the studies identified in these sources as well as a lower average quality of the studies and their reporting.

The ideal search strategy should maximize sensitivity, as this is likely to be necessary to avoid selection bias. However, a high sensitivity comes with a high number of non-eligible references that need to be read. Figure 5 establishes a parallelism between the yielding of a search strategy and the accuracy of a diagnostic test, to depict the relation between the sensitivity of a search strategy and the number of reports needed to read for a systematic review. If we assume that the gold-standard is an optimized search of all available resources, a search strategy with a high sensitivity [a/(a+c)], *i.e.*, that misses a small proportion of all eligible reports (c), is likely to have a low positive predictive value [a/(a+b)], *i.e.*, from all the studies identified only a small proportion is eligible for the review, which corresponds to a low precision and a high "number needed to read" [(a+b)/a] [38].

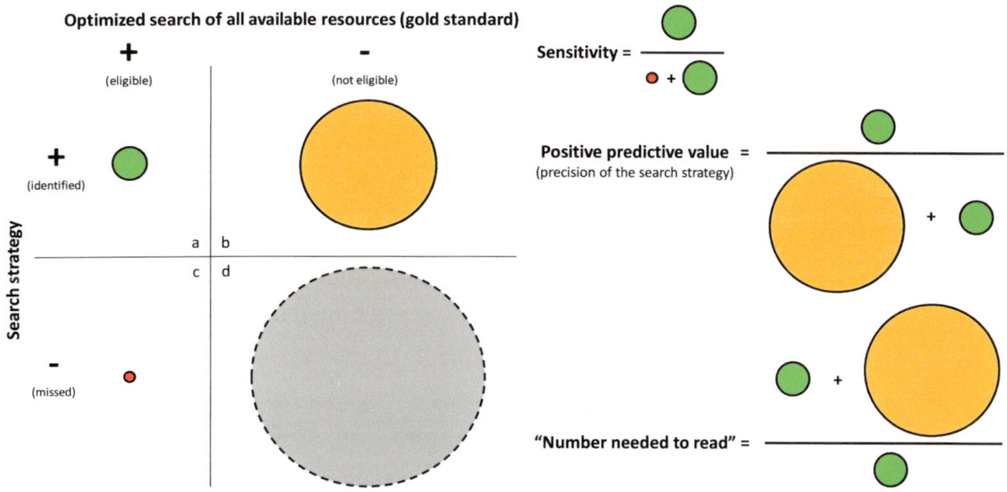

Fig. 5. Framework for assessing the yielding of a search strategy in the context of a systematic review.

Comprehensive searches of multiple sources are usually necessary to ensure that the systematic review is based on an unbiased sample of the available evidence. However, the resources available to conduct a systematic review are limited, and it is always necessary to find a compromise between a high sensitivity and a low "number needed to read". The setting-up of the search strategy for a systematic review finds a parallelism in the definition of the sampling methods for cohort, case-control or cross-sectional studies. In both cases, although the options for sampling and recruitment of the participants/studies may not be the ideal due to logistic constraints, no compromises are acceptable below a certain threshold of the study validity. However, the reasoning for the definition of the sample size in the epidemiological research in general does not apply when conducting systematic reviews/meta-analyses. In the former, the impossibility of meeting the sample size estimated for the study will probably result in the decision of not doing it or in methodological rearrangements to make it worthy. In systematic reviews, the number of available studies on a given topic is usually relatively small and the search strategy is designed to minimize bias instead of aiming a specific number of eligible reports. On the one hand, the assessment of a small sample of studies in a systematic review does not compromise its potential to provide a valid summary of the best available evidence. On the other hand, the assessment of a high proportion of all the eligible studies does not correspond necessarily to an unbiased sample, as the studies missed may be substantially different from those included in the review. This reasoning finds a parallelism with the interpretation of the participation rates in an epidemiological study, as even a high participation may correspond to a differential participation.

The screening of the reference lists obtained from different sources should be based in clear and sound criteria defined *a priori*, and both training of the people involved in the search and the independent assessment of the references by more than one researcher may contribute to reliable results in this phase of the review.

Arbitrarily defined eligibility criteria may compromise the validity of the reviews and it is not surprising that result driven decisions end up in meaningless or biased conclusions. It may be more appropriate to have broad inclusion criteria and to conduct stratified analyses than to restrict the analysis to a highly selected group of studies, which may result in missing important information.

The independent assessment of the references lists is resource consuming, and it has not been demonstrated that it is absolutely necessary to ensure reliability. We described the performances of inexperienced and experienced reviewers, in a three-step approach (Figure 6) to the screening of the reference lists, based in criteria defined in advance, and showed that the those with no previous experience may achieve food results when trained to adopt conservative selection procedures, despite consuming more time than the experienced [39].

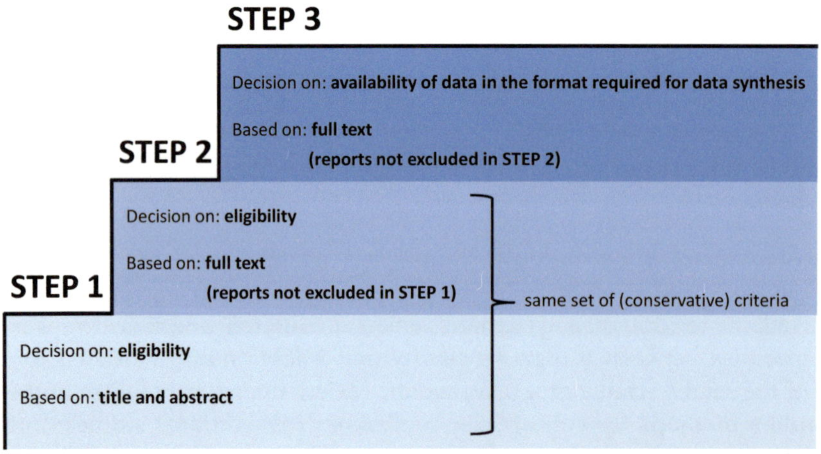

Fig. 6. Three-step approach to the screening of bibliographic references in the context of a systematic review.

In this approach to the screening of bibliographic references, the first and second steps are based in the same set of criteria for the exclusion of the studies that the reviewer can be absolutely sure that are not eligible for the review, and differ only in the amount of information that is available for the reviewer to decide. In step 1 the decisions are based only in the title and/or abstract (although it may be more appropriate not to decide on exclusions based only on the title), while in step 2 the reviewer has the full report available for analysis and a definite decision can be made. Training of the reviewers involved in this task is required for a conservative approach that ensures that only the studies that clearly are not eligible are excluded without a thorough assessment of the full report. Step 3 is also based in the full reports, and involves the assessment of the availability of data in the appropriate format for data synthesis. Although experienced reviewers may conduct steps 2 and 3 simultaneously, it may be easier to standardize the procedures and avoid errors if these are conducted separately.

Documenting all the decisions taken across these steps is essential for a proper reporting of the systematic review, since guidelines for the reporting of this type of research require information on the studies excluded according to the reasons underlying the decision, usually in a flow-chart [14].

3.3 Data extraction

From each study included in the systematic review it is necessary to collect information for the assessment of the study quality (methodological aspects that are essential to interpret the results and/or to understand the heterogeneity of the results across studies), as well as the effect measures to be summarized and corresponding precision estimates, or the information needed to compute them.

The overall quality of a systematic review/meta-analysis depends on the quality of the studies being reviewed. The synthesis of biased or confounded effect estimates yields equally invalid conclusions ("garbage in, garbage out"), and therefore the assessment of the quality of the original studies is an important component of any systematic review. Several instruments have been developed to produce summary scores of the characteristics of the studies with potential impact on the validity of the results, but the assessment of the impact of the relevant methodological aspects individually is the most appropriate way of dealing with the information on the quality of the individual studies [40-41]. Likewise, the strategies of analysis that weight the results according to their quality [42] should also be dismissed.

A large observer variation in data extraction and consequent decision on the studies to include in the review may be observed, due to different choices and errors [43]. Many reports provide several results potentially eligible for extraction and in different forms, requiring sound decisions on those to be selected, and frequently is necessary to express all the extracted data in the same format, which may easily originate conversion errors.

For example, in a replication of a previous meta-analysis on the relation between dietary calcium intake and blood pressure [44], the reassessment of the original studies showed "that data from one study had been inappropriately extracted and converted, leading to an understatement of the calcium-blood pressure relation by a factor of about 30" and "raised questions about the extraction and conversion of data from several other studies and about the statistical methods used" [45]. A study on data extraction errors assessed 27 meta-analyses that used standardized mean differences and showed that a high proportion had errors. The authors concluded that "although the statistical process is ostensibly simple, data extraction is particularly liable to errors that can negate or even reverse the findings of the study" [46]. Another investigation [43] addressed the inter-observer variation in the extraction of continuous and numerical rating scale data from trial reports for use in meta-analyses and compared experienced methodologists with PhD students. The agreement was somewhat higher among the former, but "disagreements were common and often larger than the effect of commonly used treatments" [43].

Data extraction is a demanding task and a great deal of effort is needed to ensure the validity and reliability of this procedure. On the one hand, it should be conducted following a previously defined protocol, to limit the potential for different judgements to result in different choices about the data to extract. Although there is some margin for adjustments taking into account unexpected observations, a proper understanding of the topic under study together with experience in the conduct of systematic reviews and meta-analyses should allow the definition of a protocol that requires only minor changes throughout data extraction. Most of the variability in the methodologies and reporting of data can be anticipated and taken into account in the protocol. On the other hand, the conduct of data extraction by experienced researchers is expected to contribute to minimize errors, and the independent data extraction by more than one researcher, together with consensus meetings, will contribute to identify for the errors to be corrected before summarizing the evidence.

3.4 Data synthesis

The book based on the seminal meta-analysis conducted by Glass et al [47] starts with a reference to the mathematician David Hilbert that once said "one can measure the importance of a scientific work by the number of earlier publications rendered superfluous by it"[48]. The extent to which systematic reviews provide relevant answers to their objectives depends on the accomplishment of a sound synthesis of the results, in addition to the detailed description (results and methodological characteristics) of each original study being reviewed. Figure 7 depicts a framework for deciding on the strategy for data synthesis, and the corresponding general aims of the systematic review.

Meta-analysis is a powerful tool for data synthesis, but it should be conducted only when the individual studies are homogeneous regarding their methodological characteristics, to the extent necessary for the weighted average of the results from the individual studies to be meaningful, which tends to occur more frequently among experimental studies than in those with observational designs. However, the fulfillment of this condition is not sufficient, and the homogeneity of the effect measures is also required. There are several methods available to identify and quantify heterogeneity [3, 49-50], but this will not be addressed in this chapter. Under these circumstances, meta-analysis may be a valuable option to summarize the evidence, contributing to overcome the statistical power limitations of the individual investigations.

This may be illustrated by the meta-analysis represented in the logo of the Cochrane Collaboration [51]. It shows a meta-analysis of randomized controlled trials (RCT) assessing the effect of a "short, inexpensive course of a corticosteroid given to women about to give birth too early". The first RCT was reported in 1972, and after one decade there was strong evidence that corticosteroids reduce the risk of babies dying from the complications of immaturity. However, because no systematic review of these trials had been published at that time, for several years a large number of people did not benefit from this effective treatment. Another good example is a meta-analysis on the cardiovascular adverse effects of rofecoxib [52], in which the authors conclude that the drug should have been withdrawn several years earlier. This shows the importance of using meta-analysis to obtain more precise estimates of an effect that is estimated with a very low precision in each of the individual studies because the outcome is too rare, which frequently occurs when dealing with adverse drug reactions. In both examples, the meta-analysis contributes for a more efficient use of the resources, for research and health-care.

When the participants' characteristics, study designs, exposures/interventions, or measurement of outcomes differ meaningfully across a set of studies, or when the results differ beyond the expected due solely to the play of chance, the combined estimates are likely to be meaningless, and an analytical rather than a synthetic approach is required [4].

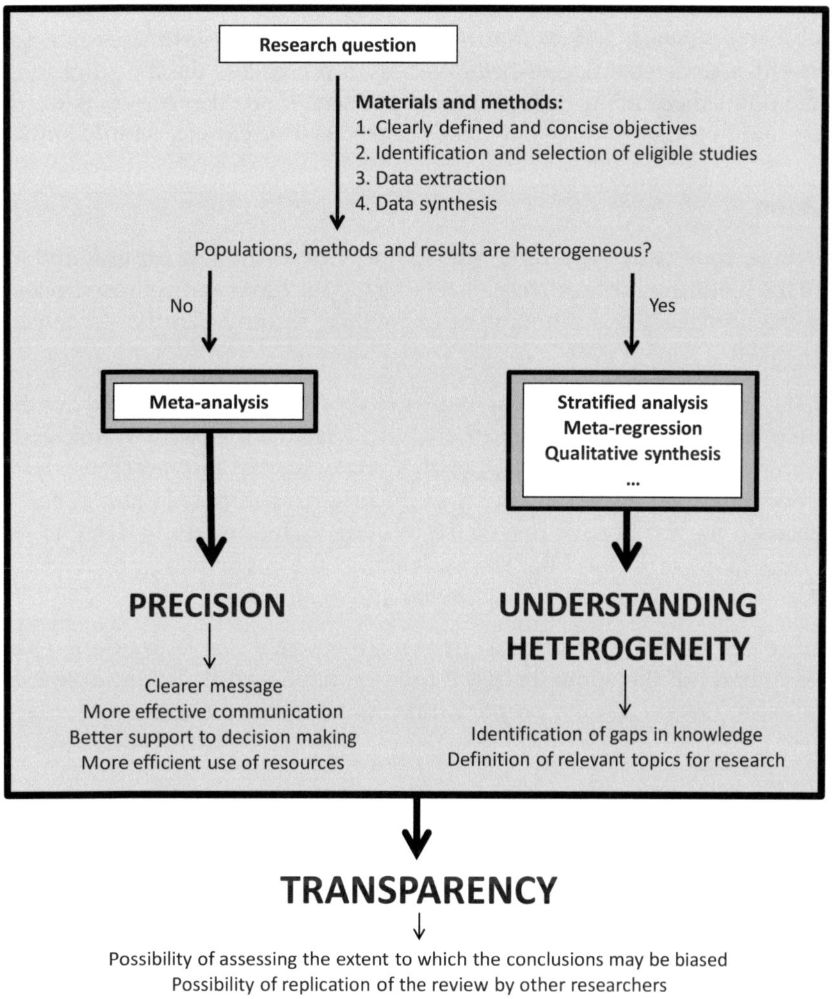

Fig. 7. Framework for deciding on the strategy for data synthesis, and general aims of a systematic review.

This strategy of analysis may be exemplified with two systematic reviews that addressed the relation between fruit and vegetables consumption and the occurrence of gastric cancer in cohort studies [53], and the relation between *Helicobacter pylori* infection and gastric cardia cancer [54], respectively. In the former, the heterogeneity of the results was explained mainly by the differences between studies in the outcome being addressed (incidence or mortality) and in the duration of the follow-up. In the latter, the heterogeneity was largely explained by the characteristics of the populations studied, with stronger association between infection and cancer being observed in the studies conducted in settings with a risk of gastric cancer. In both cases, analysis of subgroups of studies with different methodological characteristics and meta-regression were used to understand the heterogeneity.

The methods adopted throughout the whole process should aim the reduction of bias, but this may be accomplished to different extents in different systematic reviews, and the readers should be able to assess this, as in any other research design. Even when the number of studies is small and heterogeneous, and neither more precise summary estimates nor an important contribution to the understanding of heterogeneity are possible, the thorough description of the materials and methods allow its replication by others. If no other reason persists for opting for a resource and time consuming systematic review, its transparency should suffice.

4. Conclusion

There is a large consensus regarding the importance of having sound and transparent syntheses of the literature for health care providers, policy makers and researchers to be able to integrate the unmanageable amounts of biomedical information that is constantly being produced.

The objectives of systematic reviews/meta-analyses may be primarily synthetic, when aiming more precise average estimates, or analytic, when concerned with understanding the different results observed across studies, even if some overlap between these two pathways may occur, depending on the homogeneity of the original sources of data. These approaches may be placed on the top of each one of the two hierarchies of study designs proposed by Vandenbroucke [55], corresponding, respectively, to the confirmation of hypotheses when the *a priori* probability is high and to "discovery and explanation".

Understanding the place of systematic reviews/meta-analyses in modern epidemiology, and the determinants of the option between predominantly synthetic or analytic approaches for data synthesis, are crucial for a proper utilization of these resources.

5. References

[1] Hunt, M., *How science takes stock - the story of meta-analysis*. 1997, New York: Russel Sage Foundation.
[2] Petticrew, M., *Systematic reviews from astronomy to zoology: myths and misconceptions*. BMJ, 2001. 322(7278): p. 98-101.
[3] Borenstein, M., et al., *Introduction to meta-analysis*. 2009, Chichester: Wiley.
[4] Greenland, S. and K. O'Rourke, *Meta-analysis*, in *Modern Epidemiology*, K.J. Rothman, S. Greenland, and T.L. Lash, Editors. 2008, Lippincott Williams & Wilkins: Philadelphia. p. 652-682.
[5] Jenicek, M., *Meta-analysis in medicine. Where we are and where we want to go*. J Clin Epidemiol, 1989. 42(1): p. 35-44.
[6] Egger, M., G.D. Smith, and A.N. Phillips, *Meta-analysis: principles and procedures*. BMJ, 1997. 315(7121): p. 1533-7.
[7] Porta, M., ed. *A Dictionary of Epidemiology*. 5th ed. 2008, Oxford University Press: New York.
[8] Schmid, C.H., *Using Bayesian inference to perform meta-analysis*. Eval Health Prof, 2001. 24(2): p. 165-89.
[9] van Houwelingen, H.C., L.R. Arends, and T. Stijnen, *Advanced methods in meta-analysis: multivariate approach and meta-regression*. Stat Med, 2002. 21(4): p. 589-624.
[10] Greenland, S. and M.P. Longnecker, *Methods for trend estimation from summarized dose-response data, with applications to meta-analysis*. Am J Epidemiol, 1992. 135(11): p. 1301-9.
[11] Burney, P., et al., *A case-control study of the relation between plasma selenium and asthma in European populations: a GAL2EN project*. Allergy, 2008. 63(7): p. 865-71.

[12] Moher, D., et al., *Improving the quality of reports of meta-analyses of randomised controlled trials: the QUOROM statement. Quality of Reporting of Meta-analyses.* Lancet, 1999. 354(9193): p. 1896-900.
[13] Stroup, D.F., et al., *Meta-analysis of observational studies in epidemiology: a proposal for reporting. Meta-analysis Of Observational Studies in Epidemiology (MOOSE) group.* JAMA, 2000. 283(15): p. 2008-12.
[14] Liberati, A., et al., *The PRISMA statement for reporting systematic reviews and meta-analyses of studies that evaluate health care interventions: explanation and elaboration.* PLoS Med, 2009. 6(7): p. e1000100.
[15] Chalmers, I. and D.G. Altman, eds. *Systematic reviews.* 1995, BMJ Publishing Group: London.
[16] Moseley, A.M., et al., *Cochrane reviews used more rigorous methods than non-Cochrane reviews: survey of systematic reviews in physiotherapy.* J Clin Epidemiol, 2009. 62(10): p. 1021-30.
[17] Olsen, O., et al., *Quality of Cochrane reviews: assessment of sample from 1998.* BMJ, 2001. 323(7317): p. 829-32.
[18] Petticrew, M., et al., *Quality of Cochrane reviews. Quality of Cochrane reviews is better than that of non-Cochrane reviews.* BMJ, 2002. 324(7336): p. 545.
[19] Shea, B., et al., *A comparison of the quality of Cochrane reviews and systematic reviews published in paper-based journals.* Eval Health Prof, 2002. 25(1): p. 116-29.
[20] Biondi-Zoccai, G.G., et al., *Compliance with QUOROM and quality of reporting of overlapping meta-analyses on the role of acetylcysteine in the prevention of contrast associated nephropathy: case study.* BMJ, 2006. 332(7535): p. 202-9.
[21] Petticrew, M., *Systematic reviews in public health: old chestnuts and new challenges.* Bull World Health Organ, 2009. 87(3): p. 163-163A.
[22] McPheeters, M.L., et al., *Systematic reviews in public health*, in *Applied Epidemiology - theory to practice*, R.C. Brownson and D.B. Petitti, Editors. 2006, Oxford University Press: New York. p. 99-124.
[23] *World Cancer Research Fund global network's diet and cancer report website.* 9 March 2012 [cited 2012 9 March]; Available from: http://www.dietandcancerreport.org/.
[24] *The Cochrane Collaboration. The Cochrane Policy Manual.* 8 March 2012 [cited 2012 9 March]; Available from: www.cochrane.org/policy-manual/welcome.
[25] *World Cancer Research Fund International. Continuous Update Project.* 9 March 2012 [cited 2012 9 March]; Available from: http://www.wcrf.org/cancer_research/cup/index.php.
[26] Barrowman, N.J., et al., *Identifying null meta-analyses that are ripe for updating.* BMC Med Res Methodol, 2003. 3: p. 13.
[27] Moher, D., et al., *A systematic review identified few methods and strategies describing when and how to update systematic reviews.* J Clin Epidemiol, 2007. 60(11): p. 1095-1104.
[28] Moher, D., et al., *When and how to update systematic reviews.* Cochrane Database Syst Rev, 2008(1): p. MR000023.
[29] Tsertsvadze, A., et al., *Updating comparative effectiveness reviews: current efforts in AHRQ's Effective Health Care Program.* J Clin Epidemiol, 2011. 64(11): p. 1208-15.
[30] Song, F., et al., *Publication and related biases.* Health Technol Assess, 2000. 4(10): p. 1-115.
[31] de Almeida, E.A., et al., *Co-infection Trypanosoma cruzi/HIV: systematic review (1980-2010).* Rev Soc Bras Med Trop, 2011. 44(6): p. 762-70.
[32] Liu, Z., T. Xiong, and C. Meads, *Clinical effectiveness of treatment with hyperbaric oxygen for neonatal hypoxic-ischaemic encephalopathy: systematic review of Chinese literature.* BMJ, 2006. 333(7564): p. 374.

[33] Fung, I.C., *Chinese journals: a guide for epidemiologists.* Emerg Themes Epidemiol, 2008. 5: p. 20.
[34] *The Cochrane Collaboration. Glossary.* [cited 2012 10 March]; Available from: http://www.cochrane.org/glossary/.
[35] *Higgins JPT, Green S, editors. Cochrane Handbook for Systematic Reviews of Interventions Version 5.1.0 [updated March 2011]*, J.P.T. Higgins and S. Green, Editors. 2011, The Cochrane Collaboration.
[36] Hopewell, S., M. Clarke, and S. Mallet, *Grey literature and systematic reviews*, in *Publication Bias in Meta-Analysis*, H.R. Rothstein, A.J. Sutton, and M. Borenstein, Editors. 2005, Wiley: Chichester.
[37] Dundar, Y., et al., *Comparison of conference abstracts and presentations with full-text articles in the health technology assessments of rapidly evolving technologies.* Health Technol Assess, 2006. 10(5): p. iii-iv, ix-145.
[38] Bachmann, L.M., et al., *Identifying diagnostic studies in MEDLINE: reducing the number needed to read.* J Am Med Inform Assoc, 2002. 9(6): p. 653-8.
[39] Vales, C., et al., *Yielding of a systematic review: inter-rater agreement, sensitivity, specificity and workload.* Epidemiol Prev, 2010. 34((5-6 Suppl 1)): p. 157.
[40] Whiting, P., R. Harbord, and J. Kleijnen, *No role for quality scores in systematic reviews of diagnostic accuracy studies.* BMC Med Res Methodol, 2005. 5: p. 19.
[41] Juni, P., et al., *The hazards of scoring the quality of clinical trials for meta-analysis.* JAMA, 1999. 282(11): p. 1054-60.
[42] Doi, S.A. and L. Thalib, *A quality-effects model for meta-analysis.* Epidemiology, 2008. 19(1): p. 94-100.
[43] Tendal, B., et al., *Disagreements in meta-analyses using outcomes measured on continuous or rating scales: observer agreement study.* BMJ, 2009. 339: p. b3128.
[44] Cappuccio, F.P., et al., *Epidemiologic association between dietary calcium intake and blood pressure: a meta-analysis of published data.* Am J Epidemiol, 1995. 142(9): p. 935-45.
[45] Birkett, N.J., *Comments on a meta-analysis of the relation between dietary calcium intake and blood pressure.* Am J Epidemiol, 1998. 148(3): p. 223-8; discussion 232-3.
[46] Gotzsche, P.C., et al., *Data extraction errors in meta-analyses that use standardized mean differences.* JAMA, 2007. 298(4): p. 430-7.
[47] Glass, G.V., B. McGaw, and M.L. Smith, *Meta-analysis in social research.* 1981, Beverly Hills: Sage Publications.
[48] Shapiro, F.R., ed. *The Yale Book of Quotations.* 2006, Yale University Press: New Haven.
[49] Lunet, N., *Meta-Analysis of Observational Studies*, in *Applied Epidemiology and Biostatistics*, G. La Torre, Editor. 2010, SEEd: Torino. p. 207-30.
[50] Bax, L., et al., *More than numbers: the power of graphs in meta-analysis.* Am J Epidemiol, 2009. 169(2): p. 249-55.
[51] *The Cochrane Collaboration. Cochrane Collaboration logo.* [cited 2012 11 March]; Available from: http://www.cochrane.org/about-us/history/our-logo.
[52] Juni, P., et al., *Risk of cardiovascular events and rofecoxib: cumulative meta-analysis.* Lancet, 2004. 364(9450): p. 2021-9.
[53] Lunet, N., A. Lacerda-Vieira, and H. Barros, *Fruit and vegetables consumption and gastric cancer: a systematic review and meta-analysis of cohort studies.* Nutr Cancer, 2005. 53(1): p. 1-10.
[54] Cavaleiro-Pinto, M., et al., *Helicobacter pylori infection and gastric cardia cancer: systematic review and meta-analysis.* Cancer Causes Control, 2011. 22(3): p. 375-87.
[55] Vandenbroucke, J.P., *Observational research, randomised trials, and two views of medical science.* PLoS Med, 2008. 5(3): p. e67.